Promoting Positive
Practice in Nursing
Older People

Promoting Positive Practice in Nursing Older People

Edited by

Sharon Pickering MSc, BSc (Hons), BA (Hons), RGN, DipN (Lond), PGDip (HSSM)

Practice and Professional Development Manager
Northern General Hospital NHS Trust, Sheffield, UK

and

Jeanette Thompson MA, BSc (Hons), RNMH, DipN (Lond), CertEd, ITEC, PGDip (HSSM)

Manager, Community Team for People with Learning Disabilities,
Oxford Learning Disability Trust, and Lecturer,
Oxford Brookes University, Oxford, UK

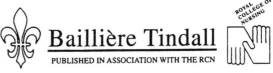

Baillière Tindall

PUBLISHED IN ASSOCIATION WITH THE RCN

London Philadelphia Toronto Sydney Tokyo

Baillière Tindall
W.B. Saunders

24–28 Oval Road
London NW1 7DX, UK

The Curtis Center
Independence Square West
Philadelphia, PA 19106-3399, USA

Harcourt Brace & Company
55 Horner Avenue
Toronto, Ontario, M8Z 4X6, Canada

Harcourt Brace & Company, Australia
30–52 Smidmore Street
Marrickville
NSW 2204, Australia

Harcourt Brace & Company, Japan
Ichibancho Central Building
22-1 Ichibancho
Chiyoda-ku, Tokyo 102, Japan

A catalogue record for this book is available from the British Library

ISBN 0-7020-2080-X

Printed and bound by Antony Rowe Ltd, Eastbourne

Contents

Section Four: Future Directions

Contributors' list

Mavis A D Arevalo MSc BSc RGN RM RHV DPSN Cert Ed, Senior Lecturer, School of Human and Health Sciences, University of Huddersfield, Huddersfield, West Yorkshire.

Janice Baker RNMS RGN CMS DHSM BA, Senior Clinical Nurse, Fieldhead Hospital, Wakefield, West Yorkshire.

Helen Bartlett BA MSc PhD RGN RHV, Professor Health Studies and Director of Research, School of Healthcare, Oxford Brookes University, Oxford.

John Brown BSc(Hons) MPhil, Director, Centre for Interprofessional Studies in Health and Social Care, University of York, York.

Gordon Evans MSc RMN RGN RCNT STD RNT, Pathway Leader (Older Person), Department of Health Studies, University of York, Scarborough Hospital Centre, Scarborough.

Michael Hall RMN CHMS, General Manager, Mental Health, Durham County Priority Services: NHS Trust.

Joy Harrison RGN RMN BA (Psych) MMedSci (Nurs.) DipEd, Senior Nursing Lecturer, University of Sheffield, School of Nursing, Sheffield.

Christine A Hunter RGN RN DipN (Lond) Cert Ed, Dip Ed, MA Counselling, Nurse Teacher, Derby Centre for University of Nottingham, Derbyshire Royal Infirmary, Derby.

Jean Hankinson RGN RCNT RNT Cert Ed MEd, Nurse Teacher, Derby Centre for Nottingham, Melbourne House, Derby.

Lee Hutchinson RNMH RGN Cert Ed BCs, Nurse Teacher, Derby Centre for Nottingham, Melbourne House, Derby.

Jillian Jefferson RMN RGN BSc (Hons) DipApp SS, Senior Nurse (Mental Health) Education and Development, Durham County Priority Services: NHS Trust, Derwent Clinic, Shotley Bridge Hospital.

Gill Johnson BSc(Hons) RGN RCNT RNT Cert Ed MISPA, Nurse Lecturer, School of Healthcare Studies, University of Leeds, Leeds.

Brenda Maslen RMN DipN Cert Ed MEd, Freelance Lecturer, Doncaster.

Aru Narayanasamy BA MSc RGN RMN Cert Ed RNT, Course Co-ordinator/Honorary Nurse Adviser (Transcultural Health Care) University of Nottingham, School of Nursing, Faculty of Medicine and Health Sciences, Queen's Medical Centre, Nottingham.

Sharon Pickering MSc BSc(Hons) BA(Hons) RGN DipN (Lond) PGDip (HSSM), Practice and Professional Development Manager, Northern General Hospital NHS Trust, Sheffield (UK).

Marc Saunders RNMH DPSN BSc(Hons) MA, General Manager, LEA Castle Centre, North Warwickshire NHS Trust, Kidderminster.

Jeanette S Thompson MA BSc(Hons) RNMH DipN (Lond) CertEd ITEC PGDip (HSSM), Community Team Manager/Lecturer, Oxford Disability Trust and Oxford Brookes University, Oxford, (UK).

Alan White MSc BSc(Hons) RGN Cert Ed, Senior Lecturer – Nursing, Leeds Metropolitan University, Leeds.

Foreword

Some years ago, in preparation for a paper I had been asked to present giving a European perspective on research in geriatric nursing (as it was then called), I analysed the main themes and trends in the nursing literature over the preceding 10 years. This was a cause for considerable personal reflection. The major focus in the literature was on the problems of old age, mainly within a hospital setting. Far less emphasis was placed on positive ageing or community care. This prompted me to call for a reorientation of nursing practice with older people so that the profession would be better placed to take the lead in developing improved services (Nolan 1994).

In urging nurses to rise to this challenge and seize the initiative, I was acutely aware of the considerable work that this would require. This remains the case. Working with older people has never been a particularly popular choice, and recent evidence suggests that nurse training reinforces negative stereotypes of old age (Stevens 1997). There is therefore a pressing need to change both the culture of care and the way that we educate nurses. The present emphasis on acute high-tech care has to be replaced with a more holistic perspective which recognises and values those individuals with on-going health care needs.

In this context *Promoting Positive Practice in Nursing Older People* could not be more timely. Even a brief glance at the contents page suggests that this book marks a refreshing departure from the majority of texts on nursing older people, a perception that is reinforced the closer one engages with its contents. From the very outset the Editors make clear their fundamental belief in the positive value of older people and the importance of transcending both intra- and interprofessional boundaries. Their aim is to produce a theoretically grounded but practice-based text that appeals not only to nurses at varying levels and working in different contexts, but is also relevant to other practitioners concerned to improve the well-being of older people. This is an ambitious agenda that the various contributors meet head on.

The result is a stimulating and challenging read which successfully deals with a number of important issues in a logical and sensitive manner. After a consideration of the values, attitudes and beliefs that should underpin care, subsequent sections move on to address factors important in maintaining health amongst older people and suggest a number of therapeutic interventions to enhance communication and reduce stress. The book concludes with a look to the future, highlighting the need for nurses to engage more fully in debates in political and policy arenas.

Given the prevailing demographic trends, ageing will affect us all, both professionally and personally. At a professional level the book is to be commended for moving us away from a pathological view of ageing. At a personal level I hope that, should the need arise, I will be cared for by a practitioner who has adopted the values which permeate *Promoting Positive Practice in Nursing Older People.*

REFERENCES

Nolan, M.R. (1994) Geriatric Nursing: An idea whose time has gone? A Polemic. *Journal of Advanced Nursing*, 20, 989–996.

Stevens, J. (1997) The education and socialisation of nurses: why a career with the elderly is a most unpopular career destination. Paper presented at the 16th World Congress of Gerontology, Adelaide, August 1997.

Mike Nolan

Editors' introduction

We chose to write this book because of our fundamental belief in the positive value of older people and our feeling that society, and sometimes nurses, do not always actively recognize this value. The particular style and format of the book was chosen because of our belief that different branches or fields of nursing were all able to contribute something positive to the area of nursing older people and our feeling that often these ideas, philosophies or therapies were not transcending the boundaries between those different areas. For this reason you will notice that the contributors are not only from a mixture of practice, management and education, but are also from adult, learning disabilities and mental health nursing backgrounds, as well as health visiting.

The book is essentially a practice-based text that is aimed at providing the qualified and pre-qualifying nurse working with older people, in a variety of settings, the opportunity to reflect upon their practice, consider other approaches that may be of value to the client group and to identify strategies or resources that they are able to use in order to introduce these approaches into their practice setting. Though this book is primarily aimed at nurses, its focus upon health, rather than illness, means it is relevant to other practitioners, within the area of welfare provision and older people.

The value base upon which this book is founded essentially places older people as equal to all others in society with the same fundamental rights, expectations and responsibilities as other adults. These rights include the fundamental right to respect and dignity, the opportunity to grow and develop and the right to have their disabilities and their differences acknowledged.

In addition, this text views the experience of ageing as a positive experience through which an individual accumulates knowledge, experience and expertise and progresses towards the elusive state of self-actualization. This is not to say any individual may have both positive and negative experiences. Often these experiences are framed by the social constructions and perceptions of society and therefore nurses need to be aware of them. It is for this reason that the first section of this book addresses the values, attitudes and beliefs that society holds and their interface with old age.

Within this context, nurses are expected to work with the older person in order to support and facilitate them in making choices regarding the interventions used or not used to meet their health and social care needs. Essential to the successful execution of this responsibility are the inter-related concepts of the nurse–client relationship and partnership with service users.

Fundamental to this partnership is the use of appropriate positive and valuing terminology. It is for this reason that this text has avoided the use of terms such as 'the elderly' as they are based upon group identity and therefore do not respect the individual and their experience.

This text has been the product of many hours of effort from a number of people. We have all learnt from writing it; we hope you enjoy reading it.

Sharon Pickering
Jeanette Thompson

1 VALUES, ATTITUDES AND BELIEFS

This section explores some of the key concepts and theories that underpin the study of growing old. The reason for this is to allow the reader to consider the impact of our belief system upon the practice of nursing. This section includes an exploration of culture and its relation to a person's experience of healthcare. There is a discussion of 'ordinary living' and ways in which it can be applied in caring situations in order to promote positive nursing practice. The importance of choice, autonomy and independence is explored in relation to high-quality nursing care in order to promote a positive quality of life. A framework of risk management is used to consider the legal implications of nursing practice.

1 Influences upon growing older

Sharon Pickering and Jeanette Thompson

KEY ISSUES

- What is old age?
- Cultural values and ageing
- Older people and physical ageing
- Chronological approaches to ageing
- Lifespan and lifecycle approaches to ageing

INTRODUCTION

The value and role of older people within our society is an issue which is not widely explored outside of the geronotological field of study. However, it is an issue which will concern each one of us at some time within our life. This concern will either be of a personal nature, in relation to friends, colleagues, family or neighbours. Alternatively, within western society, the concern may well relate to how we will decline and deteriorate physically and mentally as well as concern regarding our usefulness to society in general. This view, however, negates and fails to acknowledge the actual value older individuals do have within their own family, their community and also within the whole of society. These values have a social, a psychological and an economic focus and can be influenced by the personal and emotional attachment to one's own older relatives and friends. Other contributions include economic aspects, for example the provision of childcare and/or voluntary occupation. In addition, a more global and philosophical approach which encapsulates the belief that the continuation of the human race and its technical and scientific development relies upon previous generations and their ability to transmit and share the knowledge that they and their predecessors acquired.

This chapter will consider the definition of old age and a variety of the theories of ageing including biological, chronological and individual perspectives. In addition an exploration of how nurses can use this knowledge to improve their practice will be considered within a case study.

WHAT IS OLD AGE?

'Old age' and 'older people' are terms which are in common everyday usage. They describe a particular time in a person's life, and these words and others that are associated with old age give each of us an image and idea of what this stage in life means. Despite the frequency with which such terms are used, the actual definition of what old age is and growing old means, both to society and individuals, is problematic. Any definition of old age has more than a physical perspective; although we can define old age through certain physical changes such as the menopause and skin changes, these do, however, have a psychological impact upon an individual's life. This aspect of growing old is much more difficult to visualize and articulate, and hence is problematic for nurses.

As a society, old age is generally defined by the state retirement age of 65 years. This period of life is seen by many as one that is not productive from a societal perspective, but is more about leisure time and the space to spend time upon oneself and one's family.

CULTURAL VALUES AND AGEING

As stated, our society values work and the ability to be productive; these values dominate how our society is organized and how it operates. Every society has a set of values which give it a distinctive character that makes it different from other societies. Many societies are characterized by variations in the status accorded to people in different age groups. Within western cultures, ageing is not necessarily seen as a positive experience and as such, individuals of advancing years may not be attributed with high status or high value. Eastern cultures, on the other hand, generally believe old age means that a person has had valued experiences and therefore developed wisdom and knowledge that is useful to the

➤2, 8 rest of their society.

Victor (1994) states that most western industrial societies are dominated by the values of independence, the importance of work, progress and the youth culture. Independence and self-reliance are highly valued characteristics within western society, and as such, dependency is seen as a sign of weakness and therefore undesirable. Such individuals are often marginalized and labelled as unproductive and as 'exploiting' the state welfare system. Within our society welfare is currently funded and supported by those who are gainfully employed.

The work ethic is seen as one of the major organizing principles of western society. Within such societies much importance is placed upon individuals being fully employed and it is generally perceived that to be busy is a good thing and something to be encouraged. Cowgill and Holmes (1972) argue that the process of modernization which has occurred as a consequence of increasing industrialization has ensured that the term 'old' has acquired a negative connotation. This is the result of the more organized and controlled nature of work, post the industrial revolution, and the need for people to travel or go out to work. A natural consequence of this process has been the introduction of artificial timescales in life such as retirement age. As a result of the state retirement age, older people are largely excluded from the formal labour market and as such are not seen as part of the wider work-orientated society. Victor (1994) suggests there is a conflict between the prevailing ethos within society of activity and productiveness, and the position ascribed to older people of enforced leisure time and the perception that they are unproductive.

The emphasis that western society places upon progressing and developing stresses the future rather than the past and terms such as 'outdated' and 'old fashioned' have a highly negative connotation. This view accepts that the new is inherently better and more effective than the old. Therefore, young people who can learn and develop, are energetic, enthusiastic and innovative are more highly valued than older people who are seen as unable to learn, static and are less energetic.

This, combined with the emphasis upon the virtues of youth is a common ideology in many western societies. Within these belief systems, youth is seen as a time of resourcefulness, resilience, energy and enthusiasm and is compared with decline and deterioration, the characteristics of later life. Victor (1994) suggests that adulthood and especially old age are perceived as regressive and as a result of this many people experience a great deal of fear as they age.

OLDER PEOPLE AND PHYSICAL AGEING

Comfort (1960) describes ageing as 'an increased liability to die, or an increasing loss of vigour' . . . 'with the passage of the life cycle.' The experience of growing older is most often marked by the obvious physical bodily changes that people undergo. In asking the philosophical question as to why organisms age and die, Victor (1994) focuses upon the biological approaches to, and definitions of, ageing. A great deal of work has been carried out into how cells change as they age, and it is common knowledge that organisms are characterized by variations in the length of their lifespan. Research from the area of biological gerontology indicates that the ideal lifespan for human beings is between 115 and 120 years. However, it is believed that the reason that not everybody actually achieves this great age is as a result of different pathologies and disease processes. There have been various attempts to distinguish between biological ageing and the abnormal processes which affect the body, but they have been generally unsuccessful in identifying consistent differences.

Bond and Coleman (1992) divide the theories relating to physical ageing into programmed and unprogrammed approaches. Programmed theories identify the existence of an inbuilt biological clock which dictates the points in time at which bodily changes will occur, for example, puberty, menopause and dying. Essentially, therefore, the whole process of ageing is seen to be genetically determined. The programmed theories predominantly focus upon the Biological Clock Theory; this is based on the idea that there is an 'internal clock' governing the rate of cell activity and division. The timing of growth, decline and death is programmed into the individual from conception and as such there is very little that a person can do to prevent the changes that physical ageing brings.

Work by Hayflick (1985) further contributed to this theory, disproving the earlier work of Carrel by demonstrating that cells are only able to divide for a defined number of occasions. Hayflick (1985) showed that normal cells have a fixed lifespan which indicates that cells are programmed to age, and this programme underlies the ageing of the whole body.

It is also suggested that the amount of genetic material may play a role in the ageing process (Redfern, 1991). This is supported by the perception that people with Down's syndrome show signs that resemble accelerated ageing. In addition, the studies of families of people with Alzheimer's disease have revealed an excess incidence of relatives with Trisomy 21 (Redfern, 1991; Holland and Oliver, 1995). The suggestion within this theory is that chromosome 21 may have some relationship with the biological process of ageing.

Building upon the concept of each individual having their own biological clock and the implicit notion of time-limited cell division, are the error and somatic mutation theories. The underpinning principle of each of these theories is that during the course of cell division, errors occur either within deoxyribonucleic acid (DNA) or ribonucleic acid (RNA), thus resulting in the production of faulty cells. These cells are then reproduced through the normal processes of cell division, and over successive generations will accumulate within the individual's genetic makeup. This is seen as having the potential to interfere with the ability of the cell to maintain its biological functioning and may ultimately result in a loss of function in the part of the organism in which the error occurred.

Unprogrammed theories are based upon the belief that individuals experience physical 'wear and tear', dependent upon their lifestyle. Underpinning these theories is the idea that the genetic makeup of an individual can be influenced or damaged by external variables, for example, pollution, diet and smoking. Within these theories there is an assumption that an individual may have some personal control over how quickly and successfully they age. The unprogrammed theories that are most commonly referred to are the Error Accumulation, Free Radical, Chemical Cross-Linkage and Auto Immune theories.

Error Accumulation theory is based on the belief that environmental factors, for example, radiation or pollution, cause genetic mutation which lead to ageing through faulty cell production and proliferation. Comfort (1977) compares this with photographic reproductions, that is, if a negative is scratched, all subsequent prints from it will be flawed.

The Free Radical theory (Harman, 1968) proposed that free radicals are a central agent in the cause of the changes that can be seen with ageing at the tissue, cellular and subcellular levels. Free radicals are chemical intermediates which contain an unpaired electron and result in instability. The consequence of this is a large increase in free energy which allows these unstable electrons to attack adjacent molecules. According to this theory, free radicals damage important biological molecules, the accumulation of which leads to the decline in function that may be seen with ageing. Free radicals may be formed from materials in the diet, or in the atmosphere, or from irradation with ultraviolet light.

The Chemical Cross-Linkage theory relates to the accumulation of cross-linkages in macromolecules. This means the connective tissues such as collagen and elastin fibres form knots which reduce their elasticity. As such, the connective tissues become much stiffer and fail to function properly. An example of this may be changes within the cardiac muscle and nervous system which in turn impairs physiological functioning. There is some doubt, however, as to whether this is an effect rather than a cause of ageing (Redfern, 1991).

Finally, within the Auto Immune theory, an individual's immune response is known to decline with age and it has been suggested that it may in itself be a causative factor in the process of normal ageing. Burnett (1970) suggested that the thymus gland is central to all the changes in the ageing immune system. Thymus-mediated lymphocytes generally deal with any abnormal cells in the body by destroying them. However, the numbers of such lymphocytes are reduced with age and as such are unable to maintain their previous level of activity. This therefore results in the individual being unable to fight off disease and/or damage. Walford (1974) states that the situation may be aggravated by the production of antigens that are the result of cell mutation.

Essentially the biological theories focus upon the potential existence of a number of physical changes that take place within the human body. These include:

- Changes to the central nervous system
- Sensory changes
- Balance
- Heart and circulation
- Respiration
- Kidney and fluid balance
- Reproductive changes
- Skeletal changes
- Muscular and dermatological changes
- Homeostasis

When considering the biological theories of ageing it is easy to dismiss their value based upon the lack of concrete evidence to support them. However, it is possible that all the theories do have something to offer in the debate as to why people grow physically old. It is, however, difficult to identify just one theory that clearly explains biological ageing and it may be more useful to consider the potential contribution of each of the approaches rather than searching for the one right answer. Despite this, Strehler (1962) identified four criteria that formed the basis of ageing in the post-reproductive phase of life. These criteria include Universality, Internality, Progressiveness and Harmfulness.

For an alteration in physiology to be a part of the normal ageing process, it must happen to each member of the population, and therefore it must be 'universal'. The difficulty with this is that many conditions that are defined as a result of growing old might happen to different people at different stages in their lives and often with differing severity. Meanwhile, internality relates to processes which constitute normal ageing and must come from within the organism and not from external sources. In today's society, it is difficult to identify whether an illness is internal or as a result of environmental factors. This is particularly relevant with regard to societies' concerns about pollution and its
➤6 effect upon their nation's health.

Within the category of progressiveness, biological changes which define ageing must occur gradually over time, not suddenly. In many situations it is difficult to discriminate between acute and gradual onset, as a progressive illness may well manifest itself as an acute onset of illness. The final distinguishing feature of ageing is that the changes must have a deleterious or harmful effect upon the individual and their ability to cope with the environment.

The final result of ageing is inevitably death, which is seen as a profound loss and therefore a negative event, particularly within western cultures. In some cultures, death is seen as the beginnings of rebirth and is therefore celebrated as such. In this context ageing is not, perhaps seen as totally negative, but more as
➤2 a positive experience.

Essentially this section has considered the biological approaches to ageing and their relationship with the physical manifestations that we are faced with as we progress into later life. Biological and physical changes do not, however, take place consistently from individual to individual. It is for this reason, amongst others, that society has chosen to identify an additional system by which to categorize old age, that is, chronological stratification.

CHRONOLOGICAL APPROACHES TO AGEING

Chronological ageing is a way of measuring the value of one's life in terms of how many years a person has lived. The use of such a measure requires society to be organized in such a way that these measures are useful and beneficial. As such, each individual within society needs to have some idea of their chronological age. As already noted, physiological manifestations of ageing occur at different rates in different people. Although chronological age is frequently used to define the onset of old age, it is at best only a very inaccurate guide to the biological ageing of an individual (Victor, 1994).

Answer the following questions:

■ How old is old?
■ What is the difference between felt age and chronological age?

The use of chronology as a means of defining age is based upon a number of assumptions. The first is based upon the culture that exists within a given society. In order to understand the culture there is a requirement for the individual to have knowledge of the culture and the society. This is particularly important in relation to the social meanings that are attributed to particular ages and age groups. A further element is the use of chronological ageing to define old age. This dimension relates to the response of the Government to the perceived problems of old age.

Phillipson (1982) suggests that, increasingly, old age has become defined as the time when an individual becomes eligible to receive support from the state, or is excluded from participation in the labour market. However, Victor (1994) argues that the use of such chronological approaches is based more upon the cultural ascriptions of society than on their function as an indicator of biological ageing. Despite these limitations, chronological age is given much importance in society, especially when defining particular phases of an individual's lifespan. One important aspect of this for older people is the way in which age is used to legally determine when a person is able to work or when a person has to retire.

Society is often described as being stratified or divided along a variety of dimensions, for example social class. Riley (1971) suggests that age stratification theory uses chronological age as the defining variable. Therefore teenagers, middle-aged and older people are seen as distinctive groups within most societies. Every society divides individuals into age groups, and these groups reflect and create age-related differences in capacities, roles, rights and privileges. There are three issues which dominate this theory; these include firstly the meaning of age and the position of age groups within society. Secondly, individuals experience transitions through the lifecycle because of the social definitions of age. Finally, within such societies there are mechanisms for the allocation of roles between individuals.

Think about your roles in society; how does your age affect these roles?

Are there any differences between your roles and those of older people that you know?

Age stratification suggests that role transitions are timetabled by age norms rather than by selection. To understand these transitions we have to be aware of the process of socialization by which individuals learn to accept specific roles and role transitions. Such a theory believes that socialization is a lifelong process in which people move through a number of roles as they age. The value of this approach is that it allows us to consider any age group in terms of its demographic characteristics and its relationships to other age groups. Conversely, the classification of the age strata within society in such a way can also have inherent difficulties. These include the development and maintenance of stereotypical images of different age groups and compartmentalization of people into specific age bands and associated roles. Such a system is dynamic, and the complexity of this structure is further complicated by the inextricable link that exists with other strata such as class or ethnicity.

The age grading of roles within any age related system creates differences and inequalities. Each group is evaluated by itself and by society in terms of the dominant social values. Victor (1994) argues that this differential evaluation of roles will produce an unequal distribution of power and prestige across the age group. Thus when societies value the experience and wisdom of older people and allow them to undertake roles which capitalize upon this experience, then older people will be accorded respect. Conversely, when considering older individuals who also have a learning disability or mental health need, such a transition in societies' approach would not necessarily produce the same outcome. These individuals not only have to overcome the negative stereotypes associated with old age but also those associated with their disability.

Retirement is defined as the formal withdrawal from the labour market at a specified age. In many ways this action creates a stratum within society that is distinctly separate from the remaining adult population. As we have a society which clearly values work and productivity, this period of enforced leisure results in the retired person being disempowered and losing prestige and status within society. Phillipson (1982) suggests that individuals approach retirement in many different ways. Perhaps the most important of these is termed stable withdrawal. This situation occurs where retirement is accepted and the individual accepts the changes in life style and behaviour which follow. In many ways retirement is seen as a right of passage where people's roles within society are formally altered.

For a person who has an enduring mental health need or a learning disability this rite of passage may not be as clear cut as it is for other older people. These individuals may not have had the same experience of work. Though valued employment is the goal of many services, achieving this for each individual can be problematic and many people will find themselves only able to access valued occupation for a part of their working week. In addition the change in finances that is often associated with retirement will usually be different for this group of people. This is a consequence of their previous dependence upon the Welfare State and as such they do not always have substantial savings to fall back on. This situation creates different constraints for the person to consider in the context of managing their period of 'retirement'.

The process of transition to retirement is a complex phenomenon and Victor (1994) suggests that it is far too simplistic to divide people into the retired and the non-retired. Atchley (1976) divides the process of retirement into a series of phases; these phases are not unique to retirement but are typical of all major role transitions. The phases include pre-retirement, where expectations are formed, honeymoon, which immediately follows retirement, and disenchantment, which is as a result of failure to develop satisfying roles and routines. Reorientation is defined as a phase where stock is taken and choices are made, stability is where an individual can deal with the changes brought about by retirement, and finally, termination is where retirement is no longer of importance. This stage in life is often manifested by the onset of disability or poor health. When considering the stages identified by Atchley (1976) it is essential to consider what this may mean for those people who have an enduring mental health need or a learning disability as the labels ascribed to these individuals instantly place them in the final category of Atchley's phases.

Retirement as a formal withdrawal from society is further explored in work by Cumming and Henry (1961) who identified the concept of disengagement. Expressed in its simplest form this perspective suggests that there is a gradual but inevitable withdrawal or disengagement from interaction between the individual and the social context. Cumming and Henry (1961) argue that this withdrawal is undertaken in preparation for the ultimate act of disengagement, that is the death of the person. Whilst the individual is preparing themselves for death, society is preparing the individual for growing old, by withdrawing the pressure to interact. Central to this theory is the assumption that both the individual and society benefit from the process of disengagement. Withdrawal for the individual may mean a release from the social pressures of productivity, competition and continued achievement. For society, the withdrawal of older people permits more energetic and younger individuals to take over which is seen to make economic sense. Therefore disengagement is seen as a way of transferring power between generations in an orderly fashion.

Does the concept of disengagement have any value to those people who have not been part of the formal workforce?

You may have explored the relevance to people who have a learning disability, informal carers, people with a physical disability and people who have an enduring mental health need. Often these individuals do not experience the same demands from society in relation to the social pressures for productivity, continued achievement and competition. Disengagement for these individuals does not serve the purpose of transferring roles and responsibilities to the next generation.

Victor (1994) identifies that although there is some empirical evidence to support this theory, much of it is ambiguous as insufficient attention has been paid to the strategies of substitution and compensation used by many older people. For example, older people may replace a widespread and loose-knit pattern of interaction with more intense and local networks. Blau (1973) argues that disengagement has been used to avoid dealing with the issue of the marginalization of older people in society, whilst Fiske (1986) suggests that the existence of disengagement theory allows professionals to rationalize their own negative stereotypes. Within this, the theory of disengagement enables the erection of barriers between older people and other social groups.

An alternative view to the notion of disengagement is that which is encapsulated within activity theory (Havighurst, 1963). This idea maintains that normal and successful ageing involves preserving the attitude and activities of middle age into older age. To compensate for activities and roles the individual gives up, substitutes are found. The assumption within this is that the relationship between society and older people remains stable and the norms for old age are the same as those for middle age. Older people are rated against middle-age values, and ageing is a continuous struggle to remain middle aged. Lemon *et al.* (1972) suggest there are two further central assumptions to these ideas. These are, firstly, that morale and life satisfaction are related to high-quality social integration, and secondly, that role losses such as retirement are inversely corre-

➤6 lated with life satisfaction or dissatisfaction.

As with disengagement theory, supporting evidence is ambiguous. Lemon *et al.* (1972) found no evidence to support the above assumptions; however, Palmore (1965) demonstrated some relationship between activity, morale and personal adjustment. A further difficulty with activity theory is that there is no account of what happens to those individuals who lose the battle to remain middle aged. However, Victor (1994) suggests that this perspective is more positive than disengagement as it concentrates upon older people being integrated as full members of society.

LIFESPAN AND LIFECYCLE APPROACHES TO AGEING

Bond *et al.* (1992) suggest that the study of the psychology of ageing is best placed within the lifespan perspective. Lifespan and developmental approaches to the ideas around ageing are relatively recent in their evolution. As such, they are less clearly defined compared to more traditional psychological theories and ideas, such as intelligence and the ability to learn.

Erikson provides an alternative approach in his theory of lifestages. This approach to the human life course looks for connections between earlier life experiences and later behaviour and attitudes. Erikson (1982) felt that personality develops throughout a person's lifespan. This is in direct contrast to other psychoanalysts such as Freud, who believed that personality was determined by childhood habits and experiences. Erikson (1982) argues that at different ages, different conflicts have to be resolved. There are eight of these conflicts of which only the final one occurs in old age. This is the conflict of integrity versus despair. The goal of this final stage is ego integration – the acceptance that earlier goals have been satisfied or resolved, and there are no loose ends. His Epigenetic theory suggests that without a sense of ego integrity, ageing creates feelings of anger, bitterness and inadequacy, which reduce coping mechanisms in later life (Erikson, 1963). This lack of coping is felt to lead to a less successful experience of growing older.

Conversely, Levinson *et al.* (1978) proposed a normative theory of the life structure which consisted of a series of alternating stable (structure building) and transitional (structure changing) phases. These include the mid-life transition (40–45 years) which may herald a wish to be more oneself and more self-generating in one's actions. The successful resolution of the mid-life stage leads into another stable period (45–50 years) before another transition at around 50 and finally into old age.

The concept of the lifecycle can also be used as a way of defining old age. The lifecycle is usually seen as a progression from birth to death or from infancy to old age. Within this progression, biological, social, economic and cultural factors interact to determine the sequence of a person's life. Victor (1994) argues that from this perspective the categories of the lifecycle such as youth, middle age or old age are seen as social constructs which are based upon social cues and norms rather than a more structured approach to society.

Such an idea appears simple; however, the interaction of the above factors makes progression through the lifecycle a highly complex process. Neugarten (1974) suggests that the lifecycle has become increasingly differentiated into smaller and smaller subgroups for example, adolescence, pre-school, old age, very old age and very very old age. Laslett (1989) uses the terms 'third age' (50–74) and the 'fourth age' (75+) as ways of redefining groups of older people.

The information considered thus far indicates that considerable time and effort has been devoted to trying to unravel the mysteries of what happens to our bodies and our skills and abilities as we grow older. Writers and researchers have also tried to understand the position that older people have within society and what variables come to bear on older people, both individually and as a group, in order to create these aspects of social order. Many authors have also attempted to consider these influences from the perspective of the older person. It is not within the remit of nursing to answer any of these questions as nursing is not about finding the ultimate truth in the way that perhaps biology or psychology is. Nursing older people is primarily concerned with the individual, their personal experience and their needs. In order for nurses to address this issue effectively they do, however, need an understanding of the areas touched upon within this chapter, and others considered during subsequent chapters. Analysis of these issues will better equip nurses working with this client group to provide high-quality nursing care to individuals. The final part of this chapter considers the theories discussed thus far and associated information in the context of nursing older people.

APPLICATION TO NURSING PRACTICE

The practice of nursing does not exist in a vacuum, as an activity nursing is affected by the experience of the client, the nurse and all those others involved in a person's life and their healthcare. Within this scenario, each of the players is also influenced by both their present and their past experiences, i.e. the socialization processes they have undergone. Nurses have experienced an additional process in the form of their nurse education and the specific culture that exists within the different parts of the nursing profession (Melia, 1987). Essentially, this means that nurses are firstly subject to many of the traditional societal stereotypes about older people. They are also subject to the stereotypical beliefs that abound regarding ill older people, which are generally negative. The issue that nursing and nurses must address is how these values impact upon their individual nursing practice.

The following care study considers the experience of one lady (Maud) during a difficult period in her life. This study will, through a description of her experiences, explore some of the ideas discussed in the earlier part of this chapter. These discussions will not alway directly relate to nursing or nursing environments, nor will they be made overtly relevant to nursing. They are, however, all important for nurses to consider and reflect upon, as the actual relevance will be determined by the nature of real-life nurse-client interactions. This care study will be explored both in terms of Maud as an individual, her close relations and those who come into contact with her. Here the reader will be guided to more relevant in-depth reading of the impact of the theories that are being described.

CASE STUDY

Maud was 50 years old when we first met her. She had come to the GP surgery complaining of headaches and occasional nose bleeds. She was diagnosed as having hypertension, which was quickly and effectively managed through a combination of drugs and a low-salt diet. Her husband hated having to share this diet as he had always enjoyed plenty of salt with his food.

Kenney (1989) identifies that most older people live a normal independent life and most processes in their body appear to function adequately. Evidence, however, suggests that there are some age-related changes that occur naturally, for example those that affect the cardiovascular system. These include structural changes to the connective tissue and muscle in terms of contractility and elasticity. Of particular relevance are the changes in connective tissue matrix, which lead to stiffness of the myocardium. Redfern (1991) states that when comparing the cardiovascular function of both young and old people, it is important to ensure that the level of physical fitness is similar, i.e. heart rate, blood pressure and other cardiorespiratory parameters. In terms of blood pressure, Kenney (1989) suggests that there are increases in arterial pressure that are a consequence of age. Longitudinal and cross-sectional studies have shown an increase in systolic pressure in older people as well as a smaller rate of increase in diastolic pressure (Kenney, 1989).

There is a debate, however, as to whether this increase in blood pressure is an inevitable consequence of normal ageing processes and essentially biological in its origin, or whether there are additional external factors to be considered such as diet and lifestyle. Advocates of the biological approach to ageing see the decrease in an older person's ability to maintain homeostatic equilibrium as evidence that ageing is a process that takes place within the individual and is not influenced by external variables. Kenney (1989) highlights examples of primitive societies who do not generally show an increase in blood pressure as they age, potentially indicating that external factors can and do have an effect. These results have been replicated in people with chronic mental health problems who have grown old in protected institutional environments.

Additional perspectives may be gained by further consideration of programmed and unprogrammed theories of ageing identified earlier in the chapter.

CASE STUDY

Maud was happily married to Robert and they were coming up towards their Ruby wedding anniversary. They had one son who was married with two children. At this time Maud was preparing herself for her retirement. This was a big event for her as she had worked for many years in the local factory. Robert was still in full-time employment and had a further five years before reaching retirement age.

Both Maud and Robert were very tidy people, both in themselves and in their home. Maud would dust, polish and hoover every morning before setting off to work. Both of them had a very clear routine that they liked within their lives. A very important part of this routine was her regular visit every Saturday morning to the local hairdresser for her weekly shampoo and set, six-weekly tint and four-monthly perm. In addition to the care that she took with her hair, Maud was meticulous about her overall appearance, always liking to look her best, she paid particular attention to her skin, using well-known skincare creams to maintain the condition of her skin.

The structure of the skin is known to alter with ageing, one of the most obvious outward signs of this is the appearance of wrinkles. The precise cause of wrinkles is still unknown, however theories and ideas abound regarding this, particularly focusing upon their eradication. So much so that a multimillion-pound industry has evolved based upon exploitation of both the absence of empirical information and the abundance of speculation regarding the cause of wrinkles in skin. Those people who perceive wrinkles and other outward physical signs of ageing as purely biological in origin will search for answers in areas such as cell division, biological clock theories etc. Those individuals clearly identify ageing as something that is able to be cured, hence the popularity of both the cosmetic industry and plastic surgery. An alternative viewpoint, however, is that old age also has a social construction associated with it. This social construction is the viewpoint that is commonly espoused by members of a given culture. Typically western cultures extol the virtues of youth, which is perceived as a time of energy, enthusiasm, resourcefulness and inventiveness. In comparison later life is seen as being characterized by decline and stagnation.

CASE STUDY   Maud was feeling very positive about her approaching retirement with lots of thoughts about what she would like to do with her time, particularly as she felt that she was still a very fit and active lady. She was proud of her ability to still walk the four or five miles into town, even though it was not as far as she had been used to walking in her younger days. This did, however, allow her to continue with her favourite pastime of rambling with the local walkers' club. Maud would meet with her friends at the club each Sunday afternoon when they would go for a walk around a site of local interest or one of the nearby villages.

Fennell *et al.* (1988) suggest that retirement is an essential part of old age, particularly as it is used as a marker that old age has started. Coleman (1982) however, identifies that the lead up to retirement for many people appears to be very stressful. A key cause of this stress is seen to be the lack of understanding that individuals have about the concept of retirement and what it will mean for them as a person. Phillipson and Strang (1983) identify that for many individuals they have no clear focus and are concerned about what they will do with the rest of their lives. This may have some impact upon how they then spend their increased leisure time.

There is some overlap between the psychological and sociological approach to growing older. Within this, an individual may experience personal stress, such as worry regarding social and economic stability, as a consequence of the social institution of retirement. This may be the case even though the individual will be expecting the life transition.

CASE STUDY

Since Maud had been diagnosed as having a cataract over her left eye, Robert had begun to join her for her Sunday afternoon outings. Maud found this extremely pleasant as she was able to share the experience of the walk more thoroughly with Robert, they could talk about the little things that they saw and also problems they had at work or in the family. Robert, though he enjoyed spending the time with Maud and the other ramblers, was particularly concerned about Maud's ability to manage uneven ground and changes in daylight. As such, he felt that he could support her at these points on the walks without undermining her independence and the enjoyment of the day.

In addition, to her problems with her sight, Maud also had some degree of hearing impairment; this was the result of an untreated ear infection when she was 56. This meant that she was unable to hear what people said to her if they were not facing her, if they were in another room, or if there was significant background noise. This, on occasions, caused difficulties between her and Robert as he had sensitive hearing which meant he could not stand the television being turned up too loud. Maud, however, needs to have it relatively loud in order that she can hear all that is being said.

The incidence of deafness increases with age. Gilhome *et al.* (1981) suggest that 60% of people over the age of 70 are deaf or have severe hearing impairment. This situation means that hearing impairment is a major difficulty for many older people. Many people adjust to this loss by using strategies such as lip reading, facing people directly or turning their head to maximize the effectiveness of their 'good ear', when communicating. However, there is evidence to suggest that people with hearing loss do experience feelings of depression, low ➤9 self-esteem, and social isolation (Redfern, 1991).

These feelings might be amplified for a person who lives alone as their environment may be restricted and therefore boring and monotonous. This, combined with reductions in the effectiveness of elderly people's sensory ability, can ➤12 also result in a lack of sensory stimulation. In some circumstances, where people have health problems and are very isolated, individuals may be inappropriately assessed as being disoriented or confused. An isolating lifestyle has been shown to lead to a decrease in the capacity of the individual to learn and think; it is suggested that a lack of stimulation reduces the effectiveness of the brain.

CASE STUDY

Two months later the big day of Maud's retirement arrived; she had a number of celebrations planned, both at work and at home with her family. Maud started her final day at work with some very mixed feelings; she was excited at the thought of not having to actually get up and go to work ever again and all the time she would have for herself and her family. At the same time she felt a sense of sadness that she would be leaving a lot of very good friends, many of whom she had known a good number of years. At this time, however, the excitement outweighed the sadness, and the very busy and hectic schedule of parties and celebrations filled all Maud's time.

During the first month Maud was busy writing thank-you letters, catching up with lots of other outstanding jobs, occasionally popping into where she used to work to see her old friends and planning the holiday that she and Robert had promised themselves on her retirement. On return from their holiday in Jersey, life began to settle into a new routine. Robert still had to get up and go to work most days of the week,

Maud still got up at the same time as her husband and, as she had always done, finished the dusting, polishing and hoovering before 8.30 a.m. Suddenly the rest of the day seemed an awfully long time for her to do the washing and ironing and to get Robert's dinner ready for when he came home.

The days seemed to get progressively longer for Maud; she loved breakfast time while Robert was home, the evenings when he had returned from work and the weekends, when they still spent time together, and also with the ramblers' club. The only highlights of what Maud now perceived as extremely long and empty days were the occasions when her son and her grandchildren visited.

Adjustment and adaptation to life occur for each individual at various life stages. The ability to adapt or adjust to the changes that occur physically, psychologically and socially with increasing age, are said to be the key to successful ageing (Bromley, 1988; Bond and Coleman, 1990). It may be that individuals who adjust well have a greater sense of well-being, better self-esteem and personal motivation than those who find retirement a period of dissatisfaction. Gurland and Toner (1982) suggest that individuals who have the greatest difficulty adjusting to not working are more likely to experience depressive illness.

CASE STUDY

One day whilst Maud was out in town she bumped into an old friend from work who had also retired. Maud and Elsie went for a coffee at the local hospice shop, and whilst they were talking Maud realized that Elsie was still extremely busy, possibly even busier than before her retirement. She spent much of her time helping out at a local charity shop as well as working in the hospice coffee shop and the friends of the local theatre group. Elsie invited Maud to join her at the friends of the local theatre coffee morning to see if she would be interested in the activities of the group.

Ten days later Maud went to her first coffee morning, she could not believe how many people she actually knew. Maud spent the whole morning at the coffee morning and thoroughly enjoyed herself. On her return home, she was shocked to discover how quickly the day had passed and how much she had to talk to Robert about during the evening. Following this Maud became more and more involved with the work of the group, and soon Elsie had got Maud not only working at the theatre but also covering a few hours each week at the local charity shop.

Maud's involvement in all these activities soon began to make her feel much more positive about herself and her retirement. Her days became much fuller and almost started to feel as though they were flying past. They also provided much more for Maud and Robert to talk about and within a fairly short space of time Maud was almost as busy as she had been prior to her retirement. In addition to the shop and the theatre group she also regularly supported her daughter-in-law, by baby sitting her new granddaughter. Maud now found she had more interest in walking and often went on days other than her old Sunday slot, she also quite enjoyed the occasional shopping trip – time permitting.

Evidence suggests that society features a division of labour between the sexes (Stacey, 1981; Dex, 1985). In this, women tend to be ascribed work within the home and family whilst male responsibilities tend to lie within the paid work arena. Although this may be a generalization amongst younger women, for many older women this was seen as the norm (Fennell *et al.*, 1988). Essentially therefore many contemporary older women have never been an acknowledged part of the economic viability of the environment in which they live. This situation can be seen to be perpetuated by the number of older women who support their children by providing childcare for them without any financial remuneration. Despite this essential contribution to both their family and to society, in general older people are still frequently perceived as economically non-productive.

CASE STUDY   Life was now feeling very positive and enjoyable once again, when one day Maud received a phone call whilst working in the hospice shop. Robert had been taken ill at work and rushed to hospital. Maud rang her son immediately who left work and came to pick her up. On arrival at the hospital a doctor explained to Maud and her son, that Robert had had a serious heart attack and was very poorly, but stable. Maud and her son stayed until the evening, at which point all three of them decided that it was for the best if Maud and Jack were to go home and return the following day. Maud was unhappy about leaving Robert but could not see what else she could do. Jack asked if she wanted to come and stay with him and his wife, but Maud said she would be fine, she would be much happier in her own home.

When she got home, Maud busied herself making some tea. The house seemed very big and empty; it was the first time that she had been separated from Robert since their wedding. Bedtime eventually arrived and Maud made herself go to bed, she found it difficult to sleep, it didn't seem right, her in the big bed alone and Robert all that way away in the hospital. Just as Maud was dropping off to sleep, the telephone rang, it was the hospital asking her if she could get there as soon as possible as Robert had had a relapse. Maud rang for a taxi immediately and got dressed in a blind panic.

Maud arrived at the hospital 20 minutes later; she was, however, too late. Robert had had a second heart attack and had died without regaining consciousness. Maud was devastated, not only by the news, but also by the fact that she had not been there when her beloved Robert had passed away. How could she have gone home and left him all alone in this place? Maud stayed with Robert until Jack arrived; Jack took her downstairs to his car and took her home with him.

The next few days were the most difficult Maud had ever experienced; she found it very hard going back to her and Robert's home knowing that he would never walk through the door again. She found it impossible to organize his funeral; in fact Jack had to do most of that.

When the day of the funeral arrived, Maud got up out of bed with a determination that she was going to look her best for Robert. She put on the dress Robert had always liked her in; it wasn't black, but that didn't seem to matter. Looking back on the day, Maud felt it was a nice dignified service and one that Robert would have liked.

Bereavement is often seen as an experience that only old people have. This is based on the social construct that death is the only certainty in anyone's life and is reinforced by the belief that man will live threescore years and ten. Murray Parkes (1975) identifies that for many older people undergoing this experience, society will expect them to come to terms with the inevitability of the situation. In addition, older people are not necessarily expected to experience the same amount of grief as a younger person, if they lose a partner or friend. This is in part due to societies' acceptance of the inevitability of death and the understanding that older people are closer to this ultimate consequence of life than younger people. As a consequence it may be that the grief reactions that older people have are seen as not important and as not such a painful experience. Within this, it is possible that the period of grieving for older people is expected to be shorter than younger people.

CASE STUDY

Over the next few months, Maud felt lost and alone, the emptiness of the days reminded her of when she had first finished work. When she finally realized this Maud also realized that though she still loved Robert she had to rebuild her life and that she knew she had the strength to do it. The following day Maud went and visited her friend Elsie and they arranged to go to the next theatre group coffee morning.

The loneliness that Maud experienced is arguably the consequence of the changes that have evolved in the society in which we live. Recent years have seen the transition from the extended family model within a society that had a strong feeling of community to one of the nuclear family where people are more isolated from one another (Aries, 1983). Implicit within the evolution towards a more fragmented society has been the transition of death as a communal and public activity to a much more private, insular one.

CONCLUSION

Walker (1985), Townsend (1986) and Phillipson (1982) suggest that the values that individuals hold regarding everyday life are based upon how they have been socialized. In this way beliefs about ageing and what it is like to be old are determined by personal experiences and societies' presentation of ageing. Western stereotypes of ageing are seen as particularly negative and older people are perceived as having exceeded their usefulness, as well as being poor, deaf, immobile, incontinent, senile and generally ill.

This perception has consequences for an individual's status within society, which in turn has implications for the way in which essential services are made available to older people. For example, healthcare services for older people are identified as separate from mainstream provision as a consequence of the perception that this group of people require different care to that of a younger person who may have a similar need. It could be argued that this differentiation of service need is rooted in the belief that the older person is more dependent and therefore requires more resources.

Townsend (1986) suggests that the concept of an old person as dependent upon others and unable to maintain their own lives is a consequence of dominant economic and political forces. Therefore, experiences such as retirement, poverty, institutionalization and the restriction of domestic and community roles reinforce negative images of ageing. This situation has the potential to lead to the development of a self-fulfilling prophecy in which economic and political forces create a perception of dependence. As such therefore, services are then designed based upon these values and beliefs, and the experiences that individual people have with these services shapes them into behaving in a dependent manner. The final outcome of this cyclical process is that the older person's behaviour then reinforces the original political and economic belief upon which the cycle was founded, thus creating a self-fulfilling prophecy.

In conclusion, this chapter has briefly explained some of the influences upon the experience of growing old in western society. This has included the consequences of how old age is defined. Within this, consideration has been given to chronological approaches to ageing and the impact of the stratification of society based upon age. This chapter has also explored the effect that the outward signs of physical ageing can have upon an individual's experience of growing older. In addition the chapter has briefly looked at the lifecycle and lifespan approaches to ageing. The areas addressed do not provide an all-encompassing exploration of the influence upon old age, but some areas are covered that are of crucial importance to nurses working with this group of people, as was demonstrated within the care study.

FURTHER READING

Belsky, T.A. (1990) *The Psychology of Ageing: Theory, Research and Interventions*. Springer, New York.
This text looks at the psychology of ageing with particular reference to stereotypes and realities. In addition, there are sections looking at the ageing body, intelligence, memory and creativity as well as personality. There are also useful sections which consider the effects of bereavement and retirement.

Bond, J. and Coleman, P. (1992) *Ageing in Society: an Introduction to Social Gerontology*. Sage Publications, London.
This book is a general gerontological text which provides a broad overview of many of the theories which underpin the study of ageing. There is a section on psychological effects of ageing and also adjustment in late life which is particularly useful for practitioners.

Fennell, G., Phillipson, C. and Evers, H. (1988) *The Sociology of Old Age*. Open University Press, Milton Keynes.
This text provides a sociological perspective on growing older. There are useful and interesting sections on relevant images of old age and health and illness in old age.

Johnson, A. and Slater, R. (1990) *Ageing and Late Life*. Open University Press, Milton Keynes.
This reader for the Open University is a particularly good source of broad information which relates to the experience of ageing.

Kenney, R.A. (1989) *Physiology of Ageing: a Synopsis*, 2nd edn. Year Book Medical Publishers, Chicago.
This text utilizes an easy reading approach to explore the general aspects of ageing, the theories of ageing and the effect of ageing upon the systems. Part One of the book is useful reading in relation to homeostasis and the effect of increasing age.

Redfern, S. (ed.) (1991) *Nursing Elderly People*, 2nd edn. Churchill Livingstone, Edinburgh.
There are a variety of texts concerning nursing older people. This book is perhaps the most comprehensive as it covers not only the physical

manifestations of ageing and the related nursing care, but also the underpinning theories of ageing. There are useful chapters which consider the psychological and biological impact of ageing. In addition, Redfern does address some of the political dimensions of nursing older people.

Spence, A.P. (1989) *Biology of Human Ageing.* Prentice Hall, London.
This whole book deals with the biological aspects of growing old. Of particular relevance is Chapter One, which discusses the general effects of ageing and how chronology and biology can differ. Chapter Two is a useful overview of the general theories of ageing.

Further reading around the normal ageing process can be found in Redfern (1991), Kenney (1989) and Spender (1989).

Additional information regarding the impact of a youth culture can be found earlier in this chapter. More in-depth reading can be found in Victor (1994) and Bond and Coleman (1992).

Further perspectives on the psychological and sociological approaches can be found within the sections relating to chronological approaches to ageing, in particular disengagement and activity theories. More in-depth reading can be found in Fennell *et al.* (1988), Redfern (1991) and Bond and Coleman (1992).

Further perspectives on the issues of isolation may be derived from consideration of the theories relating to intelligence and ability, memory and learning. More in-depth reading can be found in Redfern (1991) and Atkinson *et al.* (1993).

Adjustment and adaptation can be further considered in the context of Activity theory. Additional reading in this subject area can be found in Bond and Coleman (1990).

REFERENCES

Aries, P. (1983) *The Hour of Our Death.* Penguin, Harmondsworth.

Atchley, R. (1976) Selected social and psychological differences between men and women in later life. *Journal of Gerontology,* 31, 204–211.

Atkinson, R.L., Atkinson, R. C. and Hilgard, E.R. (1993) *Introduction to Psychology,* 10th edn. Harcourt Brace Jovanovich, New York.

Blau, Z. (1973) *Old age in a Changing Society.* Franklin Watts, New York.

Bond, J. and Coleman, P. (1990) *Ageing in Society: an Introduction to Social Gerontology.* Sage Publications, London.

Bond, J., Briggs, R. and Coleman, P. (1992) The study of ageing. In *Ageing in Society: an Introduction to Social Gerontology.* Sage Publications, London.

Bromley, D.B. (1988) *Human Ageing: an Introduction to Gerontology.* Penguin, London.

Burnett, F.M. (1970) An immunological approach to aging. *The Lancet,* 2, 358.

Coleman, A. (1982) *Preparation for Retirement in England and Wales.* NIAE, Leicester.

Comfort, A. (1960) Discussion session 1. Definition and universality of aging. In *The Biology of Aging,* Strehler, B.L. (ed.), pp. 3–13. American Institute of Biological Sciences, Washington.

Comfort, A. (1977) *A Good Age.* Mitchell Beazeley, London.

Cowgill, D.O. and Holmes, L.D. (eds) (1972) *Aging and Modernization.* Appleton, New York.

Cumming, E. and Henry, W. (1981) *Growing Old: the Process of Disengagement.* Basic Books, New York.

Dex, S. (1985) *The Sexual Divisions of Work.* Wheatsheaf Books, Brighton.

Erikson, E.H. (1963) *Childhood and Society,* 2nd edn. Norton, New York.

Erikson, E.H. (1982) *The Lifecycle Completed: a Review*. Norton, New York.

Fennell, G., Phillipson, C. and Evers, H. (1988) *The Sociology of Old Age*. Open University Press, Milton Keynes.

Fiske, M.J. (1986) *Independence and the Elderly*. Croom Helm, London.

Gilhome Herbst, K.R. and Humphrey, C. (1981) Prevalence of hearing impairment in the elderly living at home. *Journal of the Royal College of General Practitioners*, **31**, 155–160.

Gurland, B.J. and Toner, J.A. (1982) Depression in the elderly: a review of recently published studies. *Annual Review of Gerontology and Geriatrics*, **3**, 228–265.

Harman, D. (1968) Free radical theory of aging: effect of free radical inhibitors on the mortality rate of LAF1 mice. *Gerontology*, **23**, 476.

Havighurst, R.J. (1963) *Successful Ageing*. In Williams, R.H., Tibbitts, C. and Donahue, W. (eds) *Processes of Ageing*, Volume 1. Atherton, New York, pp. 299–320.

Hayflick, L. (1985) The cell biology of ageing. *Clinical Geriatric Medicine*, **11**, 15–27.

Holland, A.J. and Oliver, C. (1995) Editorial: Down's syndrome and the links with Alzheimer's disease. *Journal of Neurology*, **59**, 111–114.

Kenney, R.A. (1989) *Physiology of Ageing: a Synopsis*, 2nd edn. Year Book Medical Publishers, Chicago.

Laslett, P. (1989). *A Fresh Map of Life: the Emergence of the Third Age*. Weidenfeld and Nicolson, New York.

Lemon, B.W., Bengston, V.L. and Peterson, J.A. (1972) Activity types and life satisfaction in a retirement community. *Journal of Gerontology*, **27**(4), 511–523.

Levinson, D.J., Darrow, D.N., Klein, E.B., Levinson, M.H. and McKee, B. (1978) *The Seasons of a Man's Life*. Knopf, New York.

Melia, K. (1987) *Learning and Working: the Occupational Socialisation of Nurses*. Tavistock, London.

Murray Parkes, C. (1975) *Bereavement Studies of Grief in Adult Life*. Pelican, Harmondsworth.

Neugarten, B. (1974) Age groups in American society. *Annals of the American Academy of Political and Social Science*, **415**, 197–198.

Palmore, E. (1965) Differences in the retirement patterns of men and women. *Gerontologist*, **5**, 4–8.

Phillipson, C. (1982) *Capitalism and the Construction of Old Age*. Macmillan, London.

Phillipson, C. and Strang, P. (1983) Pre retirement education. A longitudinal evaluation. Department of Adult Education, University of Keele, Stoke on Trent.

Redfern, S. (ed.) (1991) *Nursing Elderly People*. 2nd edn. Churchill Livingstone, Edinburgh.

Riley, M. (1971) Age strata in social systems. In *Handbook of Ageing and the Social Sciences*, Binstock, R. and Shanas, E. (eds). Van Nostrand Reinhold, New York.

Spence, A.P. (1989) *Biology of Human Aging*. Prentice Hall, Englewood, New Jersey.

Stacey, M. (1981) The division of labour revisited, or overcoming the two Adams. In *Development and Diversity: Bristol Sociology 1950–1980*, Abrahms, P., Deam, R., Finch, J. and Rock, P. (eds). George Allen and Unwin, London.

Strehler, B.L. (1962) *Time Cells and Aging*. Academic Press, New York and London.

Townsend, P. (1986) Ageism and social policy. In *Ageing and Social Policy*, Phillipson, C. and Walker, A. (eds). Gower, Aldershot, pp. 15–44.

Victor, C. (1994) *Old Age in a Modern Society*, 2nd edn. Chapman and Hall, London.

Walford, R.L. (1974) Immunological theory of aging: current status. *Federation Proceedings*, **33**, 2020.

Walker, A. (1985) Care of Elderly People in *Challenges to Social Policy*, Berthoud, R. (ed.) Gower, Aldershot.

2 | Cultural perspectives on ageing

Helen Bartlett

INTRODUCTION

The heterogeneous nature of old age has been highlighted in Chapter 1 through an examination of the biological, psychological and sociological aspects of ageing. However, the cultural processes in any society are also important to consider in understanding the diversity of old age. Culture refers to the distinctive language, knowledge, beliefs, customs and habits shared by a group of people. A group's culture provides members with a pattern for living together that is passed on to successive generations. The ageing experience in different cultures may, therefore, vary enormously, depending on:

- How old age is defined
- The expectations of older people
- The value placed on them
- Attitudes towards them
- The care needed and who is responsible for giving it

Even within the same culture there will be differences between people from different historical periods as cultures change and adapt to new pressures and needs.

Understanding cultural perspectives is important for health professionals working with older people, to promote culturally sensitive practices and more positive images of old age. Leininger's theory of cultural care diversity emphasizes the link between care and culture and the multicultural role of the nurse (Leininger, 1988). Although there are differences of opinion about the focus of Leininger's work, the need for transcultural awareness to understand the individual's point of view and assess their needs adequately is generally acknowledged (Wilkins, 1993). This is important for clients living outside their own culture and also for health professionals who may be working in a culture different to their own.

Older people from minority ethnic groups may be discouraged from seeking help because they are uncomfortable with the age, language and cultural differences of care providers. Intraethnic cultural variations also have implications for the delivery of care by health professionals (Valle, 1989). Within a minority ethnic group, expressions of culture may vary according to the setting, for example, at home, the workplace, or in the community. Caregivers and older people alike may exhibit ethnocultural responses to episodic crises in their health condition. The challenge for health professionals is to recognize, accept and respond appropriately to different cultural groups. It will also require them to look beyond the medical model of old age and negative stereotypes that depict old people as a homogeneous group of disadvantaged, poor, disabled and socially devalued people.

This chapter examines the significance of culture for the experience of ageing from a variety of perspectives. First, the impact of change and modernization on older people is discussed and the implications for intergenerational relationships explored. Secondly, examples of the ageing experience in other countries are used to illustrate a range of contrasting cultural characteristics influencing the construction of old age. This focuses largely on East Asian cultures where research has recently been conducted on ageing and aged care provision. Thirdly, the case study of Hong Kong is used to illustrate the impact of change and modernization on a rapidly ageing population. Fourth, the situation of older people in minority ethnic groups in Britain is examined. The chapter concludes with a discussion of the implications for nursing practice.

MODERNIZATION, CULTURE AND AGEING

Considerable attention has been paid by anthropologists to the impact of cultural change on older people, in particular the process of modernization. Cowgill and Holmes (1972) postulate that as societies become increasingly modern, the status of older people falls. The negative effects are more pronounced in the earlier stages of modernization, but the situation improves in the later stages with the availability of pensions and improved health care. A major limitation of the cross-cultural study of 14 societies undertaken by Cowgill and Holmes is acknowledged to be the linear approach to the arrangement of societies (from pre-literate to modern industrial), rather than a longitudinal design. This assumes that historically, Western industrial societies can be compared with pre-literate societies. In later work, Cowgill (1974) attributes the decline in the status of elderly people to four key aspects of modernization: the development of modern health technology, modern economic technology, urbanization and mass education. Such advances, it is argued, contribute to the ageing of the population, inter-generational tensions, devaluing of retirement and of employment skills of the old, break-up of the extended family and reduction of the power of old people.

The existence of an earlier era in which older people were venerated and cared for by the family has been strongly challenged by recent historical analysis. Convincing evidence of a 'golden age' of older people in pre-literate cultures is lacking (Victor, 1994). A different view of Britain in the nineteenth century is presented by Quadagno (1982), who argues that there was no golden age and that extended-family living was a result of economic factors and not necessarily characteristic of traditional societies. In reality, the village communities of pre-industrial Britain were characterized by grinding poverty, short life expectancy and neglect of non-productive members. A complex set of inter-related factors possibly influenced the position of older people in these societies (Victor, 1994), including:

- Contribution to economic, family or cultural activities
- The value of their experience to the society
- The status attributed to them from their previous work activities
- Their control over knowledge, scarce resources or political power

Victor (1994 p. 73) concludes that for most people, ageing was 'a time of pauperism, degradation and dependency' and that in Britain there was no time when the old were venerated for themselves. In America too, it has been argued that the status of old people was threatened long before the changes associated with modernization commenced and resulted from ideological changes related to notions about liberty, equality and individualism (Achenbaum, 1978).

INTER-GENERATIONAL RELATIONSHIPS

The twentieth century has been described as a 'cultural watershed' in relation to the traditional contract across generations and age groups in America and Europe (Bengston, 1993). According to Bengston, prospects for future relations between generations may be either negative or positive. A deterioration in age group or generational relations may result from increases in the dependency ratio (the ratio of dependent aged to the working-age population), increases in perceptions of intergenerational inequity and increased 'ageism'. On the other hand, there are factors that may reduce the potential for intergenerational conflict in the twenty-first century. For example, the current 'cultural lag' between changes in the population age structure and social structures and norms may disappear in a few decades when cultural values have evolved to reflect the changes. Bengston (1993) also argues that societal norms of solidarity, support and reciprocity, may prevail in the care of older people, and lessen the potential for intergenerational conflict. It is even suggested that new roles for the aged may emerge, such that they may be increasingly viewed as repositories of wisdom.

The debate about age-cohort conflicts in the USA has not gained such prominence in other western countries such as the UK. However, it is predicted that future age-cohort relations will be affected by recent health and social welfare reform (Walker, 1993).

In-depth interviews with residents from five different nursing homes in the UK reveal some of the value differences between generations (Bartlett, 1993). A major complaint of individuals in some of these settings, is that nurses do not talk to them and communication is difficult with young members of staff. The following comments from people in this study illustrate the point:

> You can't talk to these young ones because they haven't got the sense to know what they're talking about. They don't seem to realise that they'll be old themselves one day (p. 134).

The young ones aren't used to speaking to older people. They are in and out very quickly. If I were to speak to the younger ones about the old days, they'd think I was going up the wall (p. 134).

When you're older, people dismiss you and think you're a nitwit. They know nothing about your life. I've been all over the world ... none of the sisters even know about my life. I've never told them and they've never asked me (p. 135).

FAMILIES AND CARING

Contrary to the popular stereotypes of the old being abandoned by their family in western societies, the research demonstrates that the family is in fact still the mainstay of care provision for older people in the community (Victor, 1994). While it is true that co-residence is no longer a usual practice, this reflects the preferences of older people, rather than their neglect by families. Social isolation is a problem for some older people, particularly those without children or partners, but the majority have a supportive network of family, friends and neigh-

➤9 bours. Neglect or abandonment may be observed by health and welfare workers in the course of their work, but such problems are the exception when placed in a wider representative context (Jeffreys, 1996).

Nonetheless, residential or nursing home care of older people is one solution to the ageing phenomenon usually associated with western societies. In these settings, positive, close and stable family and social relations are still a major determinant of residents' valuation of the quality of life (Bartlett, 1993). Some residents inevitably feel abandoned by their families on admission to a nursing home and have their expectations dashed, as the following quote from a nursing home resident in Bartlett's study conveys:

I spent all my money on my family setting them up in business and now they never come to see me. You used to read about things like that and never think it would happen to you (p. 148).

CROSS-CULTURAL COMPARISONS

The characteristics of the ageing process are complex and intertwined in culture. It is therefore important that ethnocentric explanations based on one culture are not generalized. Cultural comparisons are important to obtain a fuller understanding of the range and diversity of experience in old age (Nydegger, 1983), but attempts to explain how certain cultures value old age are few. The following discussion refers to East Asian countries to illustrate the significance of a range of cultural beliefs and practices for old age.

Markers of age

In industrialized countries, old age is defined by chronological boundaries and this controls access to pensions and other special concessions. In most European countries and the United States, the official retirement age is 65. Interestingly, as life expectancy has increased and the health status of older people improved, further classifications have been introduced to differentiate 'old' into 'young-old' (under 75) and 'old-old' (over 75). A further category of 'oldest old' is also used to define those aged 85 or more. However, the use of the term 'Third Age' attempts to move away from a purely chronological definition to recognize increased social and leisure activities and later life opportunities, e.g. education through the University of the Third Age.

In Asian societies influenced by Confucian doctrines, the ageing process is also believed to progress in phases. In traditional China the sixtieth birthday marks the beginning of a new calendrical cycle and elevation to the status of elder. The age of a person is also recognized by the form of address which may be used before the age of 60. In modern Korea, the mandatory retirement age is 55 for those working in the private sector and 58–65 in the public sector. Old age pensions are only available to those aged 65 or over. In traditional Korean society, however, three divisions of age were used: 'strong', 'aged/elder' and 'weak', reflecting their ability to contribute to the national labour force. The link between age and economic production is still evident in China, where the retirement age is set at 60, but this does not apply to agricultural workers who form a majority of the population and may continue to work for many more years.

In spite of its widespread use in modern western and Asian societies, chronological age is a poor indicator of health status or physical capacity. It ignores social class, gender and role, but is linked strongly with cultural values and expectations.

Health and ageing

The medicalization of ageing in western countries has served to reinforce old age as a negative state characterized by ill-health and disease. However, modern western medicine is not necessarily the norm and other health beliefs and practices are important for professionals to understand when caring for older people.

Traditional Chinese medicine is an integral part of Chinese culture. It has a long history and a unique theoretical framework based on the interaction of the Yin and Yang, the five elements and the vital organs of the body which are connected by a system of meridians through which the essential energy of life circulates (Wong, 1991). Traditional Chinese medicine uses methods such as acupuncture, herbal medicine, moxibustion and bonesetting. In Chinese culture today, traditional Chinese medicine is widely used by the Chinese in Hong Kong, Singapore, Korea and the People's Republic of China (PRC). However, only in the PRC and Korea is it fully integrated into the healthcare system, whereas in Hong Kong and Singapore it is unregulated and exists very much outside the mainstream. Although western medicine is the primary form of treatment in Hong Kong, among women the practice of consulting a western doctor decreases with age and the use of herbalists increases (Wong, 1991). Many ethnic elders still continue to use their traditional cures and supplement their western care when they see fit. Family members play an important role in preparing special foods and performing significant rituals. In mainland China, the family is also key in providing basic nursing care for patients in hospital, although this practice is also believed to be related to the nurse recruitment policy (Olson, 1993). While the presence and involvement of relatives in giving care may be usual in some countries, this practice could be difficult and threatening for some nurses if encountered when caring for people from minority ethnic groups in a western culture (Murphy and Macleod Clark, 1993).

Determinants of status and role

In spite of the many negative connotations of ageing, in western industrialized societies it can be viewed as a time of great potential and renewal, particularly if there are no health and financial concerns. The reduction of work and family responsibility may give a sense of freedom. However, for those in the 'old-old' category, a new set of experiences involving considerable redefinition may occur (Fry, 1995). Social worlds contract, physical conditions become less threatening and social norms may be rejected if they are incompatible with physical capacity. A special status may be bestowed on long-term survivors. The Taoist philosophical tradition of many Asian countries emphasizes longevity and promotes it through the use of various medicines and lifestyle (Koo, 1987).

Society defines the position of older people according to its social structure. Treas and Logue (1986) suggest that there are four ways in which societies may define their aged:

- As a low priority
- As an impediment
- As a resource
- As victims of the development process

However, in some countries, for example China, while older people may be viewed as a resource, they are the recipients of few public resources (Olson, 1993).

Filial piety is the central tenet of respecting older people in Confucian society (Box 2.1); this may operate at both the family and societal levels (Sung, 1995).

BOX 2.1   *Characteristics of filial piety*

The typical ideals reflected in Chinese and Korean stories are:

- Showing respect for parents
- Providing physical and financial sacrifices for parents
- Fulfilling responsibilities and obligations to parents
- Repayment of debts to parents
- Devotion to care and protection of parents
- Love and affection for parents
- Sympathy for aged and sick parents
- Making parents happy and comfortable
- Harmonizing family relations around parents

- Compensation for something undone by caring parents
- Deep concern for the continuity of the family
- Saving face for family by entertaining parents' friends
- Maintaining shrines and graves of ancestors
- Following religious teachings about parent care
- Harmonizing relations with neighbours
- Carrying out difficult and unusual tasks for parents

Sung (1995)

Through the Confucian documents, the young were taught to respect, care for, and obey their elders.

As the responsibilities of children towards their parents are expected to continue after death, great importance is attached to burial and mourning for parents. The spirits of the ancestors are worshipped in their shrines and maintenance of their shrines and graves is an important filial duty, practised even today in Korea and Hong Kong.

Ikels' (1983) study of the adaptation of ageing Chinese in Hong Kong and the United States, highlights the differences between these two societies and the native China from where older people had come. The seven variables believed by Roscow (1965) to strengthen the position of older people were used to illuminate the differences:

- Ownership or control of private property on which younger people are dependent
- Command or monopoly of strategic knowledge of the culture
- Links to the past
- Kinship and the extended family are central to the social organization of the society
- The small size, stability and homogeneity of the community
- Low degree of economic productivity
- High mutual dependence among the members of a group

All seven factors could be found in traditional China, but no longer exist in America. Studies such as this can assist our understanding of the enormous change in social context experienced by older minority ethnic groups and provide important insights for health professionals in caring for such groups in community or hospital settings.

Aged care policy

There are renewed efforts in some East Asian countries, such as Singapore, China and Korea, to preserve the traditional ideals and practices of filial piety through government policies and legislation.

Korea is recognized to have the strongest of the three Confucian-oriented cultures of Korea, Japan and China. In modern Korea, legal grounds for the improvement of welfare for older people were established in 1981 through the Elderly Welfare Law. However, the principle of 'care by family first, social security second' has guided social policies for older Koreans, although the case for family and state collaboration in supporting older people is increasingly being made (Choi, 1995). Public and private initiatives have resulted in nationwide efforts such as the Campaign of Respect for Elders, Respect for the Elderly Week and the Filial Piety Prize (Sung, 1995).

While many aspects of Confucian ideology have been eliminated in Communist China, reciprocal obligations between generations are the basis for old-age support policy. The 1980 Family Law of the People's Republic of China requires spouses, parents, children and grandchildren to support their relatives who are in financial need (Bartlett and Phillips, 1995). Although the state-operated medical system provides care for the poor and childless older people, it is the social system that has the primary responsibility for frail elders. This is being reinforced in Singapore, where the Government is now promoting increased family size and has introduced legislation to enable parents to obtain maintenance from their children (Phillips and Bartlett, 1995).

The outcome of recent policy initiatives in Asia is yet to be seen; however, evidence from other countries suggests that the State cannot compel families to care physically or financially for their older parents (Walker, 1993). Indeed, such actions are hardly conducive to the development of a satisfactory caring relationship. Western societies have a non-intervention policy in the belief that if the state helps it will undermine intergenerational obligations. This view is even more deeply embedded in the USA although there is little evidence to support it. The recent policy shift to community care in the UK means that greater onus is placed on the family to care for older people, despite their limited capacity to do so. Access to services is usually as the result of a crisis situation having arisen, rather than as a support or preventative measure.

With industrialization, the growth of old age homes is increasingly evident in a number of non-western countries such as Hong Kong, Japan, Korea and China. Considerable variation in these facilities has been noted, including the accommodation, management, activities and personal freedom (Holmes and Holmes, 1995). As yet, there has been little research into the impact of residential care in non-western societies on the residents' lives, but government regulation is increasingly necessary to monitor and control rapid private sector expansion in order to protect residents and safeguard standards.

CASE STUDY

Case study of Hong Kong

An examination of age and ageing in the newly industrialized City-State of Hong Kong raises many questions and issues about cultural beliefs, caring practices and policy for the care of older people. Hong Kong is an interesting example of a bicultural community with both traditional and modern westernized sectors and for this reason it has been previously selected as one of the research sites in a four-country cross-cultural study of ageing (Keith et al., 1994).

Changing cultural practices

Hong Kong's recent economic development has been accompanied by an ageing of its population (Bartlett and Phillips, 1995), changes to the family structure and dilution of some of its traditional values. While Hong Kong's population is predominantly Chinese, the fate of older people does not always accord with traditional expectations (Ikels, 1983). The future care of older people is a concern of health and welfare professionals and policymakers alike, but cultural change is not achieved overnight and an examination of Hong Kong's situation highlights issues faced by many other countries in the Asia-Pacific region and elsewhere.

Hong Kong's senior citizens are the first generation to experience the effects of industrialization. Only 13% of the population aged 65 and over were actually born in the territory; the vast majority (84%) were immigrants from mainland China (Bartlett and Phillips, 1997) and they may speak several Chinese languages or dialects other than Cantonese. The cultural environment of Hong Kong is quite different from their homeland and consequently, differences in their expectations and those of their families are naturally to be expected. In particular, there is a reluctance on the part of the married younger generation to co-reside with their parents, illustrated by the fact that approximately 65% of Hong Kong's population live in an unextended nuclear family. In 1991 only 18% of men aged 65 and over and 36% of older women lived in an extended nuclear family (Bartlett and Phillips, 1997). Increasingly, older people are to be found living on their own or with another older person, although this is contrary to their cultural beliefs. While the importance of filial piety is still acknowledged, challenges to its practice can be seen within Hong Kong's society. The sad plight of the 'caged men', whose living accommodation comprises only a small rented bed-space, illustrates the contradictions found in a society that still promotes the practice of filial piety. Reports of abandonment, suicide (Kwan, 1988) and elder abuse (Kwan, 1995), highlight some of the negative aspects of ageing encountered in this newly industrialized culture. The following oft-quoted article from the *South China Morning Post* of 17 June 1976 illustrates what is believed to be a growing problem of abandonment during the 1990s:

> A 65-year-old woman who spent four days on the Macau hydrofoil wharf waiting for her son to return with her travel documents finally got back to Hong Kong yesterday with the help of friends. Lee Ho Min-ching was taken to Macau two weeks ago by her son and daughter-in-law for medical treatment. Once there, her son, Lee Kwong-wah (38), put her in a boarding house and gave her $200HK. The couple then took her identity card and travel documents and told her to wait for three or four days for their return. She stayed at the boarding house for ten days until her money ran out and then took up her vigil at the hydrofoil wharf.

The Government response to this situation has until very recently stated that the care of older citizens was a family responsibility. However, the ageing population and the apparent difficulty experienced by increasing numbers of families in meeting their responsibility triggered the Hong Kong Government to introduce a new policy of 'care in the community' in 1973. This was intended to supplement family care with community support and to minimize the need for residential care (Chow, 1993). The importance of preserving traditional family values in care of older people has been stressed in successive social welfare policies, and the need to avoid residential care as a solution. However, it is evident that such values are increasingly difficult to uphold as Hong Kong's social structure changes. While the approach of 'care in the community' complements traditional values such as filial piety, without adequate State support the burden of care still remains with the family, who are increasingly limited in their capacities to care for their aged members. Support networks among friends and neighbours are still secondary and unlikely to make a significant impact on the level of community care provision.

Residential care

The development of private care homes for older people is following the same trends as western countries and within some of these settings, the quality of older people's lives has been found sadly lacking (Bartlett and Kwan, 1993). In an effort to improve standards and quality of care the Government enacted legislation in 1994 to regulate all sectors of residential aged care for older people.

Further examination of Hong Kong's residential care homes for older people highlights some cultural differences about the concept of quality in these settings. In 1994, the quality of care in such care homes was evaluated using a comprehensive quality measure consisting of items organized in four key domains (Bartlett, 1994). In developing this measure, the relevance of many western approaches to quality measurement was challenged. For example, some of the outcome standards used as a basis for evaluating quality of care in Australian nursing homes (Commonwealth of Australia, 1987) were found to be unsuitable for Hong Kong. Expectations of the physical environment had to be modified, as it was unrealistic in such a densely populated territory, to expect homes to offer spacious accommodation, outdoor garden areas for residents, or single rooms. None of these facilities would have been usual under normal living circumstances in Hong Kong. The family life and living arrangements of Chinese people also question the use of concepts such as privacy in identifying quality items. Some fundamental differences in the personality traits of Chinese people also had to be taken into account when selecting items for measurement of the psycho-social dimension of the quality construct. For example, the importance of having a private place to meet visitors was not necessarily supported. Instead the view emerged that it was more important for residents to have everyone notice their family members visiting. Concerning food, a different emphasis to that found in other instruments was placed on this subject; because of its social significance in Chinese culture, questions about the provision of special food for festivals were considered important to include. Other cultural contrasts were also revealed during the course of this study, with implications for care delivery.

For example, at one care-and-attention home, staff were having difficulties dealing with an older person who persisted in taking various Chinese medicines in addition to the prescribed western medicines. In common with a large proportion of Hong Kong's population, older people regularly use Chinese medicines and the person in question was, unsurprisingly, reluctant to give up this practice. However, the young nurses demonstrated little understanding of this individual's predicament or how to handle it. At the other extreme, an older Chinese man living in another care home continued to act as a herbalist and served the other residents with the approval of the nursing staff.

These examples highlight the lack of knowledge among nursing staff about traditional forms of medicine and the dilemmas that may be created as cultural practices change. A number of other difficult intracultural issues were also revealed, including cases where individuals refused western treatment for a fracture in preference to the attentions of a bonesetter.

There are many cultural contrasts to be found between the generations in Hong Kong and only a greater cultural awareness on the part of health professionals will avoid the development of tension and conflict when differences are confronted.

CULTURE AND ETHNICITY

Older ethnic people in Britain

Cultural patterns are most visible among different ethnic groups (Box 2.2). While only 3.22% of people from minority ethnic groups are aged 65 or over, these people are from diverse minority ethnic groups, with important differences in culture, age and need. One of the problems with making general observations about ethnic groups such as Asians for example, is that while certain distinctive cultural characteristics may be shared, for example, a cyclic view of time, the importance of ancestry and emphasis on the collective good, individual and group differences can be overlooked and stereotyping encouraged. Even within groups such as the Chinese, members may come from widely different places

BOX 2.2	*Minority ethnic groups in Britain*

Just over three million people from minority ethnic groups live in Britain (OPCS, 1993). They are categorized as:

- Black-Caribbean
- Black-African
- Black-Other
- Indian
- Pakistani
- Bangladeshi
- Chinese
- Other-Asian
- Other-Other

such as Hong Kong, the People's Republic of China, Singapore, Taiwan, Korea and Malaysia. They speak a wide range of dialects, and may demonstrate different cultural practices.

Health needs

Surprisingly little is known about the needs of older people from minority ethnic groups in Britain (Age Concern, 1995a). The theory and practice of gerontology has been described as 'ethnocentric' by Blakemore and Boneham (1994). The UK's healthcare system has not been particularly responsive in meeting the needs of these groups (Age Concern, 1995b; Jones and Van Amelsvoort Jones, 1986; Murphy and Macleod Clark, 1993). Lack of attention to privacy, meals and customs are just some of the problems identified over ten years ago (Barker, 1984) and are still with us today. Few health authorities employ ethnic group development workers, target programmes or carry out consultation exercises with local ethnic groups (Morton, 1993). The 1989 White Paper *Caring for People* points out the varying needs and problems of people from different cultural backgrounds. The need for sensitivity by service providers and for consultation with minority ethnic communities in care planning is mentioned. The importance of addressing the healthcare needs of black and ethnic groups is also acknowledged in the Government White Paper, *The Health of the Nation* (1992). Under the new community care reforms there is no guarantee, however, that the services people need will be delivered.

Although research on the health patterns of older people from minority ethnic groups is limited, they appear to experience more long-term chronic illnesses than the majority of the population and their illnesses are very often associated with a poor housing and economic situation (Age Concern, 1995b). More is known about the Asian and Afro-Caribbean groups than 'invisible' groups such as Polish, Jewish and Cypriot people. For example, it is known that the mortality rate from coronary heart disease, diabetes and tuberculosis is higher among Asians (Whitehead, 1988), while strokes, liver cancer, diabetes and accidents account for a relatively high mortality rate among Afro-Caribbeans. Increasing numbers of older people from some ethnic groups are being diagnosed as having mental health problems.

Such findings on health and illness among older people of minority ethnic groups suggest considerable diversity within and between groups. Social class, gender and geographical factors are all believed to have an important bearing and while the emerging patterns are complex, the evidence points to rising inequalities in health among older Asian and black people in Britain (Blakemore and Boneham, 1994).

Improving access to and utilization of healthcare

Different patterns can also be seen in the take-up of services. For example, the use of general practitioners by older Asian and Afro-Caribbean people is higher than the majority of the population, but Afro-Caribbeans are more likely to be admitted to hospital than Asians (Age Concern, 1995b). Generally, the standard health promotion programmes do not reach older ethnic groups because they are culturally and linguistically unsuitable. Among the female population of over 50s, for example, only 10% of Bangladeshis, 15% of Pakistanis and 47% of Indians speak English (Health Education Authority, 1994).

Differences in beliefs about health and disease have important implications for community and hospital care and health promotion activities. The development of separate services for minority elders is not necessarily the solution, however. Concerns are now focused on improving the quality and targeting of ethnic health services and the NHS Ethnic Health unit was established by the Department of Health in 1994 to focus on this issue. Particular initiatives from this unit include a new guide for Good Practice and Quality Indicators in Primary Health Care (National Association of Health Authorities and Trusts, 1996). There are now examples of a number of local initiatives attempting to meet the needs of ethnic elders (Age Concern, 1995b):

■ A weekly luncheon club and health screening service for older Chinese people is run by Age Concern Newcastle and the North East Chinese Association. This not only provides an important social outlet, but also gives participants the opportunity to seek advice on health problems from someone who speaks their native language. Health promotion activities are run through a Partnership Drop In For Elders for older Asian and Chinese people
■ A Health Advocates scheme operated by the City and East London Family Health Services Authority with the aim of improving access to healthcare for people from minority ethnic groups. The advocates are bilingual and guide and refer individuals to different agencies and interpret during consultations where appropriate

Residential and nursing home care

Only 1.6% of Afro-Caribbean and 1.5% of Asian people aged over 60 are resident in hospital or residential homes compared with approximately 4% of white people aged over 60 (OPCS, 1993). The use of sheltered housing by ethnic groups is similarly low (Age Concern, 1995c). While this may be accounted for by demographics, other factors such as the inappropriateness of residential care for different ethnic groups could be a deterrent. The services may not provide culturally appropriate care that accommodates different dietary requirements, religious practices or leisure activities. Geographical location may also be a problem. For those unable to converse in English, the very limited availability of bilingual staff or translated material means that communication difficulties will not be addressed. The popular misconception that the family cares for older people from ethnic groups can mean that their needs are often overlooked.

Self-help groups or voluntary organizations may provide specialist schemes for older people that help to make services appropriate and accessible (Age Concern, 1995c).

- The Birmingham Jewish Welfare Board provides a day care centre, sheltered housing and residential and nursing home care for older Jewish people in the City. Information, advice and advocacy is also provided through home visits.
- An Asian Carers' project is run by Age Concern Wandsworth. Volunteers who speak the appropriate language are used to take over the caring role on a regular basis to give the usual carer a break.

In Australia, considerable progress has been made to increase the access of ethnic older people to existing or mainstream services. Supported by capital grants, ethno-specific hostels and nursing homes have been established, and culturally appropriate services have been developed in other hostels and nursing homes. The clustering approach has also been successfully tested, allowing the admission of people from similar ethnic backgrounds to specific nursing homes. This has provided a more flexible solution than the development of ethno-specific services (Gibson, 1996).

IMPLICATIONS FOR NURSING PRACTICE

Delivering appropriate nursing care to older people from different cultures does not require nurses to become 'expert' in the finer details of every ethnic group encountered. The development of awareness and sensitivity to cultural differences can be achieved in various ways.

Assessment and care planning

For practitioners treating older people from minority ethnic groups, the importance of assessing the degree of acculturation has been noted by Valle (1989). Three positions along a continuum mark the degree of ethnic orientation. Individuals with a strong orientation toward cultural origins and homeland exhibit the 'traditional position'. Where people divide their allegiance between their homeland culture and the current mainstream culture they are said to be 'bicultural'. When complete integration with the mainstream culture has occurred, 'assimilation' is regarded to have taken place. Those in bicultural and assimilated positions still have a minority ethnic group heritage and their needs should not be overlooked.

Information about the patient's cultural values is crucial for planning culturally appropriate nursing interventions that encourage compliance with treatment regimens. While there are a variety of cultural assessment tools available, six essential cultural phenomena have been identified by Giger and Davidhizar (1990). Essential client data include ethnic affiliation, languages spoken, religious practices, food preferences, family patterns, health beliefs and practices. Any assessment should also include information about the caregiver. Traditional healing methods are to be respected and with careful health assessment it may be possible to incorporate them in care planning if they are not harmful. The use of alternative healers may be encouraged if they are believed by the client to be beneficial. The importance of understanding and accommodating health and religious beliefs is also recognized to be crucial for effective rehabilitation involving, for example, occupational therapy, physiotherapy or chiropody (Squires, 1991). Even when the health professional has some knowledge, it may still be necessary, however, to seek further help and advice from bicultural advisors or consultants.

For nurses working with ethnic elders, understanding past patterns and relationships is crucial for the delivery of appropriate care. Used appropriately, the technique of reminiscence is recognized to be a very valuable activity for nurses working with older ethnic people and older people generally, especially in long-term care settings such as nursing homes and long-stay NHS wards. Recounting and reflecting on the past can reduce the sense of alienation experienced by those faced with a change of life. It should also be recognized, however, that past experiences may be painful and their recollection may result in the need for counselling support (Terry, 1997).

Promoting positive practice

Developing self-awareness and sensitivity on the part of the nurse is the key to promoting positive practice with older people. Some of the guidelines developed by Burnside (1988) for nurses working with older people from minority ethnic groups may be useful to consider (Box 2.3).

BOX 2.3	*Guidelines for nurses working with older people from minority ethnic groups*

- Acknowledge the limitations of one's own knowledge and understanding
- Put aside one's own biases
- Use polite forms of address and use personal names correctly
- Seek to find value in different health beliefs and practices and their perceived benefit by older people
- Understand and use non-verbal messages to communicate
- Consult the literature to increase one's cultural sensitivity
- Be aware of the vast differences within broad ethnic groups
- Become aware of a group's behavioural norms

Burnside (1988)

CONCLUSION

Reflecting the very nature of culture, the scope of this chapter has been, of necessity, wide-ranging. The numerous cultural dimensions and perspectives explored serve to demonstrate the diversity of old age and the need for nurses to develop cultural awareness and sensitivity. The value of cross-cultural studies in promoting greater understanding of the practices of different cultures has been illustrated and by using Hong Kong as a case study, a variety of important cultural dimensions with a bearing on age and ageing have been identified. Also highlighted are the potential sources of intergenerational conflict.

Ultimately, the promotion of positive practice with older people from different cultures depends on the formulation of an agenda for action by the nursing profession that addresses practice, education and research. The design of nursing curricula should reflect the multicultural composition of the older population by including core content on ethnicity/culture and health.

There is considerable scope for the development of a rigorous research programme into many aspects of culture and ageing, in particular, the care of ethnic elders. While the plight of older people from minority ethnic groups in Britain is increasingly recognized, the adequacy of cultural responses to their needs is unclear, particularly in relation to long-term care. Other issues, for example, culture and nutrition among older people have received limited attention in the literature. Also, little is known about the uptake of rehabilitation services among these groups. Despite the difficulties associated with undertaking cross-cultural research, more studies are needed to examine new issues such as intergenerational relations.

The goal for nurses working with older clients is to develop the self-awareness and cultural flexibility necessary to understand and accept older people as individuals, whatever their ethnic group or cultural background.

FURTHER READING

Age Concern (1995) *Age and Race: Double Discrimination. Life in Britain Today for Ethnic Minority Elders.* Age Concern England and Commission for Racial Equality, London.
This publication is the result of a joint initiative, between the Commission for Racial Equality and Age Concern England, to improve the quality of life of older minority ethnic groups. It comprises an informative collection of papers on a range of important issues including: housing, health, income, social welfare, education and leisure. Useful organizations are listed, in addition to further published materials.

Ahmad, W.I.U. (ed.) (1993) *'Race' and Health in Contemporary Britain.* Open University Press, Buckingham.
An analysis of the health and healthcare of Britain's black population is provided by this important text on ethnicity and health. The edited collection of chapters address the politics of research, current health issues and health policy. The care of black elders is considered through an examination of models, policies and prospects.

Ahmad, W.I.U. and Atkin, K. (eds) (1996) *'Race' and Community Care.* Open University Press, Buckingham.
This book provides a critical analysis of 'race' and community care in Britain through an examination of the historical relationship between state welfare and minority ethnic communities, family and social change. Various case studies in 'race' and community care are provided and focus on disability, mental health, cash for care, and the role of the voluntary sector.

Health Education Authority (1995) *Toward Better Health Service Provision for Black and Minority Ethnic Groups.* HEA, London.
This report describes the HEA's role in identifying the health promotion needs

of black and minority ethnic groups and outlines examples of recent strategies, research and initiatives. It provides useful demographic and health statistics by ethnic group and NHSE region.

REFERENCES

Achenbaum, W.A. (1978) *Old Age in the New Land*. The John Hopkins University Press, Baltimore.

Age Concern (1995a) *Age and Race: Double Discrimination. An Overview of Life for Ethnic Minority Elders in Britain Today*. Age Concern England and Commission for Racial Equality, London.

Age Concern (1995b) *Age and Race: Double Discrimination. Health*. Age Concern England and Commission for Racial Equality, London.

Age Concern (1995c) *Age and Race: Double Discrimination. Social Welfare*. Age Concern England and Commission for Racial Equality, London.

Barker, J. (1984) *Black and Asian Old People in Britain*. Age Concern, Mitcham, Surrey.

Bartlett, H. (1993) *Nursing Homes for Elderly People: Questions of Quality and Policy*. Harwood Academic Publishers, Sydney.

Bartlett, H. and Kwan, A.Y.H. (1993) Paving the way for effective quality measurement in Hong Kong's residential aged care sector. *Hong Kong Journal of Gerontology*, 7(1), 10–13.

Bartlett, H. (1994) Measuring quality of care: issues arising from policy reform in residential services for older people. In *Proceedings of the First South-East Asian Nursing Research Conference*, Hong Kong 5–7 December.

Bartlett, H.P. and Phillips, D.R. (1995) Aging trends – Hong Kong. *Journal of Cross-Cultural Gerontology*, 10, 257–265.

Bartlett, H.P. and Phillips, D.R. (1997) Ageing and aged care in the People's Republic of China: national and local issues and perspectives. *Health and Place*, 3(3), 149–159.

Bengston, V.L. (1993) Is the 'Contract across generations' changing? Effects of population aging on obligations and expectations across age groups. In *The Changing Contract Across Generations*, Bengston, V.L. and Achenbaum, W.A. (eds) Aldine De Gruyter, New York.

Blakemore, K. and Boneham, M. (1994) *Age, Race and Ethnicity: a Comparative Approach*. Open University Press, Buckingham.

Burnside, I. (1988) *Nursing and the Aged. A Self-Care Approach*. McGraw-Hill, New York.

Choi, S.J. (1995) Social welfare policy for elderly Koreans. In *Aging in Korea. Today and Tomorrow*, Choi, S.J. and Suh, H.K. (eds). Federation of Korean Gerontological Societies, Chung-Ang Publisher.

Chow, N. (1993) The changing responsibilities of the State and family towards elders in Hong Kong. In *International Perspectives on State and Family Support for the Elderly*, Bass, S.A. and Morris, R. (eds). Haworth Press, New York.

Commonwealth of Australia (1987) *Living in a Nursing Home. Outcome Standards for Australian Nursing Homes*. Australian Government Publishing Service, Canberra.

Cowgill, D. (1974) Aging and modernization: a revision of the theory. In *Late Life: Communities and Environmental Policy*, Gubrium, J.F. (ed.). C.C. Thomas, Springfield, IL.

Cowgill, D.O. and Holmes, L.D. (1972) *Aging and Modernisation*. Appleton-Century-Crofts, New York.

Department of Health (1992) *The Health of the Nation: a Strategy for Health in England*. HMSO, London.

Fry, C.L. (1995) Age, aging and culture. In *Handbook of Aging and the Social Sciences*, Binstock, R.H. and George, L.K. (eds). Academic Press, San Diego.

Gibson, D. (1996) Reforming aged care in Australia: change and consequence. *Journal of Social Policy*, 25(2), 157–179.

Giger, J. and Davidhizar, R. (1990) Transcultural nursing assessment: a method for advancing nursing practice. *International Nursing Review*, 37(1), 199–202.

Health Education Authority (1994) *Black and Minority Ethnic Communities: Health and Lifestyles*. HEA, London.

Holmes, E.R. and Holmes, L.D. (1995) *Other Cultures, Elder Years*. Sage, Thousand Oaks, CA.

Ikels, C. (1983) *Ageing and Adaptation. Chinese in Hong Kong and the United States*. Archon Books.

Jefferys, M. (1996) Cultural aspects of ageing:

gender and intergenerational issues. *Social Science and Medicine*, **43**(5), 681–687.

Jones, D.C. and Van Amelsvoort Jones (1986) Communication patterns between nursing staff and the ethnic elderly in a long term care facility. *Journal of Advanced Nursing*, **11**, 265–272.

Keith, J., Fry, C., Glascock, A., Ikels, C., Dickerson-Putnam, J., Harpending, H. and Draper, P. (1994) *The Ageing Experience. Diversity and Commonality Across Cultures*. Sage, Thousand Oaks, CA.

Koo, L.C. (1987) Concepts of disease causation, treatment and prevention among Hong Kong Chinese: diversity and eclecticism. *Social Science and Medicine*, **25**, 405–417.

Kwan, Y.H. (1988) Suicide among the elderly: Hong Kong. *The Journal of Applied Gerontology*, **7**(2), 248–259.

Kwan, Y.H. (1995) Elder abuse in Hong Kong: a new family problem for the old East? *Journal of Elder Abuse and Neglect*, **6**(3/4), 65–80.

Leininger, M. (1988) Leininger's Theory of Nursing: Cultural care diversity and universality. *Nursing Science Quarterly: Theory, Research and Practice*, **1**(4), 152–160.

Morton, J. (ed.) (1993) *Recent Research on Services for Black and Minority Ethnic Elderly People*. Age Concern Institute of Gerontology, London.

Murphy, K and Macleod Clark, J. (1993) Nurses' experiences of caring for ethnic minority clients. *Journal of Advanced Nursing*, **18**, 442–450.

National Association of Health Authorities and Trusts (1996) *Health Care for Black and Minority Ethnic People*. NAHAT Briefing, Issue 100, Birmingham, NAHAT.

Nydegger, C.N. (1983) Family ties of the aged in cross-cultural perspective. *The Gerontologist*, **23**, 26–32.

Office of Population Censuses and Surveys (1993) *National Population Projections 1991-Based*. Series PP2 no.18. HMSO, London.

Olson, P. (1993) Caregiving and long-term health care in the People's Republic of China. In *International Perspectives on State and Family Support for the Elderly*, Bass, S. and Morris, R. (eds). Haworth Press, London.

Phillips, D.R. and Bartlett, H.P.(1995) Aging trends – Singapore. *Journal of Cross-Cultural Gerontology*, **10**, 349–356.

Quadagno, J. (1982) *Aging in Early Industrial Society*. Academic Press, New York.

Roscow, I. (1965) And then we were old. *Transaction*, **2**(2), 20–26.

Squires, A. (ed.) (1991) *Multicultural Health Care and Rehabilitation of Older People*. Edward Arnold, London.

Sung, K.T. (1995) Measures and dimensions of filial piety in Korea. *The Gerontologist*, **35**(2), 240–247.

Terry, P. (1997) *Counselling the Elderly and their Carers*. Macmillan Press, London.

Treas, J. and Logue, B. (1986) Economic development and the older population. *Population and Development Review*, **12**(4), 645–673.

Valle, R. (1989) Cultural and ethnic issues in Alzheimer's disease research. In *Alzheimer's Disease Treatment and Family Stress: Directions for Research*, Light, E. and Lebowitz, B.D. (eds), National Institutes of Mental Health, Rockville, MD.

Victor, C. (1994) *Old Age in Modern Society*. Chapman & Hall, London.

Walker, A. (1993) Intergenerational relations and welfare restructuring: the social construction of an intergenerational problem. In *The Changing Contract Across Generations*, Bengston, V.L. and Achenbaum, W.A. (eds.) Aldine De Gruyter, New York.

Whitehead, M., with Townsend, P. and Davidson, N. (eds) (1988) *Inequalities in Health: the Black Report and the Health Divide*. Penguin, Harmondsworth.

Wilkins, H. (1993) Transcultural nursing: a selective review of the literature, 1985–1991. *Journal of Advanced Nursing*, **18**, 602–612.

Wong, T.W. (1991) *The Utilisation of Traditional Chinese Medicine in Hong Kong*. Department of Community and Family Medicine, Hong Kong University.

3 Promoting ordinary living for older people

Jeanette Thompson and Sharon Pickering

INTRODUCTION

Some of the most able minds in nursing, from both education and practice, have attempted to define what nursing is and, therefore, what nurses do. That this argument has not been successfully concluded reflects the variety of roles and contributions that nurses make as well as the continually changing face of healthcare provision. Consequently, the popular (and historical) view of nurses and nursing has tended to focus conveniently on the completion of tasks and the physical need of clients. The relationship between this, rather narrow view of nursing, and a medically dominated model of care does not need detailed examination. However, it is clear that, in these circumstances, the management of care is predominantly concerned with the absence of disease rather than ensuring a satisfactory balance between psychological, social, environment and physical health. Further evidence of this is the emphasis on interventions and invasive treatment, the central and dominant role of the clinician and the fact that the hospital continues to be seen as the principal supplier of healthcare. In addition, the research agenda has tended to dwell on biological causes and the cure of ill-health.

For the most part, the view of nurses and nursing is based on the premise that health is the polar opposite of the above, where people are only perceived as healthy when no trace of disease (i.e. no physical symptoms) can be identified. This is irrespective of how the person, as an individual in their own right, feels. However, the preventative model adopts a positive approach to healthcare where measures are taken to reduce the incidence and prevalence of illness, and, therefore, the need for illness-focused models of care. A central tenet of such an approach is the importance of health-conscious public policy.

The preventative model focuses on the health needs of individuals, groups and whole populations and recognizes the importance of mobilizing a wide range of agencies with a rich variety of expertise. Implicit in this is the need for high-quality epidemiological research which aims to understand the links between patterns of health, disease and relevant social factors alongside research that comprehensively explores the nature of health and ways in which healthcare providers can contribute to the health status of society. Furthermore, the shift in emphasis from a medically dominated to a preventative model of care has to be reflected in the fact that this care is most appropriately delivered within a community setting. Currently, healthcare policy is pursuing a significant primary care agenda (HMSO, 1996, 1997; NHSE, 1996).

➤6

When considering a sociological perspective of health, the health of individuals and communities is determined by a complex interaction between social, economic, environmental and personal factors (Seedhouse, 1986; Dunn, 1961; Peplau, 1952). Yet, by recognizing such a broad range of influences on health status we must recognize the potential to apportion blame for ill-health. Such blame might be directed at the individual, at business and industry as well as perceived deficiencies in public policy.

Furthermore, if we accept that there is a broad range of factors impacting on our own health status then we have to expect that with this comes a degree of individual and collective responsibility. Evidence of a developing awareness of health-influencing factors and the interplay between individual and collective responsibility can be found in the increasingly stringent health and safety standards (e.g. Health and Safety Commission, 1992, 1994) which go some way to ensuring that, even where the will is diminished or the commercial pressure great, the need of individual and collective responsibility is legislatively explicit.

There are clear parallels between the approach to health and the continually developing role of the nurse. Currently, these discussions tend to focus on the relative merits of technical and humanist approaches to delivery of nursing care (see Box 3.1) where the origins of technical nursing are found within the medical and curative model of health. Conversely, the humanist approach focuses upon relationships and interpersonal communication and can be equated with, for example, rehabilitative and continuing care. In brief, this is a reflection of the debate of nursing as a science or nursing as an art.

This has been widely debated both in the professional and academic arena. An abundance of literature exists, much of which is located within the discussions relating to the use and value of nursing theories and models. The speciality of nursing older people in whatever context has traditionally focused upon more humanistic approaches, fundamentally seeing interpersonal skills and communication at the heart of nursing practice. Recent technological advances in medicine have contributed significantly to the healthcare of older people, and as such have resulted in an increasingly acute/technical focus to the care of this group of people.

This chapter will consider the changes initiated by the National Health Service and Community Care Act (HMSO, 1990) that are of relevance to the healthcare of older people. The major focus will be upon the concept of ordinary living and how the principles underpinning this can be used to facilitate the maintainance and support of older people within their own home. In addition, these concepts will be explored in relation to other environments in which older people may be living, and practical interventions in support of the principles of ordinary living will be discussed.

BOX 3.1	*Technical and humanistic approaches to nursing*

It seems that the technical approaches to nursing are increasing in direct correlation with technological developments in medicine. Changes in junior doctors' hours have also had an impact upon roles within care teams, in the context of who undertakes what activity (Calman, 1996). The UKCC's documents *Scope of Professional Practice* (UKCC, 1992) and *Guidelines for Professional Practice* (UKCC, 1996) can be seen as a vehicle that nurses are able to use to respond to these changes.

Greenhalgh (1994) identifies a difference between the 'extended role' and an 'expanded role'. The extended role typically focuses upon tasks such as intravenous cannulation, and phlebotomy, roles which have traditionally been considered as part of medical practice. Nurses taking on these roles need to consider the impact this may have upon the amount and quality of nursing care which they are then able to deliver.

Humanistic nursing can be seen as being paralleled with the 'expanded role' as defined by Greenhalgh (1994). Central to this concept is that of advancing nursing practice in which nurses empower clients through the use of expert knowledge and interpersonal skills (UKCC, 1994). Essentially therefore, within this approach communication is enhanced by the tasks of nursing, rather than the more commonly understood framework, whereby the tasks of nursing are supported by interpersonal skills.

Nursing in this context is highly intuitive and only minimally supported by technical equipment. As such, therefore this could be described as the 'art of nursing', rather than the use of the scientific approach (Kitson, 1993). Operating from the humanistic perspective is often perceived as nursing at its least complex and least skilful. However, it may be argued that in reality the skills required of nurses to practice their art in this way are extremely complex, difficult to articulate and require high levels of competence.

THE IMPACT OF THE NATIONAL HEALTH SERVICE AND COMMUNITY CARE ACT (NHSCCA)

The National Health Service and Community Care Act (HMSO, 1990) was initially intended to create welfare services that were more responsive to consumer needs and in which resources were more appropriately used by targeting them to the areas of greatest demand. A number of more specific objectives exist within the Act that have particular relevance to the care of older people These include:

- Maintaining people within their own homes
- Increase in community-based care in support of this
- Growth in housing and care provision within the independent sector
- Creation of a purchaser/provider framework

Underpinning these changes are the distinctions that have been made between health and social care.

For older people, and nurses working in this area, the reforms have secured a number of benefits; however, there have also been a number of costs. The conflict that is developing between healthcare, free at the point of delivery, and social care, which has to be paid for, is creating dissonance for users, carers and also nurses working with older people. Within this Act opportunities do exist to enhance the quality of care received by older people, for example, maintaining people within their own homes, or more appropriate and homely settings. Inherent within these developments is the option for nursing to develop and expand the humanistic approach to nursing care.

ORDINARY LIVING

This chapter has suggested that humanistic nursing requires a high level of expertise, this necessitates nurses being skilled in the areas of relationship building, self-awareness, listening skills, empathizing, self-disclosure, trust and genuineness. It has to be acknowledged, however, that competence and expertise in these skills alone does not provide the nurse with a framework in which to assess, plan, implement, record, monitor and evaluate care. Nursing models have traditionally been seen as frameworks within which nurses deliver care. This chapter intends to consider some additional approaches to informing care delivery, that are evolving within areas such as learning disabilities and mental health and have relevance in working with older people in non-acute settings.

One of the key concepts this chapter will consider is 'ordinary living' (King's Fund, 1980). Ordinary living is, whether we know it or not, familiar to all of us, as a consequence of our home life and community involvement. However, this apparently simple description can be deceptive and is the cause of many of the difficulties experienced in implementing the concept. Evidence within the area of learning disabilities demonstrates that successful implementation of the concept of ordinary living requires high levels of knowledge and skill (Mansell, 1992).

DEFINING ORDINARY LIVING

The King's Fund (1980) defined the goal of ordinary living as

> to see people with a learning disability in the mainstream of life, living in ordinary houses, in ordinary streets with the same range of choices as any citizen, and mixing as equals with the other, and mostly non-handicapped members of their own community.

Ordinary living evolved during the 1980s in response to demands for the closure of long-stay learning disabilities hospitals. Central to this philosophy is that of living in an ordinary house, in an ordinary street, and having an ordinary life. In environmental terms this means people living in houses that are in keeping with the nature of those other properties in that area. For many people, particularly those who have lived in learning disabilities or psychiatric institutions, this meant moving from large ward environments in which 30 or more people may have lived to much smaller properties for five or six people. Such developments mean that the homes in which people live are not clearly defined as institutions either by label, size or architecture. People are therefore, being given the opportunity to reside in properties that are in keeping with the rest of the community.

For many older people the issues are different. Having experienced 'ordinary living', in which they may have owned their own home, have raised families and exercised personal autonomy and choice, their move tends to be into larger environments where many of the elements of the ordinary life they had, are either removed or altered. The issue for those people working with this group of individuals is to consider the value of ordinary living as a means of maintaining the quality of life experienced during their adult years.

For some individuals the transition from home (ordinary life) to institution does not always take place in one stage. In reality it may be more of an incremental process. This may mean the person will move through a whole range of services, for example, alarm button services or warden supported through to sheltered accommodation before being admitted to nursing home care. At each stage in this process a little more of a person's freedom and autonomy may be lost. The incremental nature of this transition has the potential to disguise the full extent to which an individual's personal freedoms, autonomy, choice and ➤14 control have been eroded.

List who comes in and out of the care environment in which you work throughout the day.

State the purpose of each person's visit.

Identify how much control the older person has upon the number, types and times of visits.

What does this mean to the people living in this environment?

You will probably have identified a large number of people coming in and out of the environment throughout each day. Work by Oswin (1972) identified that a large number of people were coming in and out of a ward environment caring for children with cerebral palsy. Evidence from an unpublished study in Sheffield (Northern General NHS Trust, 1992) also suggested that in an acute care setting, a client experienced contact with up to 120 different people during one episode of care. Though neither of these studies relates directly to working with older people the experiences can be seen as transferable to different environments. The situation each of these people found themselves in demonstrated a lack of control over who came in or out of the environment. Obviously, this has an impact when the identified environment is deemed to be that person's 'home'.

Control over who does or does not enter a particular environment is an important issue in the context of ordinary living. This, however, is not the only issue of importance; other areas for consideration in the context of nursing elderly people can include the experience of living within a local community and actively participating in the life of that community. Issues such as choice and empowerment, respect and dignity, status and competence, all of which are vital in this area of work. Though these are explored in a number of texts, it is our intention to consider them in the context of O'Brien's (1987) five accomplishments, which will be explored within the next section of this chapter. These accomplishments are community participation, community integration, competence, respect and choice. The essential goal within this framework is the achievement of community participation. The remaining accomplishments aim to ensure that this takes place in a valued and meaningful way.

COMMUNITY PARTICIPATION AND COMMUNITY INTEGRATION

O'Brien (1987) defines community participation as the experience of being involved in a growing network of personal relationships. Essential in the development of effective community participation is the concept of community presence. Brost and Johnson (1982) identify that people ordinarily live, work and play in communities comprising citizens of a variety of ages and who have interests and talents that encompass the whole spectrum of human beings. O'Brien (1987) refers to this as the experience of sharing those 'ordinary' places that define 'ordinary' community life. In the past, services for people with learning disability have been organized in a way that congregates the recipients of services in places that are physically separate from their community. Often this has forced people to leave their natural families, neighbourhoods and schools in order to receive the support they need.

In the context of healthcare for older people this can be seen as equating with the growing number of nursing and residential homes. Of relevance are the ways in which some of these establishments or institutions have the potential to replicate some of the difficulties experienced within learning disabilities and mental health services in the past. Essentially, within the broad descriptor of older people two different groups exist, each with different histories and different experiences. Consequently the application of the concepts of community integration and participation will need to be adjusted accordingly.

Goffman (1961) described the 'total institution' as one where people live, work and play almost exclusively within the same environment. Using this definition, nursing and residential care settings could be seen to be a perpetuation of institutional care models. Advocates of institutional care argue powerfully of their ability to keep people safe and protected and that they provide benefits to both the individual, their family and society as a whole. However, there are also certain risks implicit within such care models. The most obvious of these is the loss of control and autonomy that may be experienced by the individual in relation to their own lifestyle. This loss of independence can manifest itself in a number of different ways, including both physical and mental changes.

Many of these physical and mental changes can be ascribed to factors that are associated with the ageing process rather than the consequences of institutionalization. The difficulty for nurses, is to ensure, when applicable, that any health or social needs are attributed appropriately to the constraints of the environment or to the changes within the individual. Nurses who are able to appropriately differentiate between these causative factors are then in a position to be able to commence the skilful process of counteracting the effects of institutionalization or rehabilitating the individual.

In the context of community integration and participation, the role of the nurse can be said to be twofold. Firstly, identifying ways in which individuals are able to maintain the relationships and networks that they have. This is of importance for those older people moving from a community based lifestyle into residential or nursing home care. Secondly, nurses must further develop their focus outside of the service environment in order to identify ways of developing the networks and social contacts of older people. Fundamental to the exploration of an individual's social network is the need to consider ways of actively developing and maintaining their involvement within the community. In order

What might you consider to be your community?

Essentially, a community can be seen as consisting of (Hillery, 1955):

- A group of people
- Within a geographical area
- With a division of labour into specialized and interdependent functions
- With a common culture and a social system which organizes their activities
- Whose members are conscious of belonging to that community
- Who can act collectively in an organized manner

to achieve this it is important that nurses have a clear understanding of what is meant by 'Community'.

Bulmer (1987) argues that social ties and activities vary considerably throughout adult life and have a lasting effect upon personal expectation. Middle class or professional groups have extensive networks which are often work based whilst working class people do not. Bury and Holme (1993) suggest that this kind of variation means it is impossible to make assumptions about social activities and support through a person's life.

There are two additional concepts which are relevant for nurses to work with in the maintenance, development and promotion of community participation. These are *Gemeinschaft* and *Gesellschaft* (Box 3.2). The differences identified between *Gemeinschaft* and *Gesellschaft* represent parts of a continuum, not the picture in its entirety. It is therefore important that nurses become more skilled in not only the assessment of the individual, but also the community in which that person lives. The next section considers the fundamental principles upon which nurses can assess, plan, implement and evaluate nursing care for older people in order to more effectively orchestrate an ordinary lifestyle, irrespective of the environment in which the person lives.

BOX 3.2	*The concepts of* **Gemeinschaft** *and* **Gesellschaft**

Gemeinschaft – refers to the sense of community, the intimacy of face-to-face relationships, the sense of place (social and geographical) and belonging that comes from being brought up in a particular locality amongst family and friends and in keeping with traditional family and church values.

Gesellschaft – such a community is derived from competitive and highly mobile nature of industrial society where relationships are not an end in themselves but a means to profit and self interest. In this society neither personal attachments nor traditional rights and duties are important. Relationships between people are superficial, impersonal and calculating, are determined by bargaining and defined in written agreements.

COMPETENCE

O'Brien (1987) states that competence is related to the experience of being able to develop the ability and skills to perform functional and meaningful activities with whatever assistance is necessary. He further acknowledges that the ability and opportunity to participate in such valued activities have the potential to increase a person's power to define and pursue objectives that they perceive as personally and socially important. Essentially competency can be seen as the development of appropriate knowledge, skills and attitudes. In the context of people with a learning disability, this often equates to nurses identifying key areas for skill development and working closely with individuals to enable the acquisition of that skill or competence. In the instance of older people, consideration must be given not simply to the acquisition of the skills but more to the maintenance and continued usage of these skills.

If competence is identified as the individual's ability to function within or operate as part of society, it is important to consider what the level of ability is and what people are expected to be competent in. Whelan and Speake (1979) suggest that 'coping skills' are extremely important in society and they identify that this requires self-reliance and social independence. This is defined as the ability to carry out tasks related to independent living to a standard that does not require input from another person. It is the intention of this section to not only consider competence in the context of independence, but also with regard to mutually beneficial or interdependent relationships.

The need to achieve self-reliance and social independence is reinforced by the fact that a technical society places high value upon certain competencies and skills, for example, numeracy, the use of credit cards etc. If an individual possesses combinations of these skills, society will often make positive judgements about them; conversely, the lack of such skills may result in negative judgements. More rarely, people who are highly valued in relation to a specific competency, such as maths or science, may find that this will compensate for missing or limited competence in other areas such as interpersonal skills. A classic example of this situation is societies' reverence for the eccentric professor. A clear understanding by nurses of these issues can assist in helping the older person to maximize their own positive attributes to facilitate the person's acceptance and value within society.

French (1993) suggests that the notion of independence can be taken too far and can become a restricting force rather than an enriching experience. Often older disabled people spend inordinate amounts of time completing everyday tasks, such as dressing themselves, rather than spending that time upon more enjoyable activities related to a quality lifestyle. Ultimately, when striving towards the goal of independence or competence with a person who has a disability, the balance must be maintained between whose needs are being served, those of the disabled person or those of the carers and professionals. Norton *et al.* (1962) identified that the fundamental aim of nursing older people is to develop and maintain independent living. Therefore the nurse would not put

Assess the environment in which you work in order to identify the ways in which it promotes and restricts the maintenance and development of competence.

Explore the ways in which you assess an older person's skills with regard to competence and independent living. How do you plan to meet these needs? How could you improve this situation?

someone's shoes on for them on the basis that they would then have to do this for the rest of that person's 'life'.

In the context of French's (1993) commentary, Norton *et al.*'s (1962) philosophy appears to be less and less desirable when considering the area of self-help skills for individuals who will not return to an independent living environment. However, in the situation of people returning home, the aim of nursing must continue to be maintenance of levels of competence. Nurses therefore need to become more discriminatory in the application of some of the fundamental philosophies of nursing, particularly in regard to the appropriateness of skill development. They need to consider the issue of skill development/maintenance in the context usefulness to the individual and their quality of life.

INTERDEPENDENCE

Independence is regularly presented as the goal of nursing care. In striving to achieve this objective, nursing is potentially restricting older people and those with mental health needs or a learning disability to living in particular types of environments. Establishing criteria that people have to achieve, based upon a model of independence, will often result in a person living in a more restrictive and controlling environment than may be necessary. The person concerned may, once in such an environment, find it difficult to break free from the self-fulfilling prophecy that develops (Figure 3.1).

A more realistic model for the basis of nursing care may be be one of interdependence. Though this is not a common term in nursing language, it is not an unfamiliar concept. Interdependence is based upon models of ordinary living in which each citizen openly accepts their need to rely upon each other. Some relationships and dependencies are based upon intimate personal relationships, whilst others are based upon some form of economic exchange. Whatever the basis of the relationship the essence of interdependence is the reliance upon another person. If nursing is able to adopt this as a basis for care delivery, rather

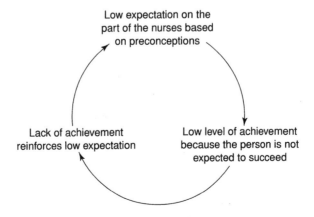

Figure 3.1 Cycle of underachievement.

List 10 things you did yesterday. How many did you do totally independently?

Your list might have included feeding yourself and your family. Think about the process of buying, preparing and cooking the food you ate. How many other people were involved in this process?

You might have thought about the growing or manufacture of the food, the retail outlets from which you purchased the food, the utensils you used and where these came from, and also the fuel you used to cook the food. As such, an activity that is normally perceived as one of the skills of independent living becomes one where we are all interdependent upon each other.

A further example of the concept of interdependence is that of movement and transport. It is an accepted part of everyday life that people will use aids to support their movements around the community. These include cars, bicycles, buses, trains, lifts and escalators. These are not considered to compromise our independence. However, think about those individuals who are reliant upon a wheelchair. Is this seen in the same way as other methods of transport? Anecdotal evidence would suggest that this is not the case as wheelchairs are frequently seen as an indicator of a persons' dependence. A difference can therefore be seen between how these different aids are perceived by members of society and how these differences influence where we place a person on the dependence–independence continuum.

than the goal of independence, then the outcome for individual clients should be a better quality of life within a less restrictive environment. In this context competence becomes the goal of care delivery because it is the wish of the older person rather than the nurses desire to make a 'disabled person' more able.

Nurses need to begin to reshape the way they approach the care situation and reconfigure the dependence–independence continuum. In doing this, assessment of client need and nursing interventions can then be placed within a context of interdependence. Fundamental to the success of nurses in implementing this concept is the need to fully understand the underpinning principles. Perhaps the most crucial of these is the need for nurses and clients to mutually respect and value one another.

RESPECT

Having respect for an individual and their way of life is seen as fundamental in terms of nursing practice. However, this is something that we may take for granted. Being respected by friends, family and colleagues impacts upon how we see ourselves and therefore upon our self-esteem. A fundamental difficulty for nurses comes from the inherent problems in teaching someone to respect themselves. The difficulties that the nurse may encounter will be different in each of the areas of nursing. In the context of learning disabilities and mental health nursing, many of the client group will have spent much of their lives without experiencing that fundamental feeling of self-respect. The problems inherent in teaching individuals to respect themselves are rooted in the fact that self-respect cannot be given by another person. In order to empower an individual to respect themselves you have to overtly and unconditionally respect that individual. This requires a culture of respect and being respectful.

Many other older people will have experienced the respect of others, and had self-respect, by virtue of their 'ordinary' lives in the community. Entering into care situations in later life many challenge this. The need for a culture of respect is as important in this context as any other. O'Brien (1987) defines respect as having a valued place amongst a network of people, and the participation in valued roles within community life. The potential difficulty in this situation is that disabled people may be confined to a narrow range of stereotypical, low-status, community roles which in turn will restrict their opportunity to be seen as valued individuals. If respect is seen as essential with regard to everyday living then it is important to explore how individual people gain respect. In society there are a variety of ways in which people achieve respect. These are class, work, learning and communication. A fundamental way in which nurses are able to contribute to developing mutual respect is through accessing people to such ◄1 opportunities and through nurse–client communication.

Argyle (1975) identifies the importance of both verbal and non-verbal communication in the giving and receiving of messages. The process of normal ageing may significantly impact upon an individual's ability in receiving and/or transmitting these messages. It is important that nurses consider the impact of ►10 altered patterns of communication upon self-respect and self-esteem. The difficulties in maintaining self-respect as a result of impaired communication skills may significantly impact upon a person's ability to interact socially and therefore upon their self-esteem. The potential of impaired communication skills is that an individual experiences a sense of social isolation that may or may not be related to environment and physical competence. This may potentially result in an older person being unable to stand up for their own rights and responsibilities in that they are unable to assert their own wishes.

In many ways this scenario reinforces the beliefs and stereotypes that society ◄1 hold about age and older people. As already discussed earlier in this book, nurses are influenced in the same way as other members of society. As such the care that we give may be based upon the idea that all older people are passive and do not want to take responsibility. This situation may again have negative effects on a person's self-esteem and the respect with which they are held. If a person has impaired communication skills then it may be seen to be the nurse's responsibility to empower them with regard to both communication and self-respect. It may be argued that without self-respect an individual will not gain respect from others. A fundamental way in which respect can be demonstrated is through providing individuals with choices within their lives.

CHOICE

O'Brien (1987) states that choice is the experience of growing autonomy from both small everyday matters through to the larger more life-defining events. It may be argued that personal choice defines and expresses an individual's total ►4 being. Therefore, the concept of choice is vital with regard to the provision of nursing care. This element of care delivery will be interpreted differently within different types of healthcare services. Whilst many services have achieved some success in the provision of small choices, the more complex decisions such as where to live, who to live with, whether to get married and have children have often been seen as irrelevant or too complex for people with learning disabilities.

In the context of older people, many will have spent their lives making choices both small and complex in nature, independent of professional involvement, but in conjunction with important family members. The changes that individuals experience as a result of the ageing process may impact upon the opportunities to make choices. This may be the consequence of the perception of relatives and friends that the older person is no longer able to make decisions. The increased involvement of professionals in the care of some older people can result in the loss of autonomy and independence in this area, often as a consequence of the belief that 'the professional knows best' (Williams, 1993).

➤14

◄1; ➤10 & 12
Choices can also be reduced as a consequence of changes in social, economic and physical status. For example, the loss of a spouse and or family and friends impacts directly on the choices a person has with regard to social experiences. The loss of the work through either redundancy or retirement also affects an individual's ability to choose. This is particularly relevant to the economic choices that an individual may make. In the physical domain, the impact of the ageing process upon hearing, for example, may prevent an individual from accessing information both about their health, about family and life events.

Brost and Johnson (1982) discuss the concept of continuous growth and learning throughout life. Central to this is the belief that individuals develop new goals, learn new skills and engage in new experiences. For people with disabilities, particularly when they are dependent upon bureaucratic and powerful organizations the common expectancy of incapacity is in conflict with the need to develop opportunities to maximize and maintain choice.

➤4
Reflecting upon the spectrum of care identified earlier in the chapter, the changes regarding the opportunities for choice can be seen to diminish significantly. For a person admitted into continuing care, the social, economic and emotional changes could be enormous. This may be as a result of both the changes in their social circle, the need to pay for care, and the loss of a familiar and well-loved home. The increased input from professionals in these situations has the potential to alter the locus of control within a person's life. Williams (1993) suggests that professionals have a great deal of difficulty allowing people that they are caring for to be self-determining. Brost and Johnson (1982) identify that all people rely on various methods to achieve and safeguard their rights as human beings. People with disabilities may have limited power to define and achieve their own aspirations and ambitions, as a result they may be especially vulnerable to choices being defined for them and therefore they will be at risk of exposure to exploitation, neglect and abuse. This is just as likely to occur within the professional care arena as in the 'ordinary' situation of everyday living.

A further consequence of increased professional input is the conflict experienced in meeting the needs of the older person alongside those of the organization. For example, at mealtimes when the constraints that kitchen staff have to operate within conflict with those of client choice. Though this may not appear to be of direct concern to nurses, such situations do impact upon the ability of people to

➤15
make choices within their home environment and therefore their quality of life.

CONCLUSION

Having explored the value of the concept of ordinary living and the ways in which this can be implemented for older people with healthcare needs, it becomes possible to consider the nursing role in two broad contexts, these are the public health focus and the clinical aspect of the role (HMSO, 1997). Within the public health focus, areas for nurses to consider and develop include promoting positive images and combatting labelling and stereotypes particularly in the context of the youth culture. From a clinical perspective it is important for nurses to consider their role in the rehabilitation of older people with healthcare needs, the promotion of positive health and facilitating effective communication.

This chapter has identified the opportunities that have arisen as a result of the NHSCCA (HMSO, 1990) in the context of nursing older people. It has used the central tenets of O'Brien's (1987) five accomplishments to provide a framework for utilizing those opportunities and for further developing the humanistic approach to nursing care delivery. In doing this the chapter provides an additional focus for the efforts of nurses by identifying ways in which they may utilize their skills to support people in maintaining those aspects of 'an ordinary life' that enhance the quality of care delivered.

FURTHER READING

King's Fund Centre (1980) *An Ordinary Life; Comprehensive Locally Based Services for Mentally Handicapped People*. King's Fund Centre, London.
Though this text is very much focused in the area of learning disabilities and is not nursing specific, it is still an extremely useful source document. This was one of the early texts to translate the concept of social role valorization, or normalization as it was then known, into a format that was understandable for practitioners. This text should be read to identify the elements that are transferable into older-adult services. The fact that it was written as a response to the impending closure of learning disability institutions to some extent dates this text. In others for example, the growth in nursing and residential homes for older people means that it is once again very pertinent.

Tyne, A. (1972) *Principles of Normalisation*. Campaign for Mental Handicap.
Again this document is routed in learning disabilities and at the time of major hospital closure programmes. This text does, however, present the fundamental principles of normalization in understandable non-technical language. As such it is good background reading for those that have not come across it before. As principles of normalization are not learning-disability specific but are about all groups in society who have the potential to be devalued, this text has considerable reference to the area of service provision for older people.

Victor, C. (1994) *Old Age in Modern Society: a Textbook of Social Gerontology*, 2nd edn. Chapman & Hall, London.
This text aims to portray the circumstances of older people within society in order to evaluate the major stereotypes attached to growing older. These are particularly useful aspects which relate to health and illness and services for elderly people. In addition, Victor explains issues which surround families and social networking.

Wenger, G.C. (1989) Support networks in old age: constructing a typology. In *Growing Old in the Twentieth Century*, Jefferys, M. (ed.). Routledge, London. *Wenger has produced a great deal of work around networks of older people. This chapter in this text is a good summary of the findings from her extensive research. This particular chapter is interesting as it specifically looks at the networks older people have and also the characteristics of these support mechanisms.*

REFERENCES

Argyle, M. (1975) The Psychology of Interpersonal Behaviour. Penguin, Harmondsworth.

Brost, M. and Johnson, T. (1982) *Getting to Know You*. Wisconsin Coalition for Advocacy, Madison, WI.

Bulmer, M. (1987) *The Social Base of Community Care*. Allen and Unwin, London.

Bury, M. and Holme, A. (1993) Measuring quality of life. In *Ageing and Later Life*, Johnson, J. and Slater, R. (eds). Open University Press, Milton Keynes.

Calman, K. (1996) *The Reduction in Junior Doctors' Hours: The New Deal*. NHSE, London.

Dunn, H.J. (1961) *High Level Wellness*. Mount Vernon Publishing, Washington DC.

French, S. (1993) What's so great about independence? In *Disability Barriers. Enabling Environments*, Finkelstein, V. French, S. and Oliver, M. (eds). Open University Press, Milton Keynes.

Goffman, E. (1961) *Asylums. Essays on the Social Situation of Mental Patients and other Inmates*. Doubleday, New York.

Greenhalgh (1994) *The Interface Between Junior Doctors and Nurses*. Greenhalgh & Co., Macclesfield.

Health and Safety Commission (1992) *Management of Health and Safety at Work: Approved Code of Practice*. HMSO, London.

Health and Safety Commission (1994) *Management of Health and Safety in Health Services Information for Directors and Managers*. HMSO, London.

Hillery, G. (1955) Definition of community: areas of agreement. *Rural Sociology, 20*, 111–128.

HMSO (1990) *National Health Service and Community Care Act*. HMSO, London.

HMSO (1996) *Choice and Opportunity: Primary Care for the Future*. 3390. HMSO, London.

HMSO (1997) *Primary Care: Delivering the Future*. HMSO, London.

King's Fund Centre (1980) *An Ordinary Life: Comprehensive Locally Based Services for Mentally Handicapped People*. King's Fund Centre, London.

Kitson, A. (ed.) (1993) *Art and Science*. Chapman & Hall, London.

Mansell, J. (1992) Contribution to conference 'Sharing for the Future', organised by Dept of Health, Manchester Business School, 3 July 1992.

NHSE (1996) *Primary Care: the Future*. NHSE, London.

Northern General NHS Trust (1992) An unpublished report on activity related to patient care. NGH Trust, Sheffield.

Norton, D., McLaren, R. and Exton-Smith, A.N. (1962) *An Investigation of Geriatric Nursing Problems in Hospital*. Churchill Livingstone, Edinburgh.

O'Brien, J. (1987) *A Framework for Accomplishment*. Responsive System Associates, Decatur, GA.

Oswin, M. (1972) *Children Living in Long Stay Hospitals*. Heinemann, London.

Peplau, H. (1952) *Interpersonal Relations in Nursing*. Putnam, New York.

Seedhouse, D. (1986) *Health: The Foundations for Achievement*. John Wiley & Sons, Chichester.

Whelan, E. and Speake, B. (1979) *Learning to Cope*. Souvenir Press, London.

Williams, I. (1993) What is a profession? Experience v. expertise. In *Health Welfare and Practice. Reflecting on Roles and Relationships*, Warmsley, J., Reynolds, J., Shakespear, P. and Woolfe, R. (eds). Open University Press, Milton Keynes.

UKCC (1992) *Scope of Professional Practice*. UKCC, London.

UKCC (1994) Registrar's letter 20/1994. The Council's Standards for Education and Practice following Registration Programmes of Education Leading to Qualification of Specialist Practitioner, 14 December 1994. UKCC, London.

UKCC (1996) *Guidelines for Professional Practice*. UKCC, London.

4 Promoting choice, autonomy and independence with older people

Jillian Jefferson and Michael Hall

INTRODUCTION

We are all faced with a multitude of choices every day. Most of us would consider ourselves to be independent and have some degree of autonomy. We are participants in a society in which there are growing expectations about choices, services and outcomes of services, based on market forces. The ability to represent one's own interests and needs is crucial, and can be affected by age, class, gender, ethnicity, knowledge, individual assertiveness and situational factors. The focus of this chapter is to explore choice, autonomy and independence in relation to older people with healthcare needs and their position when accessing healthcare services. Nurses can be influential in affecting the experience that older people have when they encounter healthcare services; the close working relationship that can develop between client and nurse supports this. It is important that nurses are aware of the issues contained in this chapter so that they can move on to challenge assumptions about the ability and eligibility of older people to make choices about their health and well-being.

CITIZENSHIP

It is important to examine the concept of citizenship in order to raise the consciousness of nurses to the political ideology which has shaped the National

BOX 4.1	*Civil, political and social rights*

Civil rights
- Legal rights
- The right to contract
- Property rights
- Freedom of thought
- Freedom of speech
- Choice in religious practice

Political rights
- Universal suffrage
- To organize politically

Social rights
- Access to welfare services and benefits
- Standard of living in line with current social expectations

Health Service. This section does not provide unequivocal reasons for this transition but aims to facilitate an awareness of the difficulties that can be experienced by some members of society when accessing healthcare.

Citizenship reaches back to the late-nineteenth–early-twentieth century and the New Liberalism movement. New Liberalism is defined as a political perspective which advocated state involvement in social issues by means of a welfare state. The overall aim was to preserve social order by providing assistance to the unemployed, poor, sick and older people, thus acting as a neutral agent between the conflicting interests of capitalists and workers. From this perspective came the legislation on national insurance, old age pensions, employment rights and eventually the NHS. This perspective has also been referred to as Fabianism, Reformism or by a modern term, Pluralism (Coombes, 1982). This view challenged the individualist political and economic thinking of the time, which was and still is characteristic of right-wing politics.

The individualist perspective sees society as consisting of people actively pursuing their own interests. Individuals are seen as rational and able to actively choose and express their preferences in an open market place. There is a strong emphasis on individual responsibility and self-help (Coombes, 1982).

The term 'citizenship' was used to define the establishment of statutory conditions whereby *all* members of society would be able to take a full and productive role in the nation's life. The work of Marshall (1951) was influential in defining the concept of citizenship. He described it as an achievement of civil, political and social rights (Box 4.1).

In pre-industrial society these rights were confined to a narrow elite determined by birth and social position. In 1940s post-war Western Europe there was unease that economic depression and Fascism could return. The extension of these rights to the working classes were meant to lead to a decline in this revolutionary class consciousness (Abercrombie *et al.*, 1988).

CITIZENSHIP AND WELFARE PROVISION

Beveridge (1879–1963) was chairman of a Government enquiry into the management of social services, which resulted in the Social Insurance and Allied

Services Report (1942), also known as the Beveridge Report. This report set out the principles that established the post-war welfare state, and was influenced by the concept of citizenship in the pursuit of the economic and social priorities of the time which were the establishment of (Webster, 1993):

- Full employment
- State investment in welfare
- State investment in industry

The ideology expressed by Beveridge defined welfare citizenship in terms of the British (white) family and aimed through the reconstruction of the 'normal' family to re-establish Britain as a powerful nation (Pascall, 1986).

Capitalism was adapted in order that social justice and liberty could be universal and not dependent on self-interest and market forces. This took steps towards addressing concerns about post-war social reorganization and moves towards a more equal society (Cochrane and Clarke, 1993). However, the conflicts between capitalism and welfare were born, a legacy which is high on the political agenda to this day. Rather than providing a short-term measure of improving the nation's health (as was intended) the welfare state has grown steadily throughout the post-war years.

Citizenship involves setting limitations based on birth and residence, whereby entitlement does not extend to everyone. Nationality tests are used to identify British citizens and therefore to define eligibility for welfare and services. The universalism of citizenship is conditional, and based on a family-orientated social and economic structure. At the forefront of this structure are men in full employment, who support their extended families. A proportion of the population exist who are excluded from paid employment and so become dependent on their families or the state by virtue of their age, gender, disability or race. Therefore, citizenship can be used as a yardstick against which certain groups are measured and identified as not being socially integrated.

The Report of the Working Group on Inequalities in Health – referred to as the Black Report (1980) – provided evidence that since the introduction of the National Health Service, access to healthcare in different parts of the UK had become diverse. Rather than showing a decline in inequality in health, there were differences in health experience occurring around the country and between different groups of people. The Black Report (1980) concluded that there was a strong association between material deprivation and poor health.

In 1989 just over 20% of all people of pensionable age were receiving income support to supplement their state pensions (Department of Health and Social Security, 1991). This may be underestimated as many older people do not claim benefits to which they are entitled. By definition these people are living on the poverty line. They often have little or no disposable income and as such can be described as experiencing material deprivation. Older people can often find themselves dependent on their state pension for all daily expenses and access to welfare benefits is necessary to supplement their income. This reliance on the state was termed 'structured dependency' by Dallos and McLaughlin (1993).

DEPENDENCY IN OLDER AGE

Older people live in a variety of complex ways, often diverse from the nuclear family, which continues to be the stereotypical norm in the UK. They often live alone, or in residential and nursing care establishments, they may be reliant on friends and neighbours for assistance, or live in extended family units. Diversity is a concept used to distinguish the expected from the real, of identifying ways of doing or being that is different from the norm. Judgements can be made about the degree of deviation from the norm and this shapes responses from social and political institutions. In using the concept of diversity, differences do not simply exist – but do so in a context where they are judged against a standard or norm (Clarke and Langan, 1993).

Diverse issues which tend to be highlighted include:

- Ethnicity – older people are often respected and valued differently within ethnic groups
- Gender – heterosexuality is the norm and it is against this that older gay people are judged
- Class – expected lifestyles on retirement
- Disability – old age and inevitable disability are considered the norm, people's worth and contribution to society are often measured against this belief

Older people find themselves legally bound to retire at a given age, i.e. 65, whether they consider it appropriate for themselves as individuals or not. Unless they have means of financial support from savings and private or occupational pensions, older people often find themselves in a position of relative poverty compared with their previous lifestyle. The twentieth century has seen the creation of a category of retired person which applies long before the onset of physical frailty and dependency. This is for many a forced dependency and a status which forces people to fall back on the family for personal support (Dallos and McLaughlin, 1993).

Early retirement is an important issue; people take early retirement for a variety of reasons, two main reasons being a planned decision and ill-health. The people who choose to retire early tend to report satisfaction in the outcome, whilst those with ill-health tend to report problems adjusting to their situation and fear for the future. An analysis of studies of early retirement suggests that the level of satisfaction experienced is dependent on class and financial security on retirement. People who choose to retire early have often planned for it and made financial arrangements in order to continue with their standard of living. Whilst those who retire on the grounds of ill-health are more likely to be working class, less financially secure and as a result of their health problems are limited as regards leisure activities. The role in society of those who take early retirement is unclear; they are neither unemployed nor properly retired. They fall into a gap between worker and senior citizen (Phillipson, 1990).

On an individual level, for many people retirement can be a welcome and enjoyable time in life. Financial arrangements built up over time can be accessed and provide for a comfortable standard of living. Whilst on a socio-political level British society, shaped in the 1980s by Conservative individualism, places greater value on the young and economically productive. The structured dependency that retirement can bring at the societal level, with a cessation of paid employment rights, and reliance on pensions, can render the older person less worthy and eligible in a society that values productivity as a measure of success.

The individualist ideals of self-help and family responsibility influence welfare policy and provision, often limiting access to services to those with other networks of support. Social policies and welfare are designed to supplement the role of the family in giving support and care and not to replace it.

How can older people be disadvantaged in respect of their civil, political and social rights?

■ You may have considered the following:

Civil rights
■ Buying goods on hire purchase
■ Securing a mortgage
■ Purchasing health/life insurance

Political rights
■ Exercising their right to vote
■ Difficulties accessing polling stations
■ Voting from hospital/residential settings
■ Accessing political organisations
■ Exercising their right to vote by proxy

Social rights
■ Low incomes/pensions
■ Failure to claim benefits
■ Means tested access to services

Social policies are developed with the interests of the majority as their basis. The values of the society and the economic strategies of the time will influence the provision of welfare and benefits. Those members of society deemed most eligible for services will reap the most benefit from welfare provision, for example the young, those temporarily unemployed and able-bodied people with short-term episodes of illness.

The welfare of other members of society who are considered less eligible, for example, the long-term unemployed, lone parent families, the homeless, and older people are increasingly seen as being the responsibility of their families. Policies which highlight this value base have the specific aim of reducing the burden on the welfare state. These policies have extended to older people, with the Department of Health Guidelines (1995) – *NHS Responsibilities for Meeting Continuing Health Care Needs*. Many social services are now means tested (charges may differ between authorities) and health services set against specific and general criteria for eligibility. The families of older people are increasingly being approached to assist in support of their relatives both financially and practically.

► 14

An important issue in the debate about welfare provision which affects social policies, is the changing structure of the family in society. People increasingly live in diverse family units which do not conform to any particular model of 'the family'. Care by the family may be difficult as people increasingly live away from relatives, and many are forced from their place of birth to seek jobs. The close-knit communities of the post-war years, when kinship and community spirit flourished, have long since been replaced by a migrant workforce and the decline of many former industrial areas. This results in many older people living alone or with their spouse. At times like these they may find themselves dependent for support on statutory services, or friends and neighbours who are often old themselves.

It is important for nurses to be aware of the political issues surrounding healthcare in relation to older people and its impact on services. The next step is to examine the values and beliefs that underpin nursing, specifically in caring for the needs of older people.

PHILOSOPHIES UNDERPINNING NURSING

Nursing models are a useful way of examining concepts that contribute to a representation of what nursing is. Because nursing is not tangible it is often difficult to appreciate the value of models. We can identify a model train quite easily because it represents the features and component parts of a real train. We can pick it up and examine it, looking for familiar features such as the engine, wheels, windows, doors and carriages. It will often be possible to identify the age and function of the train from its features enabling us to compare it with other model trains. Through a consideration of the following metaparadigms it is possible to analyze models of nursing according to their philosophical base, this can enable us to examine, compare and provide a framework for understanding what nursing is and what nursing activities are included in nursing care (Alligood and Marriner-Tomey, 1997):

- Health
- Person
- Nursing
- Environment

DEPENDENCE, INDEPENDENCE AND INTERDEPENDENCE

◄3   Many nursing models in practice take the idea that living/health is the basis of a continuum from conception to death.

As people move along this continuum their lives are influenced by physical, intellectual, emotional and social changes. It is identified that there are periods in people's lives when they cannot begin, or are unable to continue performing certain activities of living. Each person is said to have a dependence–independence continuum for each activity, along which movement can be in either direction (Roper et al., 1996). It is acknowledged that some people are unable to become fully independent in all the activities of living from birth due, for example, to learning disabilities.

Many nurses are required to assess a person's level of independence in the activities of living, plan care to assist the person to move along the continuum towards independence and evaluate the care that has been implemented against the goals that have been set. Often nurses are concerned with doing to the person or assisting them to achieve 'independence'. Within this process older people can easily become passive recipients of care who are unable to change or exercise control over their situations.

The concept of the dependence–independence continuum suggests that the two states are mutually exclusive; a person can be one or the other at any given time. By striving to promote independence as a goal to be achieved we attach a negative connotation to dependence, which when linked with our understanding of diversity portrays dependency as a deviation from the desired norm. An alternative view is that no one is truly independent, but that a state of interdependence is inevitable and desirable. Consider the businessman who relies on others to launder his clothes, or the family who employ a cleaner, or the vast majority of us who visit the supermarket each week to replenish the fridge and cupboards. We are dependent on others to provide goods and services which we are unable to provide for ourselves. This is not considered to be a negative dependency but a necessity if we are to function in our daily lives. People are encouraged to complain if services are not of the frequency or standard that is expected, this is regarded as a proper and just course of action. The essence of interdependence lies in the belief that every person is reliant on others for some aspect of their daily lives whether practically or emotionally (Johnson, 1990). Interdependency fosters co-operation and collaboration and is evident in effective team work. It is worth considering why we attach negative meanings to assistance that older or disabled people need in order to live. The 'burden of elderly care' is a common theme and is often highlighted as a social problem. This can be attributed to the political and economic position of older people in society and their potential marginalization.

Rather than perceiving the nurse as an active provider of care and the client as a passive recipient of that care, consider that nursing is a learning experience, a two-way process. From the interaction that is nursing, both the client and the nurse can benefit and learn from what is a unique experience.

In this context interdependence is fostered in the nurse–client relationship. Rather than the nurse doing for the person, or the person doing for themselves, the person works interdependently with the nurse. Within this framework the practice of nursing is a significant, therapeutic, interpersonal process, based on skills and an informed knowledge base, which grow and develop from the relationships formed with clients, carers and colleagues (Peplau, 1988). By adopting the concept of interdependence into our practice we can foster a culture in which we will be constantly faced with evaluating our values and beliefs as we encounter each experience, some of which will be stressful, painful and others providing great satisfaction.

The underlying belief is, that the experience that is the relationship between client and nurse, will be beneficial to both and free from negative stereotypical images. The organization of care into a named nurse system (Department of Health, 1991a) can be conducive with the concept of interdependence as client and nurse are identified as an alliance. A relationship based on information and trust can be fostered from the onset of the episode of care. This can prove especially important for the older person, who might often be finding themselves in a period of transition in their lives from being depended on by family and friends, to being dependent on others. The named nurse and older person can begin to build up a relationship on an interdependent basis, sharing information and experiences and meeting care needs together. The named nurse can also provide a pivotal role for including carers and significant others in the care plan with the client's consent.

If we base our practice on developing and fostering relationships with clients, carers and colleagues, in an interdependent way, we will be moving towards creating an environment in which people are encouraged to seek answers and information and thus make informed choices about care. In return each participant has the potential to grow and learn from the experience.

Who makes decisions about client care?

How is independence measured and by whom?

From whose values and beliefs are goals set?

The decisions about care are taken by and large by able-bodied experts in positions of power, within the confines of current policies and welfare provision. Dependence, independence and interdependence are interwoven in the values and beliefs about the position of older people in society, the roles and responsibilities of informal carers (often family and friends) and the current legislation governing welfare provision and services. A person's perceived position on the dependence–independence–interdependence continuum can sometimes be determined by the changing accessibility and eligibility for services and not by the person's perception of their situation. A person's need can remain unchanged, yet their eligibility for services can alter, dependent on current provision and access criteria.

The values and beliefs that underpin nursing practice, by and large stem from the societal level. Individualist ideology views people as autonomous agents making rational choices about their lives with minimal state intervention. A conflict is now evident; we strive to encourage people to make rational choices about their care, to participate in the decision-making process, because this is seen as good practice. In this respect do we subscribe to the individualist view ? It is important to highlight that this view of society is one founded on self-help, where support and care is the responsibility of the family; however, we have considered that often older people live in diverse family units. The conflict lies between market forces and welfare provision. Nurses need to be aware of the political debate as it can perpetuate the belief that older people are less worthy and eligible than younger, economically productive people. As a result older people can easily be seen as a burden on the healthcare system.

Legislation in the form of Citizen's Charters (Department of Health, 1991a) can provide a lever that people can use to affect the care that they receive. However, to do this requires a degree of assertiveness and ability that many people when faced with illness or disability are unable to utilize. Nurses play an important role through their interaction and relationships with clients in ensuring that people are represented. In this context it is necessary to consider autonomy, advocacy and empowerment and its place within nursing practice.

AUTONOMY

Collins' English Dictionary (Collins, 1987) describes autonomy as:

> The right or state of self-government especially when limited.
> Freedom to determine one's own action, behaviour etc.

Perhaps the above dictionary definition fails to accurately describe what many of us have come to understand by the term autonomy, particularly in the case of the older individual.

What do you understand by the term autonomy?

Make a note of phrases/words which currently spring to mind in relation to the word autonomy.

Revisit your notes at the end of this section and see if your perceptions have changed.

Today there is considerable emphasis placed on autonomy, be it in the area of open government, employment or individual rights in relation to specific areas of society.

The Conservative Government introduced the Citizen's Charter initiative (Department of Health, 1991d) which was aimed at ensuring individual rights:

■ The right to choice
■ The right to appropriate timely information
■ The right to voice dissatisfaction with specific situations in today's society

In the healthcare setting, the Patient's Charter, part of the Citizen's Charter initiative, came into effect on 1 April 1992 (Department of Health, 1991b). The Patient's Charter is designed to reassure the public about the quality of the health service. In addition to confirming existing rights (for example, to healthcare on the basis of need), three additional rights were guaranteed:

■ A maximum of two years' wait for admission
■ Prompt investigation of complaints
■ Details of local services, including local and national 'charter standards'

The local and national charter standards placed particular emphasis on quality, other types of waiting times, and staff respect for clients. Since the introduction of the Patient's Charter the Department of Health has sought to ensure that healthcare providers direct resources to ensure targets are achieved. A more recent development has been the introduction of the Mental Health Services Patient's Charter (Department of Health, 1996) which specifically targets the needs of people in both community and hospital settings who experience mental health problems. Areas addressed include :

■ Waiting times for first and urgent appointments
■ Information relating to single/mixed sex wards
■ The right to state a preference of the gender of the health professional involved
■ Well-publicized and readily accessible complaints procedures

The Patient's Charter (Department of Health, 1991b) and the Mental Health Services Patient's Charter (Department of Health, 1996) are two specific pieces of legislation which aim to give the individual a say in the care they receive. The legislation also places additional responsibilities on all the healthcare professions. While it is reasonable to assume the legislation represents a positive step for society as a whole, the case of older people warrants closer inspection. Given the potential for intellectual impairment or disability, accurate feedback is not always available from the individual themselves, thus necessitating the use of advocates who may or may not be the client's carer/relative.

ADVOCACY

Advocacy refers to the process of acting on behalf of another person in order to represent their interests and rights as citizens, as the individual would see them. An advocate is a person who actively pursues these interests and rights as if they were their own. Advocates hold a duty of loyalty, confidentiality and a commitment to be zealous in the promotion of the individual's standpoint.

Several forms of advocacy exist (Box 4.2). Citizen advocacy is already well established in other countries, notably the United States and Sweden, and is gaining momentum in Britain. In the United States advocates are recognized under the law, and have the right of access to information. There is a requirement that individual states establish agencies to promote advocacy. There is no legislation in Britain and the provision of advocacy schemes are largely dependent on goodwill and co-operation (Renshaw and Metcalf, 1987).

In 1982 a new organization – Advocacy Alliance – had successfully implemented an advocacy programme between hospital residents and volunteers. The Alliance fought to challenge stereotypical ideas and practices in the area of learning disability. They had to overcome many crucial problems, including persuading people that there was a need for advocacy and securing time and resources to pursue the project (Sang and O'Brien, 1984).

The recruitment and training of volunteer advocates requires time, money and commitment on the part of the organizer and the volunteer. They will have to build up a relationship based on trust with the person. Their relationship might be required to last for many years and in representing an older person, will often end with bereavement sooner rather than later.

However, these are not good enough reasons to discount citizen advocacy. The benefits can far outweigh the problems, especially to an older person who lives alone, perhaps has mental health needs, or lives permanently in hospital, in a residential or a nursing home. The basic assumption is that all people have the right to equality and respect and that this should be preserved and protected at all times. An advocate who is distanced from the providers of care and services may be in an ideal position to view those services objectively and protect the individual according to his/her instrumental competencies and expressed needs. Instrumental competencies enable people to cope with everyday life, for example earning a living, accessing training and education, being able to get from A to B, most people are able to satisfy these needs as they grow older and acquire the skills and knowledge needed through experience.

BOX 4.2	*Types of advocacy (Butler et al., 1988)*

- Citizen advocacy/lay advocacy – trained volunteers and staff work on behalf of others, independent from providers of services
- Self-advocacy – a person acts on his/her own behalf to present their own case. A degree of assertiveness and appropriate social skills are required for this to be effective
- Legal advocacy – lawyers and others trained in legal issues assist others to defend or exercise their rights
- Collective advocacy – a group of people unite on issues affecting more than one individual. Organizations campaign at national level in order to influence policy, e.g. MIND, Alzheimer's Disease Society (ADS), MENCAP

Expressed needs are emotional and include the need for love, friendship, security and the development of self-esteem. The ability to meet instrumental competencies and expressed needs are formed in childhood and developed throughout life. The desired outcome is for the person to be able to deal with everyday problems in an emotionally secure way (Gates, 1994).

The nurse has to balance their professional accountability and their contract with the employer with their responsibilities to the older person in their care. This can often lead to a conflict of interests. From this perspective it would be difficult for a nurse, as a salaried provider of care, to act as the older person's advocate in an objective way. However, Gadow (1983, cited in Gates, 1994) describes the practice of existential advocacy. The nurse acting as advocate is seen as the essence of nursing, and is based on the principles of self-determination and holism. Existential advocacy is representative of the unique nature of the nurse–client relationship. The nurse provides support and information, shares knowledge with the older person and carers, and always acts in pursuit of their rights.

Existential advocacy is summarized in Gates (1994) as follows:

- The nurse assists the person in self-determination
- The nurse gives of him/herself fully by involvement with the person's care
- The nurse assists the person by understanding their condition from an objective viewpoint

The role of advocate has been of increasing importance with the introduction of the Policy and Eligibility Criteria for NHS funded continuing healthcare (Department of Health, 1995). These guidelines specified that a range of health and social services be arranged and funded to meet the needs of the local population. Policies were developed to define eligibility for access to continuing healthcare services. The main groups of people affected by these policies have been older people, older people with mental health problems, people with dementia, adults with long-term health needs and some children. The policies included general and specific eligibility criteria and clearly defined the responsibilities of all the agencies involved.

Clear guidelines on discharge planning which were included within the document called for increased involvement of those being cared for and their carers in the planning process (Department of Health, 1995). To involve the older person and significant other in the assessment, planning and evaluation process of their care was upheld as an area of good practice. This is seen as an integral part of the role of the named nurse as a co-ordinator of care within the multidisciplinary team. The drive to include the older person's/carer's signature on nursing care plans and discharge plans has been a step towards increased participation in the planning process. Care has to be taken to ensure that this does not simply become an exercise in obtaining a name in a box – but instead reflects discussion and sharing of ideas and expectations between the nurse/older person/carer. In this respect the need for advocacy is clear. For those people whom we nurse that are especially vulnerable the role of advocate must be apparent in order to truly represent their rights and interests.

IMPLICATIONS FOR PRACTICE

The approach and attitudes of professionals, older people and their carers are crucial if decisions about care are to be shared. Some older people are reluctant to express choice, question the appropriateness of care offered or complain when they experience problems. Carers may find themselves faced with difficult decisions to make on their relative's/friend's behalf; conflict may arise when trying to act in the interests of someone else, however closely related, when issues are sensitive. In the previous section we considered different types of advocacy; now we will examine the nurse's role in practice in relation to the Code of Professional Conduct (UK Central Council for Nursing, Midwifery and Health Visiting (UKCC), 1992) and relevant legislation.

The demands on healthcare professionals are twofold:

- As individuals involved in the care of older persons, we must attempt to comply with legislation
- We must assist those in our care to exercise choice or voice dissatisfaction where appropriate

If older people are to benefit from this desire to ensure those in our care experience the degree of autonomy they should rightfully expect as citizens, health professionals must look to their responsibilities as advocates. While the rationale behind this last statement may seem reasonable, if not self-apparent, the position of the health professional as an advocate for older clients is far from straightforward. Consideration must be taken of other professional codes and legislation which, at times, may place the professional at odds with this advocacy role.

Members of the caring professions are bound by ethical guidelines or Codes of Conduct. In the case of nursing, the Code of Professional Conduct (UKCC, 1992) requires that:

Each registered nurse, midwife and health visitor shall act, at all times, in such a manner as to:

- safeguard and promote the interests of individual clients
- serve the interests of society
- justify public trust and confidence and
- uphold and enhance the good standing and reputation of the professions

As a registered nurse, midwife or health visitor, you are personally accountable for your practice . . .

The Code of Professional Conduct (UKCC, 1992) continues by listing 16 key points which develop the four main themes listed above. The UKCC (1996) in the Guidelines for Professional Practice recognizes the potential difficulties facing practitioners in the area of exercising professional accountability while striving to accept a role as advocate on behalf of his or her clients.

The guidelines place emphasis on the client's right to choose and use clauses 1 and 5 of the Code of Conduct to reinforce the nurse's accountability (UKCC, 1996):

- Clause 1: '. . . act always in such a manner as to promote and safeguard the interests and well being of patients and clients' (advocacy)
- Clause 5: '. . . work in an open and co-operative manner with patients, clients and their families, foster their independence and recognise and respect their involvement in the planning and delivery of care' (autonomy)

Who is best placed to determine the interests of individual clients?

Given our earlier discussion about the individual right to autonomy, it is surely the older person themselves. After all, the days of 'Nurse knows best' have long since gone: or have they? Where does the registered nurse stand when the needs or desires of an older person directly conflict with other members of the multi-disciplinary team, carers or society at large?

The Mental Health Act (1983) places further responsibilities on nurses, who are required to assist with, and at certain times, implement statute commonly known as sections which effectively restrict the civil liberties of an individual. This restriction may take the form of preventing an individual leaving hospital or undergoing physical treatments against their will. The nurse facing such moral dilemmas must again rely on the *advocacy* role. If they are to assist with actions which are contrary to the wishes of an individual and which could potentially undermine existing relationships, they must ensure that appropriate, timely and understandable information is given to the individual and his/her carers. While this may not prevent the breakdown of an existing nurse–client relationship, the nurse may take some satisfaction in the knowledge that every effort has been made to explain the necessity of the situation.

CASE STUDY

Given the information explored in this section, it will be useful to reflect on the story of Annie.

Annie was in her late sixties and lived alone in an old terraced house near the city centre. Her home was in a poor state of repair and lacked many of the modern amenities. Annie herself had grown frail and become forgetful, sometimes leaving her house unlocked or leaving gas appliances on. She had enjoyed a long and interesting career as a singer with a national company, but now the highlight of her day was to visit the nearby pub, in full make-up, and reminisce about her friends and roles from days gone by. Popular with the locals, Annie would often oblige with a song, and was always grateful for the drink (always alcoholic), which would invariably be offered in return.

As time progressed, Annie's alcohol consumption increased, she became increasingly forgetful and was more concerned with feeding her two cats than herself. Her condition deteriorated to the point where her long tolerant neighbours began to voice concern about Annie's safety, and the potential dangers to the neighbourhood when Annie left the gas on. In due course, Social Services and local Mental Health Services became involved. Attempts to offer assistance to Annie were many and varied, and always firmly declined.

Things came to a head when Annie started to fall while under the influence of alcohol. Following consultation between Health and Social Services it was agreed that Annie be admitted to the local psychiatric unit under a section of the Mental Health Act (1983). Annie would undergo a full mental and physical assessment and a multi-disciplinary team would then determine how and if Annie could return to her home.

Annie hated being in hospital, hated being away from her cats, hated being in a ward full of strangers, missed her friends at the pub and her evening tipple. No amount of reassurance could console her. She was convinced she would never get out of hospital, convinced she would never see her cats again. Why couldn't she return home to live her life, the way she had done for years?

Before the multidisciplinary team could plan Annie's future she suffered a fall in the ward. Sustaining a fractured femur, Annie developed a chest infection which deteriorated despite the best efforts of medical and nursing staff. Annie died on a ward at a nearby general hospital.

Had you been a member of the team involved in Annie's care how could you have responded to her anxieties about remaining in hospital?

Who do you believe was at risk by Annie remaining in the community without support?

How could Annie have been supported in the community?

Would it be possible to support Annie in the community without her consent?

You may have thought about a number of issues, for example, choice and empowerment.

CHOICE AND EMPOWERMENT

Choice can be defined as:

- The act or an instance of choosing or selecting
- The opportunity or power of choosing
- An alternative action or possibility

To empower can be defined as (Collins, 1987):

- To give power or authority to; authorize
- To give ability to, enable or permit

The word 'power' is evident in the above definitions and is an important issue in any discussion of choice and empowerment.

What is your definition of power?

Definitions of power could include:

- The exercising of control, influence or authority by a person or group over others
- Political, financial or social influence or control
- Legal authority to act for another
- Established authority

There are many definitions of power, which is often perceived in a negative way. Power is neither negative nor positive, but can be perceived as either by the way it is used and its effect on others. It has also been suggested by Farmer (1993) that nurses are an oppressed group and subject to the powerful norms and values of dominant groups in healthcare, and as a result are marginalized and devalued. If this is the case the way forward is not as easy as simply sharing power with our clients. Nurses need to examine their collective position within healthcare alongside that of older people and develop a clear understanding of the concept of empowerment in practice whilst moving towards empowering themselves in the process.

A definition of empowerment offered by Rodwell (1996) is:

> An enabling process, a partnership in which self and others are valued and decisions can be made, where responsibility is acknowledged and accepted.

Empowerment can be viewed as a process, and can be linked with citizenship, in that it is concerned with the relationship of individuals with society. It is commonly assumed that the process of empowerment involves those in society who have power, dispensing some of that power to those who have none. Underlying this idea is the discourse that renames clients as 'consumers', which is believed to be empowering. In this context the process of empowerment becomes an 'object' which can be delivered from those who have it, to those who don't (Finkelstein and French, 1993).

Rodwell's (1996) definition informs a different view which is that empowerment is an enabling process whereby people empower themselves by taking responsibility for making decisions that affect their lives. However any discussion of empowerment can be seen as empty rhetoric if it is characterized by tokenistic gestures giving the appearance of participation and empowerment rather than real changes in practice. Skelton (1994) advises caution when considering that nurses empowering themselves will automatically lead to the empowerment of clients. He states that this does not necessarily follow as nurses can often be seen as part of the problem that disempowers clients rather than the solution.

Collective empowerment is a process by which groups of people work together in a common cause (Finkelstein and French, 1993). We can recognize organizations such as Age Concern, Alzheimer's Disease Society and MIND who campaign for the rights of older people and those with mental health needs. At this structural level some professional organizations and pressure groups are in more powerful positions than others, and as such can influence policy according to their strength and support.

It is important to consider that, at an individual level, some people are better able to represent themselves and their interests amongst healthcare professionals than others (Davey and Popay, 1993).

 What factors do you consider will increase a person's ability to influence the care they receive?

Factors could include:
- Age
- Social class
- Status/past employment
- Self-assertion
- Wealth–private healthcare settings
- Medical knowledge
- Gender
- Support systems

Nurses often meet people in the course of their work who are vulnerable and who often find themselves in situations over which they have little control and limited appropriate knowledge.

Older people living alone can be especially vulnerable to the power of the expert and can easily be swept along in what is deemed to be 'for the best'. Often these decisions are made without the informed consent of the client or significant other. This is the practice of beneficence, whereby the professional knows what is in the best interest of the client over and above what the client wants for themselves. We have considered that there are times when consent is not the main issue, for example when the Mental Health Act is used; however, it is good practice to keep people informed regarding their care at all times.

An important step in the empowering process is considered to be the sharing of information with the older person regarding the options available to them; however, research has suggested that this is not always effective. Cassileth *et al.* (1980, cited in Morrison, 1991) explored the client's perception of the consent process and found that many of the people in the study, who had given consent for surgery, could not recall what had been said to them regarding the treatment plan. This research suggests that people who, through illness or need, have become dependent on healthcare professionals, show poor attention and recall of the information given to them.

Nurses are often best placed to recognize this and endeavour to build up a relationship with the person, with the aim of sharing information and involving the person in all aspects of their care. A common occurrence in caring for the older person is that through their belief and trust in healthcare services they delegate the decision-making process to professionals.

Problems can occur when considering issues of empowerment involving an older person with cognitive impairment, such as in dementia. Kitwood (1988) describes disempowerment as occurring for people with dementia when things are done for the individual which they are able to do in some fashion for themselves. A consequent deskilling and loss of agency occurs. He uses the concept of agency to inform his theory of the dementia process. He proposes that dementia does not comprise neurological impairment alone but also malignant social psychology, whereby the person loses their sense of self which he calls 'personhood' (Kitwood, 1989, 1990). He suggests that there are two conditions of self: the sense of self which evokes feelings and emotions, which is satisfied by unconditional acceptance and love (similar to expressed needs), and a sense of agency which evokes action and is characterized by inner vitality and being able to make a mark on the world. These concepts are drawn from work on 'selfhood' which was undertaken with children. The relevance to older people of these concepts is that they can easily be deprived of an environment of accepting love and care and the opportunity to maintain a sense of agency, especially when living alone or in residential care settings. Kitwood (1992) offers an observational method for evaluating dementia care called Dementia Care Mapping. This provides a means of involving clients in evaluating the care they receive and as a result has the potential to inform knowledge about dementia and effect changes in care.

Nurses not only care for the client but also support their families and friends and within these relationships there are also positions of power. It is very easy to accept the decisions of relatives on issues of care without directly involving the client. There are times when decisions might not be in the client's best interest or of their choosing.

The nurse is in an ideal position, in close contact with the client and family, to mediate in the decision-making process and convey accurate information to those who are involved.

Caring for the carers of people with dementia is an important issue which warrants discussion. It is often the carer (spouse, relative, friend, neighbour) who is left feeling bewildered and isolated when caring in this situation. As well as the physical toll of caring 24 hours a day, there is the stress and anxiety of making endless decisions about everyday events. Crisis can occur when major decisions such as respite care or day hospital attendance are presented. An effective named nurse system with a philosophy which values the well-being of carers can assist carers and support them in their role. The nurse can ensure that information about access and availability of services is available to the carer and can act as a co-ordinator of services for that family. In this way the information available should be consistent and comprehensive; the carer also has an identified person with whom they can discuss their situation.

CONCLUSION

It can be argued that to give the impression that older people have participated in the planning of their care and treatment serves only to give a token illusion of empowerment (Morrall, 1996). The sharing of information and knowledge with older people and their carers may not be enough to cause a shift in the balance of power between them and the healthcare professional, but it may enable them to take an active part in their care and influence decisions that are made.

The sharing of information and knowledge through the dynamics of the nurse–client relationship are important components of choice, autonomy and interdependence. People cannot make informed choices about their care if their voice cannot be heard. The role of the nurse is crucial in supporting older people whilst enabling them to exercise their right to make choices about factors that affect their lives.

This chapter has briefly considered some of the issues of choice autonomy and interdependence. We can offer choice by providing information and support and by valuing the older person as an equal partner in care. We accept that sometimes it is the significant carer with whom we are sharing this knowledge, for example, when a person has dementia, but this should not exclude the person themselves from exercising choice and acting for themselves to the best of their ability. In this way we move towards enabling older people to empower themselves.

FURTHER READING

Alligood, M.R. and Marriner-Tomey, A. (1997) *Nursing Theory: Utilization and Application.* Mosby, St Louis.
An up-to-date book from the USA which considers the movement of nursing theory from development to practice. It contains a useful glossary of terms used in nursing theory generation, and highlights main points in the text in distinctive boxes. Critical thinking exercises allow the reader to test out their understanding of the issues.

Bond, J. and Coleman, P. (eds) (1990) *Ageing In Society: An Introduction to Social Gerontology*. Sage, London.
This useful and interesting text provides a good introduction to issues of ageing and later life. Contributions include: ageing in the twentieth century, biological and psychological ageing, sociology of retirement, dependency and interdependency and poverty amongst others.

Gates, B. (1994) *Advocacy: a Nurse's Guide*. Scutari Press, London.
Gates provides a comprehensive and easy-to-read account of advocacy in relation to nursing. He uses case studies which help to bring the text to life for the reader. It is intended as a resource book for students and practitioners to dip into and inform, direct and guide their role as advocates. The author sets out to offer a pragmatic approach by which nurses can address the complexities of the role of advocate in their practice.

REFERENCES

Abercrombie, N., Hill, S. and Turner, B.S. (1988) *Dictionary of Sociology*, 2nd edn. Penguin, Harmondsworth.

Alligood, M.R. and Marriner-Tomey, A. (1997) *Nursing Theory: Utilization and Application*. Mosby, St Louis, MI.

Beveridge, W. (1942) *Social Insurance and Allied Services (The Beveridge Report)*. Cmnd 6404, HMSO, London.

Black Report (1980) *Inequalities in Health: Report of a Research Working Group*. Department of Health and Social Security, London.

Butler, K., Carr, S. and Sullivan, F. (1988) *A Friend in Need: Citizen Advocacy in Britain*, Paper No. 517/2, Personal Social Services Research Unit, Canterbury.

Cassileth, B.R. *et al.* (1980) Informed consent – why are it's goals imperfectly realised? *The New England Journal Of Medicine*, 302(16), 896–899.

Clarke, J. and Langan, M. (1993) *Family Life and Social Policy: Course Review*. Open University Press, Milton Keynes.

Cochrane, A. and Clarke, J. (eds) (1993) *Comparing Welfare States, Britain in International Context*. Family Life and Social Policy Series. Sage/Open University Press, London, Chapter 2.

Collins, W. (1987) *The Collins Dictionary and Thesaurus*. Collins, London and Glasgow.

Coombes, P. (1982). *Making Sense of Society*. D102 Social Sciences. A Foundation Course. Block 1, Unit 3. Open University Press, Milton Keynes.

Dallos, R. and McLaughlin, E. (eds) (1993) *Social Problems and the Family*. Family Life and Social Policy Series. Sage/Open University Press, London, Chapter 4.

Davey, B. and Popay, J. (eds) (1993) *Dilemmas in Health Care*. Health and Disease Series. Open University Press, Milton Keynes, Chapter 5.

Department of Health (1983) *The Mental Health Act*. HMSO, London.

Department of Health (1991a) *Citizen's Charter*. HMSO, London.

Department of Health (1991b) *The Patient's Charter*. HMSO, London.

Department of Health and Social Security (1991) *Social Security Statistics 1990*. HMSO, London.

Department of Health (1995) *NHS Responsibilities for Meeting Continuing Health Care Needs*. HSG(95)8 LAC(95)5. HMSO, London.

Department of Health (1996) *The Patient's Charter: Mental Health Services*. Consultation Edition, February. HMSO, London.

Farmer, B. (1993) The use and abuse of power in nursing. *Nursing Standard*, 7(23), 33–36.

Finkelstein, V. and French, S. (1993) *Disability, Citizenship and Empowerment*. The Disabling Society Series. Open University Press, Milton Keynes.

Gates, B. (1994). *Advocacy: a Nurse's Guide*. Scutari Press, London.

Johnson, M. (1990) Dependency and Interdependency. In *Ageing In Society*, Bond, J. and Coleman, P. (eds). Sage, London.

Kitwood, T. (1988) The technical, the personal, and the framing of dementia. *Social Behaviour*, 3, 161–179.

Kitwood, T. (1989) Brain, mind and dementia: with particular reference to Alzheimer's disease. *Ageing and Society*, 9, 1–15.

Kitwood, T. (1990) The dialectics of dementia: with particular reference to Alzheimer's disease. *Ageing and Society,* 10, 177–196.

Kitwood, T. (1992) A new approach to the evaluation of dementia care. *Journal of Advances in Health and Social Care,* 1(5), 41–60.

Marshall, T.H. (1951) *Citizenship and Social Class.* Cambridge University Press.

Morrall, P. (1996) Clinical sociology and the empowerment of clients. *Mental Health Nursing,* 16(3) 24–27.

Morrison, A. (1991) The nurse's role in relation to advocacy. *Nursing Standard* 5(41), 37–40.

Pascall, G. (1986) *Social Policy: a Feminist Analysis.* Routledge, London.

Peplau, H.E. (1988) *Interpersonal Relations in Nursing.* Macmillan, London.

Phillipson, C. (1990) The Sociology of Retirement. In *Ageing In Society.* Bond, J. and Coleman, P. (eds). Sage, London.

Renshaw, J. and Metcalf, M. (1987) *A Friend in Need: Citizen Advocacy in Britain.*

Discussion Paper No. 517/2. Personal Social Services Research Unit, University of Kent.

Rodwell, C. (1996) An analysis of the concept of empowerment. *Journal of Advanced Nursing,* 23, 305–313.

Roper, N., Logan, W. and Tierney, A. (1996) *The Elements of Nursing: A Model for Nursing Based on a Model of Living,* 4th edn. Churchill Livingstone, Edinburgh.

Sang, B. and O'Brien, J. (1984) *Advocacy: The UK and American Experiences.* Project paper No. 51. King's Fund, London.

Skelton, R. (1994) Nursing and empowerment: concepts and strategies. *Journal of Advanced Nursing,* 19, 415–423.

UKCC (1992) *Code of Professional Conduct for the Nurse, Midwife and Health Visitors,* (3rd edn). HMSO, London.

UKCC (1996) *Guidelines for Professional Practice.* HMSO, London.

Webster, C. (ed.) (1993) *Caring for Health: History and Diversity.* Health and Disease Series. Open University Press, Milton Keynes.

5 Management of risk situations

Marc Saunders

KEY ISSUES

- Risk
- Risk taking
- Risk analysis
- Risk management
- Dignity
- Ordinary life
- Value

INTRODUCTION

Think about your area of practice. Think about a typical day in your place of work and the number of decisions you might be called upon to make. How many might that be? However many decisions you make during the course of your working day, the chances are that you go off duty mentally rehearsing the experiences and evaluating your own performance; you ask yourself 'Could I or should I have acted differently?' or 'Did I do the right thing?'.

Risk management is the synthesis of the decision-making process, the values of the practitioner (and the organization) and the needs and aspirations of the service user. It is the recognition that with risk-taking comes dignity, and that with growth comes the exposure to greater degrees of risk. Most of us desire to see that our growth is recognized, yet collectively we often assume that the people for whom we provide a service wish for the exact opposite. We allow our need to 'care' to compromise the user's right to a service that respects their dignity.

Risk analysis and risk management is not, and should not be viewed as, a panacea for the practitioner in response to their search for a model of care that most closely reflects their values system and their approach to nursing practice. However, effective risk management processes will aid effective decision making, it will encourage multidisciplinary team working, it will contribute to the practitioner's learning environment and, critically, it will support a service that recognizes and values the rights and dignity of the service user.

This chapter reflects on a broad range of services provided to a number of client groups. Where possible, examples are developed to illustrate the application of risk management techniques to services for older people. It seems that in nursing there is a number of concepts and practices that are common across a broad span of specialties, however, the effective application of any one of these in any one area is dependent upon the skill of the nurse to develop imaginative and innovative ways of working. Risk management is one such concept.

THE RISE OF RISK MANAGEMENT IN HEALTHCARE SERVICES

Concepts of risk and risk taking are not new. Many services, particularly mental health and learning disability services, have had policies on risk taking and acceptable risk for some 15 to 25 years, maybe longer. What has changed is the sophistication of the approach.

How risk management began to intensify in our collective consciousness is open to debate. However, it is possible that a number of changing circumstances have contributed to a growth in its appreciation. The pressures for efficiency, cost effectiveness and excellence in practice was a stimulus for clinicians to draw upon a wider school of literature to support their practice. In addition, the implementation of the NHS and Community Care Act (HMSO, 1990) was also a significant driving force. The opportunity for provider units to become self-governing trusts, along with the loss of Crown immunity meant that these new organizations would need to purchase insurance services. Insurers have been keen to see evidence of risk management procedures being adopted by Trusts to help to reduce the likelihood of claims being made.

From this we can see that clinicians and service managers embrace risk management from different viewpoints. However, the cultural changes, not only in healthcare but in society as a whole, have implications for health services. There is increased expectation of healthcare providers and an increasing desire on behalf of clinicians and managers to see users explicitly central to the focus of care delivery. There also appears to be evidence of the public's willingness to seek legal redress when they feel the healthcare they received failed to deliver the outcomes they anticipated or were led to expect. As our healthcare system and our society increasingly mimics American culture, so does the apparent readiness of people to pursue compensation from service providers.

Good risk management will not guarantee a service, or an individual, is protected against the possibility of legal action. However, it can draw decision making into a multidisciplinary arena, where it is explicitly documented and where it can be clearly demonstrated that potential risks have been considered and reasonable actions taken to ensure that the benefits of a particular treatment or course of action outweigh the likelihood and severity of any harmful consequences.

Essentially, good risk management processes are synonymous with good practice. Both the Code of Professional Conduct (UKCC, 1992a) and The Scope of Professional Practice (UKCC, 1992b) define nurses' professional accountability and responsibilities. The concept of risk is implicit in both documents and is further evidence of risk being integral to our everyday practice. For example, the Code of Professional Conduct asserts that the nurse should foster clients' independence and involve them in the planning of care. To achieve this, the nurse has to consider the risks to the client, other healthcare workers and the wider community.

DEFINING RISK AND RISK MANAGEMENT

Many have attempted to define risk and risk management with varying degrees of success. It seems that no single set of words can happily absorb the spectrum

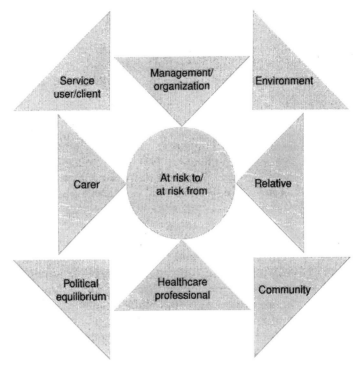

Figure 5.1   Factors affecting definition of risk and risk management.

of interpretations each can have, dependent on your particular perception. This raises the question of who or what impinges on the defining qualities of risk and risk management? Figure 5.1 illustrates one possible analysis from a human service perspective. Figure 5.1 does not explore all the potential relationships where risks may be apparent, even in human services. Similarly, the priorities may switch dependent on the situation. For example, an older person with mental health problems could well be at greater risk from self-harm than someone with reduced hearing ability who might be more exposed to environmental risk. Figure 5.1 is representative of some of the potentially 'risk-laden' relationships. For example, the service user at risk from:

- His/her own actions
- The environment
- The community
- The actions of the professional
- The actions of the significant carer

Similarly, there are other risk-laden relationships that do not focus so specifically upon the service user. For example:

- The community at risk from the actions of the service user
- The professional at risk from the significant carer
- The organization at risk from the action of the professional
- The environment at risk from the professional (e.g. disposal of sharps)
- The professional at risk from the environment (e.g. while home visiting)

Defining risk

We all accept risk as part of our everyday life, in our work, home and leisure activities. At times we actively seek out opportunities to take risks, for example, those who pursue an interest in underwater diving, or those who gamble for money. But what is risk? The answer is not as straightforward as you might at first think.

Generally, when we talk about risk we are talking about risk taking. By defining the term risk taking we can give it the degree of context it needs. *Risk taking can be defined as pursuing a course of action in order to realize one or more beneficial outcomes in the knowledge that there are consequences or outcomes that would be perceived as negative or harmful in nature should they occur.*

Carson (1988) describes two sides of a risk. Firstly, the likelihood of any particular consequence occurring, and secondly, the nature of the consequence. The example used later in the chapter will focus on these two aspects of risk. Both can be viewed in terms of the benefits realized or the costs experienced. For example, leaving later than usual to catch the morning train, there is a risk of missing the train. There is also a possibility that you will catch the train and will therefore have benefited from having an extra 30 minutes in bed. The nature of the consequence will depend upon your own circumstances. There is a chance you could lose your job. Equally, there is a possibility that nobody will notice your late arrival.

Some might argue that ensuring risk management principles are applied as part of the care planning process will effectively eliminate organizational risk. It is helpful to remind ourselves of the nature of risk and the potential combination of risk-laden relationships. It is not just service users who are subject to risk.

Defining risk management in an organizational context

We have already explored some of the origins of the concepts of risk and risk management in organizations. The following definitions serve to confirm these origins. The Chartered Institute of Public Finance and Accountability (CIPFA) suggests:

> Risk management may be defined as the planned and systematic approach to the identification, evaluation and control of risk (CIPFA, 1993, p. 2)

whilst the National Health Service Management Executive (NHSME) states:

> Risk management is mainly concerned with harnessing the information and expertise of individuals within the organisation and translating that with their help into positive action which will reduce loss of life, financial loss, loss of staff availability, loss of availability of buildings or equipment and loss of reputation (NHSME, 1993, p. 1).

Therefore, risk management in the organizational context is primarily, though not exclusively, concerned with the protection of assets (where assets refer to anything the organization holds) against a variety of risks and a range of harmful consequences. It is often associated with the concepts of quality and quality development. For example, Davis (1994) briefly explains how risk management was introduced within the continuous improvement phase of a total quality management programme.

Defining risk management in the clinical setting

Based upon the organizational view of risk management, it is tempting to believe that risk management in the clinical setting is concerned with controlling risk to minimize the likelihood of claims being made against the individual or service. In fact, it has a much more positive role to play within a service and is another method of developing and maintaining service quality.

There is a view that nurses tend to avoid risk (e.g. Grier and Schnitzler, 1979); however, this is refuted by Dobos (1992) who conducted a very small study into how nurses define risk. She goes on to argue that because of their role nurses are required to, and do, take risks.

Risk management in the clinical setting can be defined as the identification and analysis of risk combined with explicit plans to control or manage this risk, including action to prevent or decrease the likelihood of a harmful consequence, action to eliminate or reduce the extent of harmful consequences should they occur and action to increase the likelihood and quality of beneficial consequences.

RISK MANAGEMENT AND THE LAW

So far, I have been keen to accentuate the nature of risk management in terms of its relationship with good practice. However, it would be somewhat naive not to consider, briefly at least, the legal context. I have previously mentioned the

Consider your own area of practice in relation to the quality of the nursing documentation. Take a small sample of nursing documents from your area and check that it meets the following requirements:

- All entries are legible, paying particular attention to technical words that might be ambiguously represented (e.g. hypoglycaemia/hyperglycaemia)
- They are free from subjective value statements (e.g. Mr Moxon has been moody all day)
- They are free from the use of correction fluid
- They are free from abbreviations that could be misinterpreted
- Each entry is dated and includes the time of entry
- Each entry has the signature of the nurse
- They are free from crossing out which uses more than a single line, so that what was previously written can still be read

If required, would all the records be traceable within your system? Currently, there is growing evidence that a high percentage of nursing documents are not traceable within health service record systems. The pressure placed upon the nursing profession to provide high-quality nursing care is now matched by the necessity for high-quality documentation. The legal process is not sympathetic to the busy nurse, nor does it seem to be selective about where it gathers evidence in developing an argument. It does not really matter if the care provided is of the highest standard, if it can be shown that the nursing records are inadequate, the episode of care becomes increasingly difficult to defend. In short, if your records are not of a suitably high standard, how can you argue that your care is?

expectations of service users, the changing pattern of claims being made against healthcare providers and the shift in the culture of health services. Years ago, risk management as a clinical tool might have been pursued purely in the interests of good practice. However, in the late 20th and early 21st century, risk management as part of everyone's business will be essential.

Having defensible documentation is merely a shop window in your service. This is no defence if it merely disguises an unacceptable service or a service that does not focus centrally on the needs of the service user. Imagine that you are providing a service to John. John is 90 years of age, he is assertive and assumes responsibility for much of his own welfare, although he has little useful sight. He has a very supportive and involved family. Recently, staff reports have indicated that John may be developing a mild form of dementia. In spite of this he wishes to continue his daily walks to the shop (about half a mile away) and indicates this very strongly to staff.

This is the type of decision nurses will be expected to make on a regular basis. The records will show that John is experiencing a degree of confusion. In the interests of John's health and safety there is an obligation to review his daily walk to the shop. Clearly, to continue to use the shop will harbour a degree of risk for John. Nursing and other staff should consider the risk associated with continuing this activity against how much this daily walk means to John and the benefits he realizes from it.

Let us suppose that John continues with his daily walks to the shop and is seriously injured in a road traffic accident. John's family feel that care staff have been negligent in permitting John to continue to go to the shop alone. With no explicit evidence that staff have considered this issue, defence in a court of law could prove challenging.

In 1957, the Bolam Test was established. How the test came to be recognized is complex; however, for those wishing to find out more, Watt (1995) briefly describes the background to the test. The test itself refers specifically to the actions of medical practitioners, although the principle is often applied to other professional groups. The test seeks to establish whether the issue in question was managed in line with current thinking and standards of healthcare. It also establishes that successful defence against legal action cannot be guaranteed merely because the practitioner is able to find a number of others of a similar opinion.

In John's case, the application of risk management principles will go some way to ensure that John's interests have, as far as possible, been protected. The process should consider an analysis of risk (i.e. the probability of a harmful consequence and the potential degree of harm are considered) following which a decision is then made (in a multidisciplinary arena if necessary). Having done this, it is much more likely that the professionalism of the staff can be defended in a court of law than might have been possible, particularly if the best defence of the practitioner is to resort to anecdotal evidence of high-quality care.

Working within a risk management framework does not guarantee that professionals are exempted from the possibility of legal action. Nor does it guarantee a successful defence. Risk management is not a replacement for competent practice. However, it can be an effective tool which will support competent practitioners to deliver high-quality care in a contemporary health care arena.

THE INTRINSIC VALUE OF RISK AND RISK TAKING

Chapter 3 addresses the issue of 'ordinary living' principles applied to healthcare services for older people. It is my intention to revisit the concepts of social role valorization and ordinary living within the context of risk and risk taking. If we wish to provide increasingly progressive services to older people then risk and risk taking will inevitably be part of that formula. I hope to illustrate how risk and risk taking not only sits comfortably alongside the concepts of social role valorization and ordinary living, but may even be considered fundamental to their appreciation.

◄3 Risk management is not a method of systematically removing risk from people's lives. Quite the contrary. We are beginning to appreciate that with tolerable risk comes value. Society has previously required that the care of people with a learning disability and people with a mental health problem be provided in segregated and often isolated locations. Part of the motivation for this lay in the desire to feel that people were protected and safe. Arguably, while the desire was misguided, the reality for many people was anything but the haven of safety that society felt it was contributing to. Social role valorization and the principles behind ordinary living almost certainly evolved on the basis that groups of people were systematically devalued by society as a whole.

Perhaps society's devaluing of older people has not been quite so overt or so systematic, yet devaluing it has been. Clearly, the principles that underpin social role valorization and ordinary living can be applied to services for the older adult. But why do we equate risk with value?

Most likely, as a society, we value risk because it assumes a degree of choice over a given set of circumstances, and with choice there is freedom. In some cases, though not all, we place added value on those who take risks as part of their working life or during their leisure time. Additionally, to an extent, we even 'plot' the maturation of children in terms of the increasing levels of consequences associated with the risks they are exposed to. In essence, risk and risk taking is about our individual right to make a particular choice or decision, regardless of its correctness, and to be permitted to learn, or not to learn, from our own mistakes.

How can we be sure that risk and risk taking is fundamental to the concept of an ordinary life? For a number of years, services for people with a learning disability and services for people with mental health problems have striven to provide people with a quality of life that reflects the quality of life experienced by the non-disabled population. The theoretical developments in terms of ordinary living have given service providers important reference points from where to view their service, for example, the 'five accomplishments' (O'Brien, 1987) and 'an ordinary life' (King's Fund, 1980).

The five accomplishments are described in more detail in Chapter 3, but are listed here just as a reminder:

- Community presence
- Community participation
- Competence
- Choice
- Respect

It is possible to see here how risk could be viewed as elemental to each of the first four accomplishments and part of the fifth in its broadest sense. Similarly, if we look briefly at the three main principles underpinning an ordinary life (King's Fund, 1980); asserting human value, the right to live like others in the community and the recognition of individuality then risk and risk taking is, once again, an implicit theme.

We want older people to experience a valued life, we want them to have choices, to take control of their lives and to have many and varied experiences. If this is genuinely so, then we have to be willing to accept that attached to this desire is an element of risk; for the service user, for their relatives, for the professional and for the organization. Empowerment is about a shift in the power bases within care services so that the user is more able to control his or her own destiny whatever the level of their need. The question is, are we willing to accept that risk? Almost without exception, service users will be.

RISK AND RISK TAKING: WORKING WITH SERVICE USERS

Until now we have attempted to define risk and to put it into a familiar context as well as to establish why an appreciation of risk and risk management is important from a perspective of good practice and from a legal point of view. But such an appreciation is of little value if it cannot be effectively operationalized. Clearly, it would be every clinician's (and every manager's) nightmare if risk was invited into our services unconditionally. However, there is, as we have seen, inherent value in risk.

Before we can make use of our insights into risk and risk taking it is important that we are able to identify with the various components of risk. Rather like a sentence or phrase can be divided into its component parts of speech, so can risk be similarly analyzed. It is my intention to examine risk in its component parts and to place each in the context of services for the older adult.

As previously stated, Carson (1988) identified that a risk has two significant aspects:

- Likelihood
- Consequence

In these terms, the likelihood refers to the possibility (or the probability) that a particular event will occur and the consequence refers to the nature of the outcome, i.e. whether that consequence is desirable or harmful. Later in this chapter, there is an example which addresses these components of risk.

Before going on to look at these in more detail it is important we make sure that we place risk and risk taking into a therapeutic context. The specific work of clinical staff focuses on achieving identified goals in partnership with the service user. Risk and risk taking ought therefore to complement nursing interventions and where particular risk consequences jeopardize the quality of these interventions then the clinician and the service user should, where possible, identify appropriate action. Briefly, risk taking is not external to nursing but is central to its effective practice.

Identifying activities or courses of action with, or on behalf of, service users that incorporate an element of risk will be familiar to all clinical staff. The development in our understanding of risk and managing risk will not make such decisions any easier or any less painful. However, it can support clinicians in making a decision. One of the benefits of this is that it enables the decision process to become explicitly articulated, often in a multidisciplinary context. It also enables the values that underpin a decision to be explicitly identified. Therefore, it is helpful if the team or service have agreed in advance its particular value orientation. This is usually seen as a fundamental part of team development but should frequently be revisited in order to ensure that the views are consistent and current.

The principal activity/course of action

The principal activity or course of action is the focus of the risk analysis, which can be divided into three options:

- To pursue a new or revised activity/course of action
- To continue with a current activity/course of action
- To discontinue a current activity/course of action

For each option, it will be necessary to identify the specific risks involved, and the variables underpinning those risks that are external to the individual in question as well as the variables that might be described as internal. The variables might effectively contribute to the likelihood of a particular consequence; they may also have an impact on the extent to which a particular consequence is harmful or beneficial. Some examples of external variables are:

- Accommodation
- Access to and use of equipment/aids
- Location
- Financial support
- Local circumstances
- Support systems
- Relationships
- Community/attitudes of the local community

Some examples of internal variables are:

- Physical health
- Mental health
- Physical ability/disability
- Personality/personal qualities
- Previous experience

Neither of these lists is exhaustive, particularly the former where the circumstances of the issue in question would significantly impact upon what those variables might be. More definite variables can be identified in the following case study.

CASE STUDY   Geoff is 87 years old. He lives in a nursing home in the UK with 15 other people of whom there are three he gets on particularly well with. Geoff is, for the most part, healthy, although he has epilepsy and experiences tonic-clonic seizures on about six occasions each year. Most of these occur early in the morning and Geoff can usually predict their occurrence shortly prior to the seizure actually happening.

Geoff has little contact with his relatives who live in Australia. He has a number of friends who live locally although most are older than Geoff and are generally in poorer health. All of them are much more reliant on other people than Geoff is.

Geoff was originally admitted to the home following a spell in the local general hospital where he was admitted for treatment of testicular cancer. Geoff did not recover well from surgery and, at that time, a nursing home placement seemed to be most appropriate. Geoff has had a long and active career working in financial services and has been able to prepare well for the time when he was no longer able to work.

Geoff is very able, although staff have been concerned that at times he is becoming confused and disoriented even in familiar surroundings and with familiar people around him. Recently, Geoff has expressed an interest in moving away from the nursing home placement in order to live a little more independently. He has not really considered what the best options will be and is fairly open-minded about any move he might make. The staff team at the nursing home feel that they have a helpful relationship with Geoff but are anxious that he does not jeopardize his health or his safety in moving away from the home.

Clearly, Geoff wishes to make a significant change in his life, and, as is often the case with life changes, there is a risk in pursuing this course of action. The case study suggests a committed staff team who wish to support Geoff in not only making a decision that is in his best interests but also one that reflects his wishes about how he would like to spend the next few years of his life. It is all too easy to imagine how, in years past, such a desire might have been dismissed out of hand. If the staff team have their philosophy clearly identified for themselves and their users, it provides a useful foundation to the decision-making process.

Analyzing the risk

Before going any further, it is important to establish that while the whole process of risk management can be particularly valuable when you have service users who are unable to easily articulate their views and wishes, this should not and cannot mean that the process is removed from the service users' sphere of influence. This has to be a collaborative process. This will be helpful to Geoff and will ensure that rather than a decision being made on his behalf he will become actively involved in the process and, indeed, may even lead it.

One of the first jobs that Geoff and the staff team may wish to do is to spend some time considering what the internal and external variables are in this particular situation. Geoff is expressing a wish to live somewhere else, therefore, a number of variables are pertinent to his circumstances (Box 5.1).

The internal and external variables are not set in stone and can be added to or manipulated as required. The variables identified are not exhaustive as far as Geoff is concerned. Remember, both the internal and external variables can impact on the likelihood of a particular type of consequence (harmful or beneficial) as well as impacting upon the quality of a consequence by increasing or decreasing the beneficial aspects or by increasing or decreasing the harmful aspects of a particular consequence.

Identifying these variables may be the job of an individual in conjunction with the service user, more usefully this can be done with the support of the nursing/multidisciplinary team. Ideas storming, as a technique, can often prove useful when doing this.

Once this part of the analysis has been completed, the next phase is to establish what are the potential consequences of pursuing the principal course of action and what action may be taken as a result of identifying these consequences. This part of the example reflects the process described by Carson (1988). In Geoff's case, moving to a new home will be the principal course of action. Before we can do this, Geoff and the team need to be more specific about what particular option he wishes to

BOX 5.1	*Variables and suggested ranges for Geoff*

External variables

- Accommodation: type- bungalow/house/flat/different nursing home/residential home/caravan
- Location: name of area/name of street/shop nearby/suburban/rural
- Relationships: who/regularity of contact/where they live
- Nutritional: cooking arrangements/aids or help required/training
- Toilet arrangements: upstairs/downstairs/aids or help required
- Personal hygiene: bath/shower/aids or help required/specially designed bath
- Staff support: full time/morning or evening visits/on call/none

Internal variables

- Current and predicted confusion
- Personality: determined/people oriented/considerate/assertive
- Physical health: currently good
- Epilepsy: seizures at known times of day/predictable/controlled with medication

pursue. Looking again at all the variables may well provide ideas or inspiration. In the interests of developing this example let us assume that Geoff has decided that he wants to live in a bungalow, not far out of town, on his own. It is now possible to identify the benefits that Geoff will (or possibly will) experience if the principal course of action is made a reality. Once again, it is important that Geoff is involved and that as many benefits as possible are identified. The potential benefits of moving to a new bungalow would be:

- Increased dignity
- Increased privacy
- Access to local amenities
- Extra opportunities for socializing
- Less institutional than the nursing home
- Time and space to be alone
- Feelings of independence
- Able to invite people back
- Can be untidy if wishes
- Able to watch any programmes on the TV
- Not affected by other people's confused behaviour
- Somewhere to put whisky collection
- Possible to own a pet

The nature of risk is that where there are benefits to be realized there is also the possibility of harmful consequences. It is important that these are explicitly identified. Do not be concerned with identifying unusual possibilities at this stage. Write down everything that comes to mind. As far as Geoff is concerned there are a number of potentially harmful consequences:

- Occurrence of a seizure whilst no one else is around
- Increase in the number of seizures
- Injury resulting from confusion, domestic accident/road traffic accident

- Subjection to local crime
- Fire hazard from cooking
- Poor diet/decrease in the quality of diet
- Loneliness
- Boredom
- Forgetting to pay bills
- Dispute with neighbours
- Illness that is not communicated to someone else
- Death

The benefits/harmful consequences can be revised over time to reflect changing circumstances. For example, if Geoff were to decide that moving to a bungalow was too difficult to arrange, he may decide that moving to a house or a flat are new options. That decision made, the consequences of Geoff's move may need to include the possibility of Geoff sustaining an injury from having to use stairs.

The decision regarding Geoff's move does not have to be made instantly. Once the possible consequences of Geoff's move have been identified, Geoff and the staff team need to spend some time considering how likely it is that each of the consequences could become a reality. Such an exercise will be relatively subjective, however, having them detailed means that each can be considered on its own merit and an overall view obtained. Once this part of the process has been embarked upon it may not be immediately clear whether to pursue the principal course of action or not. That is, if the benefits do not sufficiently outweigh the likelihood or severity of potentially harmful consequences.

The important issue at this point is the balance between the beneficial and the harmful consequences and the likelihood that each might occur. Clearly, in order to make it worthwhile the benefits need to outweigh the harmful consequences by some degree. In Geoff's case, the benefits can be considered of sufficiently high priority to justify exploring the proposed course of action. Equally, the identified harmful consequences which could occur are of a suitably severe magnitude to indicate that some work is required to ensure that the benefits consistently outweigh the possible harms.

This is not a paper exercise. It is not about adding extra benefits to the list or crossing out harmful consequences regardless of their remote likelihood. This is a much more active part of the process and is, to all intents and purposes, the management of the risk. In Geoff's case, he and the team will want to revisit the benefits to see if they can find ways to ensure that Geoff will experience those benefits as well as making specific plans to ensure that the identified harmful consequences do not become a reality. It may well be helpful to construct an explicit action plan to deal with these points. Box 5.2 shows just some of the actions that Geoff might wish to pursue with the aid of the staff team. They may decide, having developed the plan, that the actions are insufficient and that the risk remains unjustified. Equally, the team may decide to pursue the course of action with Geoff but to increase the level of staff support that Geoff receives. This may decrease the amount of privacy Geoff is able to experience, but it may make the difference in terms of Geoff achieving the move he wishes to make. Should the move go ahead, extra measures may need to be put in place to reduce the possibility of harmful consequences still further. It is important to remember that the key motivation is not the complete elimination of risk but to ensure that benefits outweigh the costs.

The flow chart in Figure 5.2 illustrates the process of risk management in a clinical setting.

BOX 5.2	*Geoff's action plan*

■ Ensure that the bungalow is near to local shops as well as within walking/bus ride distance of a local pub
■ The bungalow should be close to friends
■ Choose a cat and identify someone to help take care of it
■ Keep a record of seizures to ensure stability
■ Invest in a pager system linked to the telephone so that someone can be contacted from anywhere in the house should the necessity arise
■ Fit bungalow with robust window and door locks of a suitable standard
■ Enrol in the local meal delivery service
■ Obtain a microwave oven
■ Keep a written record of dietary intake
■ Enrol in at least two local activity groups
■ Investigate the possibility of fitting smoke detectors linked to the telephone system with a direct link to the fire service

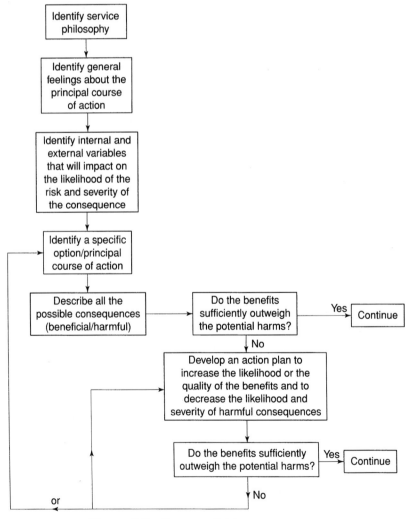

Figure 5.2   Process of risk management.

Using other data

It is clear that some of the judgements are subjective. However, they are explicitly identified so that the thought processes are there for all to see. Remember, that for some risks it is possible to identify a little more scientifically the possibility of certain consequences. For example, in Geoff's case, we know that he experiences six seizures every year; therefore, we know that if Geoff will be living on his own he will, on average, have to deal with a seizure every two months. Someone who has disturbed sleep patterns, for example, somnambulism, will have a care record that may well point to triggers or times when this is most likely to happen. Such evidence of cause and frequency could provide useful information when analyzing particular risk situations.

Research may also contribute to the analysis. From a legal point of view, particularly in light of the Bolam Test, being able to show that current research was taken into account during the decision-making process is likely to be looked upon favourably. Macmillan (1994) has identified seven headings, each with a number of factors that contribute to a 'risky discharge', each of which is relevant to the context of Geoff. Therefore, staff would pay particular attention to medical factors, mobility, social surroundings, personality, habits, social support and external factors.

RISK MANAGEMENT IN AN ORGANIZATIONAL SETTING

We have already taken time to define risk management in terms of its application within an organizational setting. We now need to explore how this is operationalized. As with risk management when it is applied to clinical situations, it is generally considered the pursuit of best practice in an organizational setting when the best interests of the service user are the prime focus of activity as well as the organization as a whole. A great deal of discussion surrounds the concept of risk management in this context; is it a science or an art? Most nurses would find this interesting as much the same debate has surrounded nursing for a number of years. Arguably, the effective implementation of risk management principles requires an ever varying degree of both empiricism and artistry (rather like nursing).

Before looking at risk management in an organizational setting in more detail, we should first discuss where risk management in the clinical setting finishes and organizational risk management begins. It is easy to appreciate how supporting someone to live in their own home is a clinical issue and addressing potential fire hazards in linen stores is an organizational concern. But what about infection control? Is this a clinical or organizational issue? In terms of the needs of a single user, the practitioner would have a particular interest because of their role in relation to that individual. However, if there was evidence of a particular infection across the whole organization then it is easier to appreciate how applying effective risk management principles to prevent further cross-infection would benefit the whole organization (in reduced need for treatment, increased bed availability, no damage to reputation and so on).

Clinicians may feel that risk management in an organizational context is of less importance to them and is more the role of the manager. The definition by ◄p. 75 the NHSME (1993) clearly discredits such thoughts. Risk management in an organizational context is concerned with, for example, minimizing waste, saving time, protecting employees' health and safety and reducing treatment side effects. The principal motivation is to preserve resources for use in the treatment of service users. There are, almost daily, stories on the radio or in the newspapers, about measures being taken to ration healthcare delivery, yet we so often look on while resources are least effectively used in paying for remedial treatment, compensation for avoidable errors and replacing wasted equipment and consumables.

It is not possible, nor my intention, to provide a detailed exposé of risk management and its application in an organizational setting. There are many texts and journals devoting a great deal of space to this subject. However, I intend to give a flavour of some of the ideas and techniques behind organizational risk management.

Risk management in an organizational context is about protecting assets. Once given some thought, it starts to become clear just how broad a subject area this is. Consider your work place in terms of the following:

■ Fire safety/fire precaution awareness
■ Accidents to staff
■ Accidents to service users
■ Infection rates
■ Stolen property/security
■ Assaults on staff
■ Drug administration errors
■ Computer data security

If your organization can improve in any of these areas then it would benefit from a risk management programme. In this context, the principles of risk management centre around the following process (NHSME, 1993, p. 4):

■ Risk identification
■ Risk analysis
■ Risk control
■ Risk funding

The first issue is what to focus upon. Many organizations (especially in industry and insurance services) now have Risk Managers and a Risk Management Group. There is a range of methods that you can use in order to isolate one or more topics for investigation, for example:

■ Listening to staff
■ Listening to service users
■ Monitoring complaints
■ Monitoring incident reports
■ Reviewing records
■ Monitoring reports
■ Carrying out audits

Whether you use one or more of these methods an important part of the process is to attempt to identify any patterns in the data you have, any trends and any clues that could indicate where changes could be made. Risk management in an organizational setting is less about reacting to incidents once they have occurred but more about creatively identifying those situations before they occur and taking positive action in advance of any harmful consequences.

Creating the culture

Whether referring to risk management in an organizational or clinical setting the culture in which the staff team is operating is important. For example, let us assume that, as part of a risk management programme, incidents in relation to medication administration errors are being examined. Clearly, the goal is to reduce the number of errors by using the reports of incidents to establish any patterns, should they exist. However, this can only happen if the staff team feel that they are able to report any such errors. The legal and professional implications are complex, but is there any defence for failing to identify and correct the practices and procedures that could potentially be harmful to service users?

Incidents as indicators

Healthcare providers are highly complicated organizations. People generally receive a sophisticated range of services regardless of the basis upon which that treatment is provided. A programme of risk management will be enhanced if there is a clear mechanism for identifying and analyzing incidents within a service and a method for introducing change in order to prevent repetition and the possibility of service users, staff or the organization experiencing harmful consequences.

Such a mechanism should be accessible to all staff, particularly staff in the clinical setting, who must feel that they are able to report incidents. Clinical staff should also be able to suggest areas and topics for further investigation where there can be a concerted effort to identify relevant incidents and improve practice accordingly.

Generally, the Risk Manager is looking for a pattern or trends in the available data and may find these in reports on, for example:

■ Accidents to staff
■ Accidents to service users
■ Reports on equipment that has malfunctioned
■ Reports on theft of property
■ Evaluative work on clinical practice (e.g. audit)
■ Complaints

This does not negate the need for swift action following a single incident where the consequences were, or might potentially have been, severe. For example:

■ The death of a member of staff
■ The death of a service user
■ A fire outbreak
■ An outbreak of food poisoning

It is not always obvious within the collected data what the trends or patterns are. The creative role of the Risk Manager in the organizational setting lies in their ability to ask the right questions of the data or to conduct data collection in a way that relevant information is accessed.

The role of insurance services

As previously stated, risk management is designed to protect the assets of an organization whatever they may be. However, it is not always possible (nor desirable) to eliminate every risk. Therefore, the organization will be expected to insure against those risks it is unable to manage effectively.

The insurance industry is far more active in the process of risk management than this might indicate. They clearly have a vested interest in minimizing the possibility of claims being made against healthcare providers and actively support organizations in developing effective risk management programmes. Many insurance companies employ staff who are trained in risk management and quality and will give advice as part of the package of services offered.

CONCLUDING COMMENTS AND RECOMMENDATIONS

We recognize that all of us are exposed to varying degree of risks. Usually we are happy to accept the opportunities for growth that accompany exposure to risk. We also need to ensure that the people we work with receive a service of the highest quality. This does not mean the elimination of risk. It means working with older clients to maximize benefits whilst maintaining potential risks at a tolerable level.

The social and legal pressures for accountability within services have increased dramatically over the last decade as has the political drive for ever more efficient and cost-effective services. Arguably, it is now more important than ever for service providers to be able to articulate the thought processes behind their decisions. This is particularly true where decisions are being made with, or on behalf of older people, where an outcome which is wholly beneficial to the service user cannot be guaranteed.

There remains a great deal to be achieved if staff and older people are to benefit from the application of risk management processes whatever the setting. Not least, an appreciation of risk and risk management should be built into the education programmes of clinical staff. There may also be some value in all organizations developing risk management procedures for local implementation. This is relevant in the context of older people, as risk taking implicitly contributes to improvements in care delivery and quality of life. Quite possibly, the biggest challenge facing us all is to convince ourselves that risk and risk management is part of all our roles and should be embraced for the benefit of all.

FURTHER READING

Carson, D. (1988) Taking risks with patients – your assessment strategy. *Professional Nurse*, April, 247–250.
When this article was published, it was a significant landmark in enabling nurses to consider how risk management could effectively be absorbed into the care planning process. This is a very practical article on risk management and is the basis for the approach described within the chapter. It touches on issues of consent and some of the ethical implications of exposure and non-exposure to risk situations.

NHSME (1993) *Risk Management in the NHS*. Department of Health, London. *This text focuses very specifically on risk management and how it might be applied in an organizational setting in the NHS. It explores the background to risk management in this context as well as chapters on direct patient care risk, indirect patient care risk and health and safety. It is a helpful guide, particularly for those who manage a service and who wish to find out about risk management in this context.*

REFERENCES

Carson, D. (1988) Taking risks with patients – your assessment strategy. *The Professional Nurse,* April, 247–250.

CIPFA (1993) *Guidance on Risk Assessment, Management and Insurance.* King's Fund, London.

Davis, B. (1994) Risk management: one component of a quality strategy. *Journal of the Association for Quality in Healthcare,* 1 (suppl.), 30–34.

Dobos, C. (1992) Defining risk from the perspective of nurses in clinical roles. *Journal of Advanced Nursing,* 17, 1303–1309.

Grier, M.R and Schnitzler, C.P. (1979) Nurses propensity to risk. *Nursing Research,* 28(3), 186–191.

HMSO (1990) *NHS and Community Care Act.* HMSO, London.

King's Fund (1980) *An Ordinary Life: Comprehensive Locally-Based Residential Services for Mentally Handicapped People.* King's Fund, London.

Macmillan, M.S. (1994) Hospital staff's perception of risk associated with the discharge of elderly people from acute hospital care. *Journal of Advanced Nursing,* 19, 249–256.

O'Brien, J. (1987) A Guide to Lifestyle Planning Using the Activities Catalogue to Integrate Services and National Support Systems. In *A Comprehensive Guide to the Activities Catalogue,* Wilcox, B. and Bellamy, I. (eds). Brooks Publishing, Baltimore.

NHSME (1993) *Risk Management in the NHS.* DoH, London.

UKCC (1992a) *Code of Professional Conduct.* UKCC, London.

UKCC (1992b) *The Scope of Professional Practice.* UKCC, London.

Watt, J. (1995) Bolam v. Friern Hospital Management Committee. *Clinical Risk,* 1(2), 84–85.

2 OPTIMUM HEALTH

The principle objective of this section is to enable nurses to promote positive health for the clients with whom they are working. This commences with a brief overview of many of the theories that underpin health and health promotion. The issues that are directly included have been selected because of their relevance not just to physical health, but also to the mental health and well-being of older people. The particular areas included are sexuality, spirituality, religion and personal social networks.

6 Promoting the health of older people

Mavis Arevalo

INTRODUCTION

As nurses, a major element of our role involves the promotion of good health and the prevention of ill-health. This is reinforced through the competencies we require to qualify in Rule 18 and Rule 18A (Statutory Instruments, 1979, 1983, 1989) and through our Code of Conduct (UKCC, 1992). It has also been highlighted as of major importance by the World Health Organization (WHO, 1978) and the Department of Health (1991, 1992) here in the United Kingdom. In order to undertake these activities, however, it is essential that we have an understanding of the meaning of health, the factors that influence health, including healthcare provision, and the theories that underpin health promotion. In relation to nursing work with older adults, there is a particular need to explore these very general ideas and theories in the context of ageing and in society's view of older people.

This chapter will explore the theories relevant to the above areas, drawing on the work of authors from a range of disciplines. It will then consider the relevance of these ideas to nursing practice with older adults. To achieve the latter, and provide suggestions for a systematic approach to health promotion for older adults, three case studies from my work as a health visitor will be examined. It is hoped that these will demonstrate the importance of individual beliefs about health to the practice of nursing and the promotion of health.

The chapter is composed of two major sections. The first, health, will provide a consideration of the concept from both theoretical and lay perspectives and the second, health promotion, will use one framework as an example of the usefulness of a systematic approach. Examples of links to nursing practice with older adults will be provided following the discussion of each theoretical perspective and the case studies will be used to emphasize the need for nurses to appreciate the health beliefs of their clients. In view of the complex nature of the theoretical material, a list of further reading is provided at the end of the chapter.

CONCEPTS OF HEALTH

According to Seedhouse (1986, p. xi) 'health is indisputably to do with people', but beyond this he argues that 'the word health is used to mean many different things'. This is supported by Aggleton (1990, p. 2) who states that there is 'little consensus about what health is ... still less is there agreement about the means by which it can be achieved'. He also states that 'the situation is further complicated by the fact that some people may be healthy according to some criteria but not others'. Seedhouse (1986, p. xii) argues that 'health is one of a number of words which are constantly in use which are so rich in meaning that they cannot be explained fully without invoking controversy'.

In relation to our work as nurses, it is important that we are aware of the various meanings of the word health as these may influence decisions that our clients make. They are also important as they may also affect the decisions that we make as healthcare workers about the interventions that we use. Beliefs about health can influence a range of human behaviours, but they invariably arise within a cultural context – beliefs about health and the nature of medical practice are culturally determined. As Lau (in Squires, 1991, p. 43) states, 'people have strong desires or needs to make sense of how diseases are caused or spread, and frequently they classify illness within the rubrics of the common lore of their culture'. He also goes on to point out that 'culture is a determinant of the incidence of disease ... this influence is exerted through the effects of culture on diet, occupation, lifestyles, healthcare habits, mating patterns and other psycho-social factors'.

Jang (1995, p. 103) supports this view, suggesting that 'the individual who becomes a patient brings to the health care setting not only his disease and trauma but also his needs, values, and life style founded on personal history and experience'. He further states that 'the culturally-derived concepts and perceptions of a society will influence the reactions and attitudes of people towards the order of the universe, health, illness, the behaviour of a sick person, education, work, play, family roles and relationships and the like'. From this perspective, health beliefs, health action and the practice of medicine are seen to develop from the beliefs and values of the originating culture. In fact, utilizing the above arguments, for health care to have any effectiveness it must have relevance for the members of that culture.

Within any culture, health beliefs can be broadly separated into two groups; theoretical perspectives on health presented by professionals; and lay beliefs, ideas expressed by members of wider society. It is important to consider both these groups, as the former may be influential in policy making and in care provision, whilst the latter may influence lifestyle, and therefore behaviour, and also affect an individual's response to health promotion strategies. As nurses, therefore, we may be influenced at a personal level by beliefs originating in our own culture, but in our work as healthcare professionals we are likely to approach the health of others from one or more of the theoretical perspectives.

THEORETICAL PERSPECTIVES ON HEALTH

Medical approaches to health

Medical approaches to health have been, and still are, very influential in determining beliefs about the nature of health. This perspective seeks to equate health with a series of clearly definable and measurable qualities. Sidell (1995, p. 4) for example, suggests that 'biomedical explanations relate to the physical body and health is explained in terms of biology'. It is argued that each body is essentially alike and so health is related to normality; deviation from these norms would represent pathology or a diseased state. Describing normality is problematic as physiological parameters change with age. If the young adult is taken as the reference point then most individuals over the age of 30 could be described as deviating from the norm, as happens, for example, when women over that age become pregnant for the first time.

From this perspective, health is seen as an absence of disease; however, should disease occur, health can be restored through the use of appropriate treatment. Medical intervention focuses on the disease, the tendency being to concentrate on discrete organs and tissues or, more recently, biochemistry and genetic influences. This narrow approach limits the attention paid to the interaction of the various elements that constitute the whole being. It has also generated the view that health is a commodity which can be bought and sold. As Aggleton (1990, p. 11) suggests 'restoring an individual to health is little more than a technical matter – something to be performed by experts through the administration of drugs or by surgical intervention'.

The views of biomedicine have their origins in the so-called Cartesian Revolution of the 17th century. Prior to this time, it was believed that the body was the seat of the soul and that to damage the body was to damage the soul. This also generated the belief that disorder of the soul would be demonstrated by disease of the body and that cure would come through prayer and divine intervention. Mind and body were therefore seen as being inextricably linked. Descartes (1596–1650) postulated, however, that God created two classes of substance that make up the whole of reality. One class was thinking substances, or minds, and the other was extended substances, or bodies (Microsoft, 1994). This came to be described as mind/body dualism or 'the ghost in the machine'. This theory paved the way for the development of modern medicine by providing the impetus to see the body as a physical entity, separate from the mind, and subject to damage and disease in much the same way as a machine may be damaged.

These ideas were further consolidated by the work of Pasteur and Koch in relation to germ theory and the causation of disease, and Darwin in relation to genetic transmission of physical qualities. The combination of these ideas generated the 'doctrine of specific aetiology' (Dubos, 1959), the argument that all disease occurs within the physical body and that once aetiology is known, a cure can be found. This has since come to be known as the biomechanical or medical model. The overall effect of this has been to define health in terms of physical function as an absence of disease where disease comprises 'deviations of measurable variables from the norm' (Blaxter, 1990, p. 3).

A number of problems have arisen, with the concept of norms against which human beings can be measured. This is evident in the wide variation demonstrated in basic physical parameters such as height, weight, and blood pressure. There are also difficulties in relation to definitions of health which focus only on the physical dimension. We know, for example, that psychological stress produces a measurable physiological response identical to that produced when there is physical stress, thereby providing evidence that separating mind from body is not appropriate.

It is important to recognize that other aspects of the human situation are also important in relation to health. As Sidell (1995, p. 4) states, 'biomedicine with its emphasis on the functioning of individual bodies has little to say about emotional and psychological health … yet the separation of mind and body in explanations of health is a fairly recent phenomenon … in earlier historical periods in western society and in some contemporary eastern cultures mental and physical health are inseparably linked'. Nevertheless some of the commodities offered by medicine can, and do, treat acute disease and may therefore improve physical health, but this approach is not sufficient to solve all the problems encountered in working to treat chronic disease and to increase health.

The approaches of biomedicine are problematic in relation to older adults where 'later life is portrayed as a time of declining strength and increased frailty as organs and tissues wear out or succumb to disease and degeneration' (Sidell, 1995, p. 4). The philosophy of cure has created a commodity of cosmetic surgery that will seek to limit the physical signs of ageing through repair and replacement of damaged tissue. It has also directed research into the ageing process in the hope of being able to slow down the physical deterioration at a genetic level. This has generated the idea that ageing is a disease process and can be cured. The close ties between medicine and nursing have also meant that many nurses have come to view health in terms of an absence of disease, but adopting a curative approach is problematic in relation to many areas of medical and nursing work, areas where care is more important than cure.

This difficulty is exemplified by the example of a 92-year-old woman called Gladys. She lived with her daughter but was a very active lady for her age and very mentally alert. Having had a severe chest infection during the summer which required hospitalization she told her GP that she had no wish to 'go through all that again' and, should the infection recur, she wanted 'to be left in peace'. The infection did recur some six months later and Gladys remained adamant that she would take no medication. She died within six hours of being seen by the same GP. Speaking afterwards he said he felt very uncomfortable

To what extent does the medical model influence your own care area?

You might have considered the emphasis on physical care or a tendency to see physical disease and medication as being more important than psychological and social needs.

with the idea that the patient refused treatment but he accepted that she had the right to make such a decision and die in comfort at home. Not all nurses and GPs would feel comfortable with this, and, in hospital, allowing this choice could be even more difficult. It also poses serious ethical questions about an individual's right to sacrifice their physical health in order to obtain mental or spiritual health.

Health as ideal state

Some of the earliest moves to change the narrow view of health proposed by biomedicine originated with the WHO in their constitution (1946) and reiterated at Alma Ata (WHO, 1978) where the ambition to achieve 'Health for all by the year 2000' was expressed. Their oft-quoted definition that 'health is a state of complete physical, mental and social well-being and not merely the absence of disease and infirmity' has come to typify the idea that health is an ideal state, a Socratic absolute of supreme well-being. Whilst this kind of definition is commendable because it considers wider issues than infirmity and disease, it has been criticized for its idealism. Seeing health as positive and enhancing, it sets high targets to be achieved, but it specifies a state of being which is almost impossible to attain. It also puts forward a rather absolute view of health by suggesting that we are all unhealthy unless we have attained complete physical, mental, and social well-being (Aggleton, 1990; Seedhouse, 1986).

According to Dubos (1979) health in these terms can be seen as a mirage, a utopian view. He argues that this is a myth which seriously distorts the true nature of health stating that 'unless men become robots, no formula can ever give them permanently the health and happiness symbolized by the contented cow, nor can their societies achieve a structure that will last for millennia'. Nor does this view face up to the many controversies regarding what is well-being, particularly mental and social, as definitions of well-being vary between cultures and groups. It can be argued that people have different bodies, ages, backgrounds and talents, and therefore the optimum state of existence for each person is bound to be different.

The aims of the WHO can be said to be admirable but unrealistic. It could even be argued that this approach is detrimental to the study of health as it sets a goal so patently unachievable that individuals and/or groups may be demotivated by the disheartening belief that each of us is permanently unhealthy. Even for the young the achievement of 'health' could only be a temporary state, for older adults this ideal state becomes progressively less achievable. Nevertheless this definition has acted as the impetus for further study in relation to health, and has to some extent weakened medical domination of discourses on health.

 The 'Health for all by the year 2000' targets are being implemented across Europe and the response of the British government has been the 'Health of the Nation' document (Department of Health, 1992, 1993). What influence, if any, have the targets of 'Health of the Nation' had in your work environment?

Health as social functioning

The importance of the concept of social functioning in relation to health has been explored in depth by Parsons (1964), who stated that 'health may be defined as the state of optimum *capacity* of an individual for the effective performance of the roles and tasks for which he has been socialised' (p. 274). Therefore health is defined 'with reference to the individual's participation in the social system' but that there are 'qualitative ranges in the differentiation of capacities' and sex, age and education are mentioned as potential factors.

Health is seen in relation to an individual's ability to 'fit in' with the norms and expectations of their society and to fulfil their designated role within that society, a process learned through socialization. Exemption from fulfilment of their role can only be permitted if the individual adopts the 'sick role', a state for which they are not responsible but for which they are obliged to seek professional help. It is also suggested that the individual is under an obligation 'to prevent threatened illness where this is possible' (Parsons, 1964, p. 275).

Aggleton (1990) argues that this perspective has its origins in the view that health is an important factor for the smooth running of society: 'too low a level of health, or too high a level of disease or illness, is likely to be dysfunctional for society and must therefore be kept in check' (p. 9). He also suggests (p. 10) that 'it implies that ill-health is something that is intrinsically bad for society', but there have been occasions when ill-health has acted as a powerful force for social change. The poor physical health of conscripts for the Boer war, for example, formed one of the first planks in the construction of the welfare state, and ill-health in certain industries has generated legislation to protect the health and safety of workers. However, without physical health an individual will be unable to take an active part in society. This view therefore, whilst demonstrating the importance of the need of individuals to fulfil their social role and of society's need for a healthy workforce, provides only a partial insight into the concept of health.

In working with older people this view of health has several problems. In stressing the need to perform specific social roles, this approach centres on the structure of society and the values and beliefs of that society. In traditional societies 'the elders' were seen to be the wise and were often consulted in relation to decision making. In modern western societies, whilst certain professional groups and higher office in government permit the presence of older people, for the majority, departure from the work role is enforced. After a lifetime of socialization into a work role, this loss of role can be problematic for the individual; it can also cause difficulties in relation to general perceptions of the group by wider society. It is often envisaged for example that older people are dependent on the State for their survival, that they represent 'a major social problem' (Fennell *et al.*, 1988, p. 43). However, what may be ignored in this approach is the hidden role that many older adults play in supporting the economy through their role within the family and in child care in particular.

It is also important to consider the extent to which this approach confers

What are your views on the fixing of a retirement age, and what do you believe to be the social role(s) of older adults when they no longer have a work role?

power on the medical profession to legitimate sickness and to define competence. Older people may, for example, be subject to medical assessment in relation to their ability to drive, their ability to operate machinery and even their right to remain in their own home. Although this power has been weakened in recent years by the increased use of multidisciplinary assessment, the medical profession continues to inform debate on physical normality, and the ability of the individual to function as a member of society.

Humanistic approaches to health

According to Seedhouse (1986, p. 36) there is a group of theories viewing health as 'a personal strength or ability'. He argues that these 'can be united under a general humanist banner'. This group of theories views health as either an 'unquantifiable resilience', or as 'an ability to adapt positively to the inevitable problems and sufferings that life throws up'. Health is seen as a way of responding appropriately, and not only in biological ways. Seedhouse (1986, p. 36) suggests that 'health is thus a means towards further and greater ends – if a person can resist or adapt positively to problems of different kinds then she has a position from which she can develop her potential to the full'. He argues that 'this group of theories recalls the position of 200 years ago where health was thought of only in holistic terms ... not something which can be precisely defined ... a way of living – a whole rule of life'. These theories have as their intention a move away from defining health as the physical body or as performing a designated social role towards health as a personal attitude or ability, including ideas of resilience, achieving potential or achieving successful adaptation to changes.

Health as resilience

Theories relating to health as resilience propose that the ability to resist disease or to cope with the problems of life is an intrinsic property of individuals but that these abilities can be developed or can be lost. Aggleton (1990, p. 11) suggests that 'sometimes the emphasis may be on the physical strength or the ability to resist disease and cope with illness ... on other occasions the emphasis may be on mental strength – an attitude or outlook on life which helps the individual cope with adversity'.

Health as achieving potential

The notion of health as achieving personal potential is exemplified in the oft-quoted statement from the work of Katherine Mansfield: 'by health I mean the power to live a full, adult, living, breathing life in close contact with what I love ... I want to be all that I am capable of becoming' (quoted in Naidoo and Wills, 1994, p. 21). From this perspective health is seen as the ability to achieve one's own desired goals. This view is expanded by Seedhouse (1986, p. 61) who argues that 'a person's optimum state of health is equivalent to the state of the set of conditions which fulfil or enable a person to work to fulfil his or her realistic chosen and biological potentials'.

The problem with the above theories is that they are both very vague, the nature of strength or reserve is not well defined and the issue of personal potential remains a difficult one. As Aggleton (1990, p. 12) suggests it is 'not entirely clear what personal potential is taken to be'. It is also uncertain whose view of achievement would dominate, as the issue of personal values and aspirations would complicate the picture. Because of this, he argues 'the notion of personal potential remains a little mystical', perhaps no more easily attainable than the ideal state proposed by the WHO. He also states that Seedhouse 'provides little guidance about the range of factors that might count as foundations for achievement'. The above definition does, however, guide us towards a theoretical perspective of health which encompasses the idea of conditions needed to permit health. The implication being therefore that health is not just a function of individuals but also a function of society.

In relation to work with older adults, these two approaches can be seen as useful because they move attention away from the physical towards the development of coping mechanism and the achievement of personal goals. This introduces the concept of quality of life to the discussion of health. It can be questioned as to whether an individual is aware of their own potential, and to what extent limitations in physical ability may limit expression of that potential. It is problematic that these theories suggest that health is composed of nebulous non-physical qualities that are somehow unrelated to the physical body, because developing appropriate assessment and intervention strategies is more difficult.

To what extent are these theoretical perspectives on health reflected in the practices of your work environment?

Examples of negative practice might include encouragement of dependence and limitations of personal choice, whilst positive practice could include enhancement of appropriate coping mechanisms and quality of life.

Health as the ability to adapt

Aggleton (1990, p. 11) suggests that health can be viewed as 'the ability to adapt to changing circumstances'. He argues that 'Renee Dubos ... has suggested that it was the human capacity to adapt to new situations, and not the advent of vaccines and drugs, that resulted in the decline of epidemic diseases in Europe in the nineteenth and twentieth centuries'. As Dubos (1959, p. 25) states, 'health and happiness cannot be absolute and permanent values, however careful the social and medical planning ... biological success in all its manifestations is a measure of fitness, and fitness requires never-ending efforts of adaptation to the total environment which is ever changing'. Dubos's argument that health is an ability to adapt recognizes that health is not an absolute, specific, uncontroversial end in itself. It is not a permanent, definable target for which successive generations of human beings, whatever their circumstances, can strive. For Dubos, health is an ability to respond positively to the different challenges which arise in people's lives.

This can be seen as a useful view in relation to older people. The ability to adapt positively to the changes, both physical and socio-economic, that occur during later life is associated with increased lifespan and better quality of life. This ability to adapt is also supported by a lifetime of experience, but it does imply a lack of control over events. The person can be seen as a passive player, having to adapt to whatever comes along, rather than being in control of the changes that occur. For the older adult there is the also the difficulty of a decreasing ability to adapt physiologically, rendering the individual less able to withstand stressors of a physical origin. Another problem is that there may be a need to make multiple adaptations within a very short space of time, thereby testing the individual's ability to adapt positively. This may be compounded by the need for professional intervention by healthcare workers which has the potential to generate dependence and to further impede appropriate adaptation.

Seedhouse (1986, p. 40) argues 'medical science *impedes people's ability to adapt autonomously* ... improved health (decreased disease) has arisen mainly as the result of social measures designed to correct the ills of industrialisation, to provide better nutrition, better housing and better work conditions'. He suggests that the causes of many of the degenerative diseases currently causing problems may be directly related to modern life which does not allow man sufficient time in which to adapt. This view was also previously presented by Illich (1976, p. 273) who argues that 'health designates a process of adaptation ... it is not the result of instinct, but of an autonomous yet culturally shaped reaction to socially created reality'. He suggests (pp. 33–34) that the health professions 'destroy the ability of people to deal with their human weakness, vulnerability, and uniqueness in a personal and autonomous way ... *cultural iatrogenesis* is the ultimate backlash of hygienic progress and consists in the paralysis of healthy responses to suffering, impairment, and death'.

To what extent do the interventions used in your nursing practice enhance or impede individual ability to adapt to changes?

Health as equilibrium

Many traditional eastern systems of health beliefs and healthcare practices differ radically from those of western science, as the issue of equilibrium, or harmony, is of prime importance. Balance within the person is seen to be as important as balance between the individual and the physical and social environment. It is interesting that the idea of balance has not been explored in relation to western theories as it is an idea well known in physiology. One of the basic concepts in the study of how the body works is homeostasis, the dynamic equilibrium that is essential to maintain the internal physiological parameters necessary to life, despite the changes wrought by the external environment or the activity of the body. Ideas about balance and harmony, although used at a biochemical level, do not appear to have been taken to their logical conclusion that balance is required in all aspects of life.

The view of health as balance or equilibrium provides a useful insight into issues pertaining to the health of older people. Given the fact that the ageing process produces alterations within the physical body, it is important that the individual accommodates these changes without becoming over-focused on any one single dimension of their health. An attempt to maintain a perfect physical body could lead to problems in relation to the individual's mental health, just as over-indulgence in social activities can produce serious physical repercussions. It is also important that the individual is in balance with their environment, and able to cope with their surroundings. How many individuals are unable to eat a healthy diet, not because they are unable to eat or unable to cook, but because they cannot get to shops with a wide range of reasonably priced products? The issue of balance can therefore be seen to have relevance when considering the health of older adults and it is an area which could well benefit from further research.

LAY PERSPECTIVES ON HEALTH

According to Aggleton (1990, p. 16) 'lay beliefs about health are the consequences of people's attempts to make sense of the various sources of information to which they have access ... popular perceptions of health arise from the attempts people make to seek order where often there is often [sic] chaos and confusion'. As such, he argues, 'lay beliefs are *syncretic* (quoting Fitzpatrick, 1984), drawing on a wide and disparate set of sources ... they are also pragmatic, in that they enable us to cope with the complexity of health issues and to make apparent sense of our lives'. Quoting a variety of sources, Siddell (1995, p. 3) states that 'researchers into lay health beliefs show that definitions of health vary not only in terms of gender, class and ethnicity but that individuals are not necessarily consistent in their own explanations of health and illness'. She argues that 'they may use different explanations depending on their current circumstances and their definitions might change through the life cycle ... what research has shown is that people draw on a mixture of official and folk accounts to weave their own explanations of health'.

Blaxter (1990, p. 16) analyzing data from her survey, suggests that there are three 'states' of health commonly identified: freedom from illness, ability to function, and fitness. Freedom from illness aligns closely with the biomedical model of health discussed earlier and it was found that 25–50% of respondents used this to describe the health of others. It was less commonly used to define own health, however, with less than 20% using this description. For self the more common definition was 'functionally able to do a lot' which approximates more to the concept of health as social functioning. In relation to fitness, both physical and psychological were considered. Physical fitness was seen to be important to the young, but this decreased with age. Psychological fitness was more consistent across the age groups, but was more likely to be used for self rather than for others.

In relation to the 60+ age group it was found that although 'never ill' was used for others (34–35%), psychological fitness (men 36%, women 44%) and functional ability (men 43%, women 34%) were ranked more highly for self. It is interesting to note that the above rankings are reversed for men and women. Case study one typifies the importance of psychological fitness and functional ability to older people. For Alice and Bill their diseases were a fact of life, but their need to be able to care for themselves and to function effectively was their main priority.

CASE STUDY

Alice (76) and Bill (81) moved into a warden-controlled flat in a tower block (10th floor) six years ago. When I met them, Bill had not been out of the flat since they moved in as he could only walk very short distances due to chronic obstructive airways disease. Alice had fractured her hip a year before in a fall, and, although now able to walk a short distance, had not been out of the building since the accident. The building possessed lifts to all floor, but access to the nearby road and to public transport was only for the able-bodied, being a steep hill.

In order to assess this couple and to provide appropriate interventions it was essential to understand their perceptions of the situation in which they found themselves. Their main concern was the extent to which they were becoming isolated from social interaction, and this was coupled with a concern that they were dependent on others to meet their basic needs, for example the purchase of food. Their health beliefs centred on being able to care for themselves and to cope effectively with their problems. The issue of disease was not seen to be important other than as a reason for their difficulties.

The couple did not wish to enter residential care as they associated this with a failure in relation to self-care, but a compromise was negotiated that they might benefit from a new scheme which offered sheltered housing with full care support (meals provided, cleaning staff, care assistance). The couple were fortunate in that they were able to secure the last available flatlet in the new building, and moved in within a matter of weeks. A short time later I was surprised to meet Alice in the town centre. She told me that Bill was enjoying mixing with the others as meals were provided in the dining room. She was also pleased by their new life as she could get 'out and about' more.

Added to these predominant views, Blaxter (1990, p. 16) also states that the idea of health as a 'reserve' has been found to be very prevalent. In exploring this idea she has found that this reserve 'can be diminished by self-neglect and accumulated by healthy behaviour ... it is largely determined by heredity, influenced by childhood and traumatic events'. There is also the suggestion that once spent, it leaves generalized weakness or vulnerability, and it can be exhausted, with some implication of irreversibility. Thus 'good' health is the power of overcoming disease, even if that disease is actually present: 'bad' health is being at risk, the loss of resistance, even if disease is absent.

Other broad categories of lay beliefs (Blaxter, 1990, pp. 20–29) include health as behaviour, health as 'the healthy life', health as energy or vitality, health as social relationships, and health as function. These general categories were also demonstrated in the study carried out by Brannen *et al.* (1994, p. 72), in relation to beliefs about health held by young people and their families. They state, however, that 'agreement within households concerning definitions of being healthy is the exception rather than the rule ... compared with young people, parents are more likely to emphasise negative statements of health, notably not being ill, while more young people dwell on healthy lifestyles and fitness'. Blaxter (1990, pp. 30–31) supports this, suggesting that not only are there differences between the sexes in relation to concepts of health, but there are also differences through the life course.

A further complication arises in relation to the fact that 'health beliefs also appear to reflect material inequalities ... those who have fewer material resources are more likely to see health as outside their control than are those with greater resources' (Brannen *et al.*, 1994, quoting Blaxter and Patterson, 1982, and Pill and Stott, 1986). Brannen *et al.* (1994, p. 69) also state that 'research in France found that positive definitions of health, expressive of personal wellbeing, were much more likely to be held by more educated non-manual workers and the financially more secure' (quoting d'Houtard and Field, 1984) and that 'research in a working-class area of London has shown the importance of "coping" to lay definitions of health; being healthy is about being able to carry on with one's ordinary everyday activities' (quoting Cornwell, 1984). These lay beliefs present further evidence for the cultural origins of health, and in particular the effects of socio-economic factors on those beliefs. It can be argued therefore that the aspirations of individuals are constrained or enhanced by the subculture within which those individuals have been socialized.

Brannen *et al.* (1994, p. 72) also found that 'given that absence of illness is the most common definition of health, we might predict that illness would emerge as a significant threat to health … but in an open-ended interview question, aspects of lifestyle, together with environmental problems, figure more prominently than illness as a threat to health'. These health beliefs demonstrate that although disease continues to remain to the fore in the thoughts of the general public, there appears to be an increasing shift away from biomedicine, particularly in the young. This could also be a function of the fact that 'young people are one of the healthiest social groups, as judged by indicators such as mortality and hospitalisation rates' (Brannen *et al.*, 1994, p. 69). Nevertheless, Stanway (1979) suggested that 'meditation, ways of controlling the mind, oriental religions, a greater interest in healthy eating, greater awareness of the problems of pollution and a growing sense of Man [*sic*] as a part of a larger world are all enjoying a wide public following'. He also stated that in spite of this 'the western medical profession continues to plod the never ending and increasingly frustrating path of orthodox health care'.

The problems that may arise when lay beliefs and professional views differ are demonstrated in case study two.

CASE STUDY   Rebecca (83) is a widow of many years who lives alone and has been housebound for the last year due to severe osteoarthritis. She nevertheless feels that she has good support from her family and her neighbours and does not feel lonely. One issue that did come forward in our discussion, however, was that she misses being able to read books. As a healthcare worker I saw this as a problem which had a potential solution so I put forward suggestions about the availability of domiciliary eye testing and possible new spectacles, and about large print books and the mobile library facilities.

Rebecca went along with me in this discussion, obviously feeling that she should allow me to undertake the requirements of my professional role and seek a solution. Eventually the real problem was finally acknowledged, however. Rebecca no longer had an adequate concentration span to read even a page as, when she reached the last paragraph, she could not remember what had happened in the first. Rebecca did not really want a solution, she just wanted to mourn the loss of an ability that she valued, but my simplistic approach almost prevented her from doing this.

In this situation my professional view of health tended towards the reduction of problems as a way to maximize potential, whereas Rebecca was attempting to adapt to the changes that she was experiencing. Our goals were different and this could have created a scenario where my intervention could have made the situation worse. This conflict is even more evident when the beliefs of the biomedical approach are used to address problems experienced by older adults. Case study three highlights the complexity of health beliefs and demonstrates how both complementary and conflicting beliefs can be held simultaneously. When considering the need to promote health the issue is therefore very complex as differing health beliefs require differing approaches.

CASE STUDY

Irene (60) was extremely distressed when only eight weeks short of her own retirement her already retired husband, to whom she had been married for 37 years, died very suddenly while visiting a relative. They were a childless couple who lived for each other but had close ties with other family members and friends. They had never prepared themselves for potential loss; as Irene admitted, she had refused to let her husband even mention the possibility.

Following her bereavement, Irene developed a range of physical as well as psychological problems, and, being unaware of the physical pain of grief, believed herself to be physically ill. Irene's beliefs about health were very much those of biomedicine in that a pain must mean physical disease, and she was very distressed when told by the GP that there was nothing wrong with her and that she needed tranquillizers. She felt that this implied she was 'making it up' and that somehow she had 'failed' to cope with the situation. This added to her already massive burden of grief, and the guilt that she felt because she was not with her husband when he died.

She was therefore in a situation where grieving used up all her available resources including her energy/capacity to respond to situations. She was left unable to participate in any aspect of living (physical, social, mental) for almost two years, suffering marked physical as well as emotional symptoms. The approach of biomedicine in this scenario was to offer medication, but this was rejected because it conflicted with Irene's perception of her situation. Irene's need was met by being allowed the opportunity to explore her feelings, and to deal with her emotions, on a frequent and regular basis, until she felt able to participate again in her social group and family. This need could only be met from outside her normal circle because they were too involved to offer the support she needed and had in fact started to tell her to 'pull herself together' within a short time of her loss.

Is the role of the healthcare professional to change the client's health beliefs or to work with their existing beliefs? What might be the problems when these beliefs are in conflict?

THE NEED FOR HEALTH PROMOTION

The 'Health of the Nation' document (Department of Health, 1992, 1993) states that 'many people die prematurely or suffer debilitating ill-health from conditions which are to a large extent preventable ... the way in which people live and the lifestyles they adopt can have profound effects on subsequent health'. The document also suggests that 'disease prevention, health promotion and health education are as much public concerns as medical matters'. There is an increased need for healthcare professionals to develop skills in the activities of health promotion and disease prevention. From the preceding discussion, the complexity of the task facing those whose intention is to promote health becomes apparent. The focus within the NHS tends to be dominated by biomedicine, but there are increasing moves towards a wider view of health. The targets set by the WHO (1985) have had some influence on broadening the scope of research into factors implicated in the health of nations and into appropriate healthcare systems. It is hoped that this will lead to an improvement in overall health, but in order to achieve this there will be a need to develop strategies for health promotion and a range of specific interventions.

According to Ewles and Simnett (1995) 'there has been much debate since the mid 1980s on the use of the terms *health promotion* and *health education*'. Prior to the 1980s the practice of health education was 'almost exclusively located within preventive medicine or, to a lesser extent, education' (Naidoo and Wills, 1994, p. 62). The focus of this practice was to change attitudes and behaviour, seeing health problems as the result of individual lifestyles. With criticism that this approach was too narrow and focused too much on individual lifestyles, the term health promotion came to refer to a movement which 'challenges the medicalisation of health, stresses its social and economic aspects, and portrays health as having a central place in a flourishing human life' (Downie *et al.*, 1990, p. 1). As Bunton and Macdonald (1992, p. x) state 'health promotion has emerged in the last decade as an important force to improve both the quality and quantity of people's lives ... sometimes termed "the new public health" it seeks to support and encourage a participative social movement that enables individuals and communities to take control over their own health'.

This is supported by Tones and Tilford (1994, p. 6) who suggest that 'health promotion might be described as any deliberate or planned attempt to foster health or prevent and manage disease'. Health education forms a part of health promotion activity but it needs to be supported by other measures related to environmental issues so that 'the healthy choice becomes the easy choice' (Tones and Tilford, 1994, p. 7). The scope of health promotion will now be considered, and in order to facilitate the discussion, the approaches suggested by Tones and Tilford (1994) will be explored in relation to promoting the health of older adults.

Tones and Tilford (1994) suggest there are three approaches to health promotion, each generating distinct goals. These are referred to as the preventive, the empowerment, and the radical approaches. The three represent distinct beliefs and values or ideologies, and it is important to analyze the origins of each in order to understand its expected outcomes in relation to healthcare. It is also important to consider that there is considerable overlap between these approaches, but as nurses we need to be aware of the beliefs inherent in the approaches that we use. As Tones and Tilford (1994, p. 45) suggest, practitioners who opt for one or other approach 'are, consciously or unconsciously, revealing what for them are important values and/or different ways of constructing their personal realities'.

The preventive approach to health promotion

This approach to health promotion has its origins in the biomedical model discussed earlier and particularly in the physical body. The underpinning beliefs are that health is an absence of disease and that individuals should, wherever possible, seek to prevent disease occurring (Tones and Tilford, 1994, p. 12). The tendency is to see individuals as rational beings who are responsible for their own health, and to see the healthcare professional as being the person to judge needs and provide advice. It is indeed argued that society expects professionals to take this role.

The goal of the approach is to persuade people to take responsible decisions, to adopt behaviours that will prevent disease and to make appropriate use of services. Success is judged in terms of behavioural outcomes with people adopting healthier lifestyles or complying with advice, the emphasis being on the ability of individuals to control their own health, rather than on the environment as shaping and constraining this (Brannen *et al.*, 1994, p. 67; quoting Research Unit in Health and Behavioural Change (RUHBC), 1989).

Arguments supporting the use of this approach suggest that experts have the knowledge which enables them to know what is in the best interests of their clients and that the individual is able to do something about their health. It is suggested that people seeking advice and help expect to be told what to do and that some people are unable to take responsibility for their own decisions. This approach tends to use persuasive or paternalistic methods (Ewles and Simnett, 1995), and on occasion resorts to coercion, to ensure that people comply with recommended procedures and lifestyles. The 'experts' can be wrong, and the assumption that one message is appropriate for everyone is problematic.

According to Brannen *et al.* (1994, p. 68), 'the lifestyle approach to health has been criticised by sociologists of health and illness for its philosophical assumptions of individualism, which obscure the social and material conditions in which people live ... the notion of individual "choice" over health-related behaviour leads, moreover, to blaming the victims'. As Ahmad (1993, p. 12) states 'biomedicine depoliticises and individualises ill health ... it diverts attention away from the production of ill health to its distribution among individuals and, by relating it to their lifestyles, perpetuates the ideology of victim blaming'. The ideology of victim blaming is therefore firmly entrenched within medical practice and consequently within the NHS. Brannen *et al.* (1994, p. 68) suggest it reflects 'the way in which market forces increasingly translate health into an item for consumption'.

When evidence demonstrates socio-economic factors are implicated in the development of disease, this is often seen as a result of poor cultural practices transmitted via socialization, rather than a problem of structural inequalities (Townsend *et al.*, 1988, p. 316). This tendency to blame individuals and their culture is problematic in relation to health promotion activity as it implies that individuals have full control over their environment and lifestyle. It is also compounded by the fact that doctors 'regard themselves as professionals, and you as the lucky recipient of their knowledge and skill ... they fail to realise that it is *you* who are ill, and who ought to have the last word about what treatment you need' (Campbell, 1984, p. 12). As Tones and Tilford (1994, p. 15) state, 'the preventive model of health education may be likened to the rearranging of the deckchairs on the Titanic' as it is an ultimately futile activity.

The empowerment approach to health promotion

A second approach to health promotion suggested by Tones and Tilford (1994, pp. 24–25) still retains the focus on the individual but suggests that empowerment is a method to remedy factors within the individual that 'militate against freedom of choice'. This approach argues that people have a right to make their own decisions but that they may need help to understand their own beliefs and values. They may also need skills to carry through the decisions they make into health action, but invariably in this approach change is by choice. The beliefs about health underpinning this approach fit broadly within the humanistic group with achieving potential seen as being an important element.

Arguments supporting this approach focus on the ethical nature of freedom to choose and individual rights. Empowerment is also regarded as developing high self-esteem, self-efficacy and a repertoire of social skills (Tones and Tilford, 1994, p. 29). It is suggested that, because the individual identifies their own priorities for health, interventions are more likely to be successful. Clients are valued as equals with a right to set their own agenda (Ewles and Simnett, 1995), the role of the healthcare professional being one of facilitation. The overall goal of the approach can be said to be one of fostering informed choice, and interventions include one-to-one counselling, advocacy, and group and community work.

The approach can be criticized, as it continues to carry a risk of victim blaming if the individual does not choose to change. It also ignores the obstacles that may prevent free and informed decision making. In particular it may fail to address 'the powerful effect of environmental factors in facilitating or hindering freedom of choice' (Tones and Tilford, 1994, p. 32). The approach is also difficult for healthcare workers as it involves relinquishing the expert role, and is problematic to evaluate in relation to effectiveness as it is a process rather than an outcome (Naidoo and Wills, 1994, p. 90). Nevertheless empowered individuals might have a better chance of influencing their environmental circumstances.

The radical approach to health promotion

A third approach suggested by Tones and Tilford (1994, pp. 16–17) is the radical approach. The beliefs underpinning this approach focus on the role of the physical and social environment as a determinant of health, and the inequalities that result based on social class, gender, age, race and ethnicity. It holds some similarities with the ideas of social functioning described earlier, but takes these further by allocating a much more important role to society itself. Sometimes referred to as the social change approach (Naidoo and Wills, 1994; Ewles and Simnett, 1995) the overall aim is to change society, rather than the behaviour of individuals, and to 'make health choices the easier choices'.

Arguments supporting this approach relate that previous public health successes demonstrate its effectiveness. It is also suggested that it addresses the real causes of ill-health through the building of healthy public policy and environmental improvements. The methods utilized are those of the political arena; setting up pressure groups, critical consciousness raising, and campaigning and lobbying to influence policy making and the development of legislation. As

Naidoo and Wills (1994, p. 91) suggest, however, 'for most health promotion workers, the scope for this type of activity will be more limited'. They also state that the necessary skills 'may not be included in professional training', and that working in such a way may be 'beyond the brief of the job, too political or someone else's remit'.

There are also other problems with this approach as it is argued that it reduces individual choice in relation to behaviour because of the level of social regulation required. It is also further suggested that it discourages individuals from taking responsibility for their own health. It is felt that raising the consciousness of individuals to a problem, only for them to find that they are unable to produce change, is more damaging to self-esteem and more dangerous than the ideology of victim blaming already discussed (Tones and Tilford, 1994, p. 21).

In fact there is a need for all three approaches to operate together to ensure progress towards meeting the targets of the WHO and of 'the Health of the Nation'. There is a need for preventive services that focus on disease processes and offer relevant screening programmes to detect disease in its early stages when it is more susceptible to treatment. There is also a need for people to take back control over their health in order to improve their self-esteem and their self-efficacy and to generate a better quality of life for themselves. Both preventive and empowering approaches will only be possible however, if the physical and socio-political environment are appropriate and support these enterprises. A 63-year-old woman of limited income can only choose (empowerment) to undergo mammography examination (preventive) if the screening service is available to her within the NHS (radical). Currently a woman over the age of 64 is not eligible for this programme unless she specifically requests it.

THE ROLE OF THE NURSE IN HEALTH PROMOTION

According to Tones (in Wilson-Barnett and Macleod Clark, 1993, p. 9) 'if nursing is to take health promotion seriously it must be actively concerned with the empowerment of clients and patients'. He also asks 'to what extent can nurses legitimately be involved in political action to promote health?' He goes on to suggest, however, that the functions of policy and education are complementary: 'a hospital which seeks to promote health through empowerment must have a sound policy'. As nurses, therefore, we are already involved in issues of policy making at a local level and, as such, involved in political action. This means that we are already in a position to utilize the three approaches discussed earlier but we need to be aware of how and why we use them. A systematic approach will now be used to consider the health promotion needs of the older people described in the preceding case studies.

The three case studies demonstrate that complex approaches are required in order to promote the health of older adults. In relation to Alice and Bill (case study one) we were very fortunate with the timing of our application for the special sheltered housing, but this facility was quickly filled and now has a considerable waiting list of other individuals whose long-term health would benefit from this environment. It is apparent that access to this new development made going out easier for the couple, but perhaps, more importantly, energy freed from the basic tasks of living could now be invested in other social/leisure activities. The question can be asked: what are the priorities for each individual?

Many may wish to retain their 'independence', but this may be at a cost to other aspects of their lives, and may also be a conditioned response rather than what they would really like to do. This is once again evidence of the complex nature of health promotion. It also demonstrates that working with individuals can only go so far and, without support in relation to the socio-economic environment, full achievement of an individual's health potential is unlikely.

Which approaches to health promotion were utilized in this situation and were there any other possible solutions?

In the case of Rebecca (case study two) I adopted a straightforward preventive approach, looking for problems in order to generate solutions based on my perceptions of the situation. In fact the preventive approach, although problematic in relation to the reading, did work in relation to another issue highlighted by Rebecca. She needed domiciliary chiropody as her family could no longer manage her thickening toenails and this was arranged for her. However, a radical approach is needed to ensure that a funded service is available to meet the chiropody requirements of older people.

Do all people who tell you their problems actually want a solution?

For Irene (case study three), the level of support needed to enable her to avoid medication was quite high, and whilst it was agreed that her circumstances were rather extreme and merited such input, for many others the cost of such a level of counselling would not be deemed to be appropriate. There is a way to provide such support for less cost, and that is to empower individuals through a support group. In this situation the role of the healthcare professional is to support and facilitate, thereby enabling the members of the client group to develop their own potential. It is important that the group members are allowed to take control of the situation, with input from the professionals when requested, as self-esteem is enhanced if the group feels a sense of personal achievement.

A major energy commitment may deplete energy from other aspects of living. Is it possible to generate more of this 'capacity to respond' or if not, how can these other areas be supported until there is free energy available?

CONCLUSION

One of the problems for nurses and other healthcare professionals, however, relates to their access to older adults who may be in need of health promotion or who are vulnerable. In a hospital or other institutional environment, nurses have close contact with the people for whom they are caring and can hopefully devote time to health promotion activity. They are also in a position to have some control of the environment within which care takes place and can thereby take the opportunity to use all three health promotion approaches. For the older person at home, however, access to even a basic preventive approach may not be available. The GP contract now requires that all people over the age of 75 years are offered a yearly check, and this could provide an opportunity to undertake health-promoting work. Greater access to health promotion will be particularly important in relation to achieving the targets of 'The Health of the Nation' (Department of Health, 1992, 1993) as some of these particularly apply to people in this age group.

A preventive approach is useful in relation to the avoidance of disease and, for some people, may help them change their lifestyle. An empowerment approach, on the other hand, puts the individual in control of their life and the radical approach ensures that they are able to make health choices. In order to undertake these activities, however, we need the ability to carry out an assessment not only of an individual's health status, but also the beliefs they hold about health, about what is important to them. It is important that the model of nursing that underpins our work reflects the importance of the individual's beliefs about health. We also need a range of interventions that we can implement in relation to these approaches, and tools to evaluate whether these have been effective. As nurses we need to develop skills in all of these areas if we are to enable older adults to achieve the level of health that they deserve.

 How might you assess an individual's health beliefs?

FURTHER READING

Health

Aggleton, P. (1990) *Health*. Routledge, London.
Provides a very useful exploration of the concept of health, considering the work of a range of authors.

Blaxter, M. (1990) *Health and Lifestyles*. Routledge, London.
Describes the health and lifestyles survey and explores a range of lay concepts of health as suggested in the survey.

Brannen, J., Dodd, K., Oakley, A. and Storey, P. (1994) *Young People, Health and Family Life*. Open University Press, Milton Keynes.
Explores health beliefs, particularly as they relate to young people and their families.

Hart, N. (1985) *The Sociology of Health and Medicine*. Causeway Books, Ormskirk.
Considers medical practice and its impact on beliefs about health and illness, in particular the links between societal factors and falling disease rates (rather than medical practice) are addressed.

Seedhouse, D. (1986) *Health: the Foundations for Achievement.* John Wiley & Sons, Chichester.
Explores a wide range of beliefs about the nature of health, including lay concepts. The author also puts forward his own definition of health.

Siddell, M. (1995) *Health in Old Age: myth, mystery & management.* Open University Press, Milton Keynes.
Addresses a wide range of issues relating to the maintenance of health in old age, in particular considers the influence of the medical model.

Health promotion

Downie, R., Fyfe, C. and Tannahill, A. (1990) *Health Promotion: Models and Values.* Oxford University Press, Oxford.
Describes a comprehensive model of health promotion which can be related to nursing practice.

Ewles, L. and Simnett, I. (1995) *Promoting Health: a Practical Guide,* 3rd edn. Scutari, London.
Provides a slightly simpler model of health promotion which is useful in considering individual practice.

Naidoo, J. and Wills, J. (1994) *Health Promotion: foundations for practice.* Baillière Tindall, London.
Considers a range of models and approaches to health promotion, providing a comprehensive overview of the subject useful for all areas of nursing practice.

The role of the nurse in health promotion

Wilson-Barnett, J. and Macleod Clark, J. (eds) (1993) *Research in Health Promotion & Nursing.* Macmillan, Basingstoke.
The authors have compiled a range of health promotion activities as carried out by nurses and these provide a range of ideas to enhance nursing practice.
    It is also essential however, that nurses consider the model of nursing underpinning their practice to ensure that the requirement to address health promotion forms a central element of the model.

REFERENCES

Aggleton, P. (1990) *Health.* Routledge, London.

Ahmad, W. (ed.) (1993) *'Race' and Health in Contemporary Britain.* Open University Press, Milton Keynes.

Blaxter, M. (1990) *Health and Lifestyles.* Routledge, London.

Brannen, J., Dodd, K., Oakley, A. and Storey, P. (1994) *Young People, Health and Family Life.* Open University Press, Milton Keynes.

Bunton, R. and Macdonald, G. (1992) *Health Promotion: Disciplines and Diversity.* Routledge, London.

Campbell, A. (1984) *Natural Health Handbook.* Apple Press, London.

Department of Health (1991) *The Patient's Charter.* HMSO, London.

Department of Health (1992, reprinted with corrections 1993) *The Health of the Nation.* HMSO, London.

Downie, R., Fyfe, C. and Tannahill, A. (1990)

Health Promotion: Models and Values. Oxford University Press, Oxford.

Dubos, R. (1959) *The Mirage of Health.* Harper & Row, New York.

Dubos, R. (1979) Mirage of health. Extracts reprinted in *Health & Disease: a Reader,* Black *et al.* (eds). Open University Press, Milton Keynes.

Ewles, L. and Simnett, I. (1995) *Promoting Health: a Practical Guide,* 3rd edn. Scutari, London.

Fennell, G., Phillipson, C. and Evers, H. (1988) *The Sociology of Old Age.* Open University Press, Milton Keynes.

Illich, I. (1976) *Limits to Medicine.* Calder & Boyars, London.

Jang, Y. (1995) Chinese Culture and Occupational Therapy. *British Journal of Occupational Therapy,* **58**(3), 103–106.

Microsoft (1994) *Encarta '95.* Microsoft Corporation, USA.

Naidoo, J. and Wills, J. (1994) *Health Promotion: foundations for practice.* Baillière Tindall, London.

Parsons, T. (1964) *Social Structure and Personality.* Free Press of Glencoe, New York.

Seedhouse, D. (1986) *Health: the Foundations for Achievement.* John Wiley & Sons, Chichester.

Siddell, M. (1995) *Health in Old Age: myth, mystery & management.* Open University Press, Milton Keynes.

Squires, A. (ed.) (1991) *Multicultural Health Care & Rehabilitation of Older People.* Edward Arnold, London.

Stanway, A. (1979) *Alternative Medicine: a Guide to Natural Therapies.* Penguin, Harmondsworth.

Statutory Instrument. (1979) *The Nurses, Midwives and Health Visitors Act.* HMSO, London.

Statutory Instrument. (1983) *The Nurses, Midwives and Health Visitors Rules Approval Order* (no. 837). HMSO, London.

Statutory Instrument. (1989) *The Nurses, Midwives and Health Visitors (Registered Fever Nurses Amendment Rules and Training amendment Rules) Approval Order* (no. 1456). HMSO, London.

Tones, K. and Tilford, S. (1994) *Health Education: Effectiveness, Efficiency and Equity* 2nd edn. Chapman & Hall, London.

Townsend, P., Davidson, N. and Whitehead, M. (1988) *Inequalities in Health.* Penguin, Harmondsworth.

UKCC. (1992) *Code of Professional Conduct.* United Kingdom Central Council for Nursing Midwifery and Health Visiting, London.

Wilson-Barnett, J. and Macleod Clark, J. (eds) (1993) *Research in Health Promotion & Nursing.* Macmillan, Basingstoke.

WHO (1946) *World Health Organization Constitution.* WHO, Geneva.

WHO (1978) *Alma Ata 1978 Primary Health Care.* WHO, Geneva.

WHO (1985) *Targets for Health For All – Targets in Support of the European Regional Strategy for Health for All.* Regional Office for Europe, Copenhagen.

7 Sexuality and older people

Gordon Evans

INTRODUCTION

Sexuality is an important part of the total composition of each individual's essential being. As such it is of fundamental importance to a person's health. Healthcare professionals therefore need to consider this issue when involved in the assessment, planning, implementation and evaluation of nursing care. From an historical perspective much confusion has existed between what is meant by sexuality and sexual health, thus resulting in little or no attention being given to this area within clinical practice. This can, to some degree, be seen as the consequence of the Victorian attitude to sexuality whereby sex was not an issue that was openly discussed. This attitude has contributed to the continuing sensitivity which surrounds the concept of sexuality both in everyday life and within health care. If nursing is to move towards a more holistic approach to care, the area of sexuality, and all the difficulties inherent within this, must be addressed. Within this, there is a clear need for nurses to face the challenge of sexuality in their own lives, to enable them to provide more effective care.

Whilst the issues that surround sexuality have for many years been left to the individual and the family, growing interest is now visible within the political arena, as demonstrated through the inclusion of sexual health within the Health of the Nation targets (Department of Health, 1992). However, Hobson (1994) identifies the lack of acknowledgement of older people and their sexuality within this.

This chapter will acknowledge the complex nature of sexuality and sexual health, and in doing this it will address the inter-relationship between these issues and the sexual act. In addition, it will demonstrate that older people are not asexual. This will be underpinned by an exploration of issues that inform and affect clinical practice in the area of nursing older people, including the physiological aspects of sexual health, sexual orientation and altered health status. In addition, the sexual stereotyping of older people not only by themselves but by others, including healthcare professionals, is considered.

WHAT IS SEXUALITY?

In the context of care planning in the area of sexuality, the observations and comments made in nursing records often reveal much more about the attitudes and beliefs of the nurse who has written that part of the document. As a consequence of this there is a need to challenge the nurse's understanding of sexuality, particularly when documentation includes information such as 'patient wears his or her own teeth', that 'their jewellery is in the ward safe' or the section is discarded as 'not applicable'. When considering Roper's view (Roper *et al.*, 1983) that sexuality is an important dimension of personality and behaviour the above responses can only be seen as underestimating the value of this area of a person's life. A number of complex facets exist within the concept of sexuality. These include the following key elements:

1 The capacity to enjoy and control sexual and reproductive behaviour in accordance with a social and personal ethic.
2 Freedom from fear, shame, guilt, false beliefs and other psychological factors inhibiting sexual responses.
3 Freedom from organic disorder, disease and deficiencies that interfere with sexual and reproductive function.

(WHO, 1986)

These elements highlight a number of areas for discussion. As the above suggests, sexuality is more than our sexual orientation, it is about our feelings and relationships with others. Our beliefs, values and lifestyles all reflect a complex range of elements that in turn are based upon personal experiences, including

Whilst acknowledging that we develop at different stages of our lives there are a number of elements that influence this development.

Consider the stages of sexuality development pathway which may have informed the development of today's older individuals, then produce a short list at each stage of factors that may have influenced their sexuality.

	Infant	School years	Adolescent	Adult	Old age
Culture					
Social pressures					
Learnt behaviour					

Discuss your list with a colleague.

You may have identified, amongst other things that babies and young children are often dressed in different colours, i.e. pink and blue, and different styles. In addition, each sex is given different types of toys when young. Figure 7.1 illustrates how culture and learnt behaviour also impact on the development of one's sexuality as one grows older.

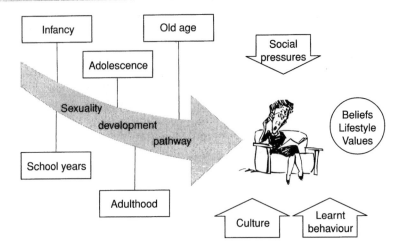

Figure 7.1   Sexuality development.

pressures from others at different times of our lives, and the culture to which we have been exposed. The development of our own individual sexuality is built upon at each stage of our lives, and we expect that our control over stimuli and experiences will be more within our own reach as we age (Fig. 7.1).

Webb (1994) highlights, how during the 20th century, we have seen many changes relating to the concept of sexuality, not least that of increasing sexual freedom. In western cultures, there remains a reluctance to see sexuality as important to older people and at times a clear reticence to discuss sexual issues across generational boundaries. However, Caplan (1991) describes the values placed by eastern cultures upon the concept of sexuality, whereby women are often seen as property to be traded and promised in their younger years.

As already stated, sexuality comprises a number of inter-related facets; whilst sex is what you do, sexual health is often linked to the sexual act. Nurses themselves may find it difficult to discuss such issues as traditionally they have not been educated to address this area. If nurses and other healthcare workers are not aware of their own beliefs and biases, they may be less effective in helping others; this is particularly evident when nurses are faced with situations that are outside their normal experience.

People's perceptions of sexuality, including nurses', can be fundamentally challenged by single-sex relationships. Male homosexuality can be seen as threatening male solidarity, as some men take on what are thought of as female characteristics. Lesbianism is also seen by some men as equally threatening, as the male appears not to be needed. However, two women in a relationship together in old age are more likely to be seen as nothing more than companionship. This failure to acknowledge the sexual nature of their relationship can create difficulties both in terms of sexual and mental health and well-being.

A challenge is often seen when caring for members of the gay community; predictions estimate that there are in excess of 400,000 homosexual men over 60 years of age in England and Wales (Gibson, 1992). This figure should be viewed with caution as many people are heterosexual and homosexual. Opportunistic sexual activity may occur in many settings, but as the individual gets older their

➤9   social networks often become limited. Many are secretive about these sexual pref-

Consider the following outline case profile. What would you do when faced by such a situation, and how might this be affected by your views of sexuality and those of your colleagues?

A 72-year-old gentleman is seen by staff in the nursing home, where he now lives, going up to a fellow male resident and intimately touching him. The staff are shocked, and avoid leaving him unsupervised. He is referred and quickly seen by a local hospital psychologist. He is described as exhibiting inappropriate behaviour.

As a nurse, what action might you take in response to the above situation:

- For the benefit/development of the staff?
- For the older people in that home?

The inappropriate behaviour might be seen as that of the nursing home care staff for not providing privacy, dignity and meeting their clients' needs. The care staff's actions might by some be seen as overzealous, and seriously lacking in communication to both gentlemen. In this situation the nurses may also feel that their own sexuality is challenged. Reflection on each nurse's own feeling to this situation would be essential in order to further develop nursing skills and competence in this area.

erences because they were brought up in the pre-1967 era of illegality, where homosexuality was seen as deviant. As a consequence, they are often less likely to be open about relationships taking part in chance encounters, often in public toilets.

A number of older men visit 'known' public toilets for such encounters. Problems occur when the male lacks mobility or his range of contacts is limited, for example when he is admitted to a nursing or residential home. It is easy to see how men who have sex with men and are still involved in a heterosexual relationship often lack the support and understanding of the gay community or the remainder of society. It is important for healthcare staff to have knowledge and understanding of those with different lifestyles to their own (Weston, 1993).

The inclusion in the 'Health of the Nation' document (Department of Health, 1992) of objectives for sexual health and HIV means that nurses can no longer ignore the above issues. This document provides the impetus for nurses to explore the wider perspectives of sexuality. Hicken (1994) suggests that there is a clear need to identify and overcome both personal and professional barriers to ensure high-quality care is offered relating to sexual health. This is further reinforced when considering the underpinning philosophies of primary nursing and the concept of the named nurse, both of which centre upon the partnership between the nurse and the client. Wright (1988) argues that closed attitudes amongst nurses to different expressions of sexuality might mean in some situations that we are unable to effectively fulfil this partnership.

HISTORICAL LANDMARKS INFLUENCING SEXUALITY IN OLDER PEOPLE

The basis of many older individuals' beliefs regarding sexuality may be placed in an historical context. Whilst a number of interesting landmarks exist, which produce fascinating reading, much of today's stereotyping as expressed by older people originates from Victorian England. Stroy (1989) confirms that for some older individuals the stereotypical images of this time of their lives include one of asexuality. However, whilst many younger individuals may wish to support this perception it is not necessarily a view supported by all older individuals themselves (Hodson and Skeen, 1994). This is made more difficult as often young people provide care in formal health and social care settings.

The Victorian era has clearly made a major impact upon current ideas of sexuality held by many older people. There is a widely held belief that the 20th century witnessed a move from an era of sexual repression to one of permissiveness. Sexuality is now generally seen as a positive force in our lives; consequently, there needs to be a clear challenge to what we within society view as normal for older people. Many older individuals today remember and have their views influenced by the fact that gay relationships were illegal; such individuals were seen as deviant and were not accepted in the armed forces. It is against this backcloth that many older people themselves form and hold stereotypical views (Gibson, 1992).

SEXUAL STEREOTYPING AND OLDER PEOPLE

Older people may sometimes find sexual intercourse difficult either because the woman experiences vaginal discomfort, or the man requires more stimulation to produce an erection. However, in terms of nursing practice there is a need to examine more than the mechanical problems involving the sexual health of older people. Thought should be given towards what constitutes acts of affection and pleasure. The assumption that sexual behaviour and sexuality at this stage of human development is inappropriate, abnormal, repugnant and impossible must be dismissed, particularly as, at times, this leads to older people themselves accepting such ageist constraints without question (Reiss, 1988).

However, with average life expectancy in Britain for both sexes increasing, attitudes towards sexuality and older people are changing. It is difficult for many younger people to imagine their parents, let alone their grandparents, being romantic, making love or having sex. Media campaigns make use of the young to portray and enforce products, supported by makeup and glamour, irrespective of the target audience. There is now a move towards promoting a positive regard for self-worth and esteem in old age. Magazines are making use of older people to promote products, by using many positive images of old age; however, many of these products are solely aimed at the older market.

For older individuals with a learning disability and or mental health problems, issues may well be different as a consequence of previous life experience. Individuals who have learning disabilities may not have experienced sexual relationships nor been encouraged to develop sexuality. This creates the potential for increased difficulties in older life. The nurse working with this group of individuals therefore needs to be aware not only of the stereotypes that exist regarding older people, but also those relating to people who have a learning disability or a mental health need. It is from a comprehensive understanding and assessment of this baseline that the nurse must begin when identifying interventions in support of a person expressing their sexuality.

The implementation of the National Health Service and Community Care Act

(Department of Health, 1990), has challenged the previous *status quo*. This is particularly relevant for those individuals who, in the past would have been admitted to a long-stay ward, but now are able to continue to live within their own home. For these individuals it may be that their social networks are restricted. The development of opportunities to meet new members of the opposite sex produces new challenges for both older individuals and the supporting care staff. It is the responsibility of the nurse to ensure that individuals are encouraged to display feelings. There is a clear need to emphasize that old age and vulnerability do not necessarily go together, but a degree of learned helplessness may be promoted by nursing staff. Challenging underpinning of stereotypes will ultimately improve the status of such marginalized individuals.

➤9

PHYSIOLOGICAL ASPECTS OF SEXUALITY RELATING TO AGEING

There is a need to promote a positive image of growing old; however, what are often the inevitable effects of ageing upon the human body are viewed by some as an indication of moving towards a state of decrepitude. It is the normal effects of ageing and how they are perceived by the individual that may affect their image of their sexuality. Degenerative changes along with the effects of ageing linked to the reproductive organs may be viewed as having a primary and secondary effect on sexuality. Whilst the primary effects are those that directly influence the reproductive organs, secondary issues are those which relate to other body structures which in turn may influence the individual's view of themselves, their image and in turn their sexuality.

◄1

The female reproductive system ages ahead of any of the other body systems. It has been found that a decreased level of oestrogen leads to a shrinking of the female sexual organs, particularly the uterus and fallopian tubes, along with drying and keratinization in the vaginal outlet. In the mammary glands there is a loss of adipose tissue, coupled with degenerative changes in the connective tissue. This also leads to the development of drooping flaccid breasts (Kennedy, 1989). The menopause often occurs over a span of several years, usually between the ages of 45 and 60.

Men do not normally experience a sudden decline in reproductive function compared to the menopause in women. It has been found that sperm production reduces with age, particularly after the age of 50, along with its viability and motility. Despite the number of sperm being reduced by 30%, males often retain the ability to be fertile up to the age of 80 (Christian and Grzybowski, 1993).

One change often seen in males is the enlargement of the prostate gland along with a significant decrease in prostate secretions. The contractability of prostate muscle also reduces, leading to an inability to force the remaining secretions into the urethra. Micturition problems such as a poor urine stream, regular and frequent voiding patterns of small amounts of urine are often early indications of deterioration of the prostate gland. This may lead to a reluctance by such older individuals to get involved in sexual activity and to a perceived loss of personal sexual worth.

A number of features may be regarded as having a secondary role in relation to the expression of a person's sexuality. In old age, changes in these areas may include:

- Reduction of skin elasticity
- Reduction of hearing
- Altered body posture and gait
- Changes in hair colour
- Loss of hair
- Loss of teeth

◀1; ▶12; ■ Reduced levels of sensations

Although the climacteric is not a universal phenomenon, most women and even men experience a range of symptoms in the years immediately after the menopause. For women, these symptoms include vasomotor instability, most commonly described as hot flushes. This may also be coupled with outbursts of sweating, tachycardia and chills. Physical phenomena may at times be coupled with episodes of mental ill-health, including emotional outbursts, bouts of depression, and less frequently, withdrawal from the family. The later stages of life place a challenge upon an individual's perceptions of their sexuality. Warmth, affection and companionship are accepted rather than the sexual act as an approach to meeting their own needs and those of partners.

ALTERED HEALTH STATES AND SEXUALITY

◀1

Whilst a number of changes that occur in later life may be physiologically based, there is a need to consider the adjustments an individual may need to make to cope with altered body image. This is compounded by the belief of many older people that 'if I am old, sexual dysfunction can only be expected'. The arena of sexual health as an inter-related component of sexuality raises a number of key issues for individuals in old age (Figure 7.2). These include issues to do with youth culture, and the effect this has on an individual's self-esteem. In addition, the physical and psychological adjustment that people may have to make, as a result of acquired disability, need to be considered.

Examples of such adjustments may include living with colostomies, mastectomies and indwelling urinary catheters. Whilst key information is made available about the working and maintenance of such prostheses, careful support is needed for the individual in adapting their life activities and should also be made available to their partner.

An example of an area where the above assumptions need to be challenged is the myth that incontinence produces a loss of sexuality and sexual activity. Where nurses do not have a positive regard for individuals, a lack of dignity and respect may develop. This may adversely affect the ability of nurses to work effectively with older people and their partners. Older people and their partners can, with imagination and determination, create a number of different approaches to coping with incontinence, so that they may retain a sexual relationship. A solution includes the folding back of the urinary catheter and covering both this and the penis with the sheath.

A further area where caution is needed is with individuals who have heart disease, and their resulting lifestyle. Heart disease should not be seen as a barrier to sexual activity in old age, neither should it be viewed as an opportunity to con-

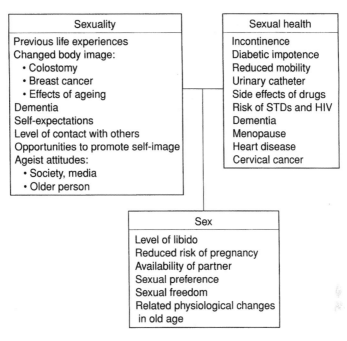

Figure 7.2 Influencing factors in old age.

firm debilitation upon an individual. Care should, however, be taken to reduce the level of exertion experienced during such an activity.

The notion of asexuality may also be seen when educating individuals following gynaecological operations. Whilst the need for individuals' education following such surgical intervention is well accepted, this is not always related to all age groups. Booth (1990) found that nurses working in such specialist areas did not always provide older people with the same advice, particularly relating to sexual health and sexual functioning, as younger age groups, believing that it was irrelevant.

Further challenges to what can be done and what is permissible in terms of maintaining sexual health centre on the use of polypharmacy for multisystem problems. Those involved in the care of older people will readily acknowledge the existence of polypharmacy for a range of multisystem problems. What is often less evident is the range of common side effects that may be experienced which affect an individual's sexual function. Many may impinge less directly upon sexuality; these include corticosteroids that will alter an individual's

Great emphasis is placed upon the role of nurses in the promotion of health. However, it has been noted that much supportive material is written with a focus upon younger age groups.

Look around your area of work at the health promotion advice information leaflets and booklets that are available. Identify the material that:

- Is produced specifically for older people
- Is produced for all ages, but has a specific section that relates to older people
- How much of the information relates to sexual health and older people?

appearance, and hence self-image. One surprising inclusion in the range of drugs that may affect an individual sexually is digoxin, as it is claimed, particularly in long-term use, that it may alter an individual's testosterone level (Rousseau, 1986). The following list includes a range of drugs which can affect a person's sexual health, and may lead to impotence:

- Antihypertensives
- Betablockers (especially propanolol)
- Bendroflurizide
- Methyldopa
- Reserprine
- Spironolactone

Webb (1985) does, however, attempt to balance the perspective on drugs and sexual drive by concluding that the suppression of the symptoms of illness can contribute to enhanced feelings of well-being and improved self-image by restoring the body image to a more positive one. Possibly one of the main mental ill-health scenarios to be linked with sexual problems is endogenous depression. Loss of libido is an early sign observed in depression and is one of the last symptoms to be resolved. This might in part be due to a general lack of feelings of well-being, but they may also be linked to the chemical changes that occur in the brain (Bancroft, 1983). Other illness-related manifestations include mania or hypomania which might increase sexual drive, but not necessarily sexual functioning.

Impairment of sexual desire and performance has been linked to most of the psychotropic drugs, such as phenothiazines and haloperidol. It is seen as difficult to separate out the effects due to the psychiatric condition and those originating from therapeutic drug regimes.

An area in which notable inroads are being made to address sexuality in old age is that of impotence in diabetes. It has been estimated that up to 50% of men with long-standing diabetes will go on to develop impotence. It has been found that few men seek help despite attending clinics regularly, although several treatments are now available (Mackinnon, 1993). Impotence is often seen as a hidden problem but may be the cause of many marital difficulties. Failure to gain an erection may be due to nerve damage, poor circulation or psychological factors. After assessment, treatment options often utilize a range of interventions which includes counselling, vacuum devices, self-injections of 'Papaverine' and penile implants. The enthusiasm and creativity demonstrated in the area of impotence and individuals with diabetes are a lesson for other areas of nursing.

ETHICAL ISSUES

Nurses who are involved in the care of older people may find themselves presented with both moral and ethical dilemmas as a result of a lack of clear guidelines. A number of such issues surround sexuality and sexual health. The emergence of the human immunodeficiency virus (HIV) and acquired immunodeficiency (AIDS) has led to individuals in all age ranges being challenged as to their sexuality. Many older people, despite having a high-risk life style may not be seen as at risk to HIV or AIDS either by society or themselves. HIV is clearly an 'equal opportunities' virus that will infect any social class and age group who place themselves at a risk (Pratt, 1995). Although the median age range of diagnosis is around 30 years of age, people over the age of 55 years of age contract the virus in small but significant numbers. It has been estimated that 10% of all those known to be infected by the virus in the UK are over 50 years of age (Rickard, 1995), though it is difficult to obtain a realistic picture of HIV and AIDS within this age group. It might, however, be reasonably predicted that this level could increase as the population itself ages, coupled with the potentially increasing life expectancy of someone with HIV, due in part to developing drug regimes (Sims and Moss, 1995).

An additional indication of 'unsafe' sexual activity in older people can be seen in the level of attendances for sexually transmitted diseases at departments of genito-urinary medicine. Butler (1993) identified that 242 patients aged 60 or above attended such clinics in two south of England cities in 1988–89. These figures may be due in part to older people themselves adopting a view of 'why bother, we are getting old anyway' and not accessing healthcare advice and support. This issue necessitates nursing interventions that not only challenge such a false belief but also inform older people. Whilst older people may feel that they are not in an age range or participating in activities where they may find or place themselves at risk of contracting HIV and other sexually transmitted diseases, it has been found as a result of these beliefs many individuals are participating in unprotected sex (Hinkle, 1991). As a result, healthcare professionals must challenge the myth that sexually transmitted diseases only affect younger age groups. The perpetuation of this belief is both incorrect and dangerous, and older people may find themselves in situations where they might be both infected and affected by any of these diseases (Allers, 1990).

Debates that focus upon the costs of care for older people also relate to the sexuality arena, with questions asked regarding the provision of such care being value for money. The provision of impotency clinics for older people with diabetes is one example. It is important for the practitioner to consider their own role when providing care; this may particularly require them to review their ◄4 position on advocacy. An extensive debate is needed to clarify thinking and views within nursing regarding this topic. What might be considered as standard good practice by one individual may be an area that requires the implementation of advocacy to improve choices and care by another. For each exponent of the view that nurses routinely act as advocates for clients, there is an equally strong supporter of the opinion that independent advocates are required and are the only realistic way forward.

A lack of understanding can also lead to the individual's health being placed at risk where healthcare professionals do not appreciate different lifestyles and the resulting health issues. Nurses are in a position to assist the older person in making adjustments; this might include a review of feelings towards a lifestyle or risk activities (Kaufman, 1993). The older person may remain sexually active by paying for sex, from prostitutes or rent boys. This may be due to the loss of a partner or partner's sex drive. Additionally it might be seen that the older person is linked to multiple partners of the same sex. Coupled to this might be a low self-esteem, resulting in a lack of assertiveness regarding safer sex with casual partners.

However, it is often the need to come to terms with the sexual orientation of a younger family member that proves most challenging. Older individuals may not understand prevention campaigns aimed at the young as they do not invoke a frame of reference for relating messages to their own lifestyle. Consequently

Mr Williams is 68 years of age and has strict moral views based in part on his religious and family upbringing. He entered the army for National Service and stayed on, working his way through the ranks, until he left 12 years later as a sergeant. His wife died two years ago, since then he has remained single, enjoying independence.

Mr Williams's upbringing and life to date has been strict, and in an area that is not supportive of individuals with a marginalized lifestyle.

Following the death of his wife, Mr Williams is now beginning to consider the possibility of a new partner. For Mr Williams, part of this process of finding someone able to share his life in the way that his wife had done may necessitate 'playing the field'.

■ What health promotion advice would you give to Mr Williams?
■ How would you maximize the possibility that Mr Williams would listen to the information you provided, considering his strict upbringing?

there is a need to target older people with health promotion and health education material. It might be found that a same-sex relationship in old age acknowledges latent feelings that are only now given opportunities to come to the fore (Waltz, 1987). The latter may well be a challenge to staff within community and continuing care settings. Rose and Platzer (1993) highlight the need for health and social care staff to be more aware and understanding of the different lifestyles where a same-sex relationship is adopted. A lack of such knowledge can lead to inappropriate questions being asked during nursing assessments.

PRACTICAL APPLICATIONS

We must not lose sight of the fact that sex is good for all of us, including older people. Persson (1980) found that older men and women who remained sexually active slept better, were more relaxed and had a better level of mental activity. Women retained their previous levels of emotional stability, experienced lower levels of anxiety and generally had better mental health.

Requests made to either health or social care agencies to fund such activities could present a fundamental challenge, not only to the individual professional but also to the organization. Nurses need to have addressed their own feelings and beliefs in this area in order to work with the individual concerned in a positive and non-judgemental manner, particularly as such situations may result in a nurse having both a personal and professional dilemma. From a professional perspective it is essential to balance the motivation to care for an individual with the professional safeguards outlined within the Code of Conduct (UKCC, 1992).

There is a need to return to the original concept of sexuality which addressed three elements, that of sexuality, sexual health and the process of sex itself, all of which are inter-related and cannot be considered alone. There is a need to consider our own area of practice, reflecting upon both practices and policies but more pointedly reviewing our own beliefs.

Durie (1987) asserts that anyone involved in the care of patients should ensure that they are aware of all the effects of any given therapy, and supports the view that sexuality is as much an aspect of well-being as having a stable personality or a normal blood pressure.

Review your own area of work and consider in what way sexuality is both positively and negatively addressed:

	Staff	Clients
Attitudes		
Care practices		
Information leaflets		
Health issues		

Discuss your responses with a colleague, then develop an action plan for overcoming at least one of the negative areas identified.

Activities in the clinical area should include the following.

An audit should be completed in relation to meeting the needs of clients in relation to sexuality. This should consider aspects such as care planning and ageist attitudes held by staff and the organization. Whilst a model may underpin the philosophy and approach to care delivery, a key question is whether it includes sexuality.

It is important to determine your colleagues' understanding of the concept of sexuality. It might be necessary to take time to ensure that they appreciate the issues that surround sex, sexual health and sexuality that relate to clients. This may include developing action plans and agreed protocols for situations that the team may reasonably expect to meet relating to sexual health.

There has been an increase in recent years in the number of educational events available to nurses and social care staff. A clear need exists for both commissioners of such events and educationalists to ensure relevant sexuality issues are reflected in the indicative content of such events.

Whilst acknowledging the role played by nurses in promoting health, there is a need to review literature handed out to clients for its equity and appropriateness to older people. Large-print leaflets that include pictures of older people would emphasize the relevance to such an age group. Additionally the content should be reviewed and adjusted if needed to include sexuality issues and the older person .

A strong case must be made for the inclusion of sexual history, as appropriate, during the routine admission assessment. To do this, nurses need to be much better equipped with the appropriate knowledge and expertise (BOR, 1994). This should lead to a reduction in embarrassment by both the nurse and the client, coupled with a heightened thoroughness of the admission assessment, ensuring that issues are not omitted and that an accurate diagnosis is reached.

An issue to explore in a clinical area is the environment in which such an assessment interview might be conducted. Effort must be made to retain confidentiality (UKCC, 1996). One might be described as optimistic in supporting the view that nurses are comfortable with their own sexuality and discussing issues of sexuality with others. There is a clear need for the nurse not to be seen as a sex therapist, but rather as a professional who is able to combine sexuality and sexual health into a holistic assessment schema when caring for clients. The skilled assessment can then be transferred into appropriate interactions centred on teaching and counselling that must be seen as the cornerstone of all nursing practice.

CONCLUSION

When considering sexuality it might not be seen to command the same urgency as areas such as tissue viability and continence promotion, both of which may save money when implemented effectively. The discussion surrounding sexuality in general and more specifically relating to older people persists. To continue to fail to address individual's sexuality leads to their basic human rights being ignored and older people not being respected and valued (Jones, 1994). This chapter has focused upon discussing what is meant by sexuality, psychological and physical changes have been considered alongside stereotypical images of sexuality in old age. The impact of body image and acquired disability has been identified as an important factor in a person's perception of their sexual health. The ethical dilemmas that face nurses as a consequence of gay and lesbian relationships, dignity and privacy and sexually transmitted diseases have been highlighted. It is hoped that this chapter has provided some practical strategies to facilitate nurses in empowering clients in terms of their sexuality and sexual health.

FURTHER READING

Caplan, P. (1997) The Cultural Construction of Sexuality. Routledge, London.
Addresses the background of sexuality based on culture; a good general overview that attempts to grapple with concepts from a social anthropology perspective.

Hicken, I. (1994) *Sexual Health Education and Training*. English National Board, London.
Can only be described as compulsory reading for those engaged in the provision and commissioning of education. A useful structure to guide the inclusion of sexuality and sexual health within education programmes. An interesting element is the worked-through older person component based upon the model provided.

Pratt, R. (1995) *HIV–AIDS: a Strategy for Nursing Care*. Edward Arnold, London.
An interesting overview of HIV/AIDS drawing on current literature in the UK and Europe. Regarded as a set text for those exploring HIV/AIDS.

Savage, J. (1995) *Nursing Intimacy*. Scutari, London.
Chapters 7 and 8 have interesting accounts of the unspoken skills of nurses, relating to the therapeutic effectiveness of nurses' interactions with patients, including symbolism and the need by all for personal space.

Webb, C. (1994) *Living Sexuality, Issues for Nursing and Health*. Scutari, London.
Contains an interesting and easy-to-read chapter on historical landmarks of sexuality.

REFERENCES

Allers, C. (1990) AIDS and the older adult. *Gerontologist,* **30**(3), 405–407.

Bancroft, J. (1983) *Human Sexuality and Its Problems.* Churchill Livingstone, Edinburgh.

Booth, B. (1990) Does it really matter at that age? *Nursing Times,* **86**(3), 50–52.

Bor, R. and Lewis, S. (1994) Are sexual issues discussed with patients? *Nursing Times,* **90**(49), 11.

Butler, R.N. (1993) AIDS: older people are not immune. *Geriatrics* **48**(3), 9–10.

Caplan, P. (1991) *The Cultural Construction of Sexuality.* Routledge, London.

Christiansen, J. and Grzybowski J. (1993) *Biology of Ageing.* Mosby, Toronto.

Department of Health (1990) *National Health Service and Community Care Act.* HMSO, London.

Department of Health (1992) *Health of the Nation – Sexual Health.* DoH, London.

Durie, B. (1987) Drugs and sexual function. *Nursing Times,* **83**(32), 34–35.

Gibson, H. (1992) *The Emotional and Sexual Lives of Older People.* Chapman & Hall, London.

Hicken, I. (1994) *Sexual Health Education and Training.* ENB, London.

Hinkle, K.L. (1991) A literature review: HIV seropositivity in the elderly. *Journal of Gerontological Nursing,* Oct 1991(10), 12–17.

Hobson, K. (1994) The effects of ageing upon sexuality. *Health and Social Work,* **9**(1), 25–35.

Hodson, D. and Skeen, P. (1994) Sexuality and ageing, the hamerlock of myths. *Journal of Applied Gerontology,* **13**(3), 219–235.

Jones, H. (1994) Mores and morals. *Nursing Times,* **90**(47) 54–58.

Kaufman, T. (1993) A crisis of silence: HIV, AIDS and older people. Age Concern Greater London.

Kennedy, R. (1989) *Physiology of Ageing.* Year Book Medical Publications, Chicago.

Mackinnon, M. (1993) *Providing Diabetic Care in General Practice.* Class Publishing, London.

Persson, G. (1980) Sexuality in a 70 year old urban population. *Journal of Psychosomatic Research,* **24**, 335–342.

Pratt, R. (1995) *HIV–AIDS: a Strategy for Nursing Care.* Edward Arnold, London.

Rickard, W. (1995) HIV/AIDS and older people. *Generations Review,* **5**(3), 2–6.

Reiss, B. (1988) The long lived person and sexuality. *Dynamic Psychotherapy,* **6**(1), 79–86.

Roper, N., Logan, W. and Tierney, A. (1983) *Elements in Nursing.* Churchill Livingstone, Edinburgh.

Rose, P. and Platzer, H. (1993) Confronting prejudice. *Nursing Times,* **89**(31), 52–53.

Rousseau, P. (1986) Sexual changes and impotence in elderly men. *American Family Physician,* **34**(5), 131–136.

Sims, R. and Moss, J. (1995) *Palliative Care for People with AIDS,* 2nd edn. Edward Arnold, London.

Stroy, M. (1989) Knowledge and attitudes about the sexuality of older adults among retirement home residents. *Educational Gerontology,* **15**(5), 515–526.

UKCC (1992) *Code of Professional Conduct.* UKCC, London.

UKCC (1996) *Confidentiality Guidelines.* UKCC, London.

Waltz, T. and Blum, N. (1987) *Sexual Health in Later Life.* Lexington Books.

Webb, C. (1994) *Living Sexuality, Issues for Nursing and Health.* Scutari, London.

Webb, C. (1985) *Sexuality, Nursing and Health.* Wiley, London.

Weston, A. (1993) Challenging assumptions. *Nursing Times,* **89**(18), 16–29.

WHO (1986) *Concepts for Sexual Health.* EUR/ICP/MCH 521. WHO, Copenhagen.

Wright, S. (1988) *Nursing the Older Patient.* Harper and Row, New York.

8 Religious and spiritual needs of older people

Aru Narayanasamy

INTRODUCTION

This chapter introduces the concept of spirituality and its significance to older people. Within this an examination of the differences between spirituality and religion and a review of personal growth and development related to spirituality is offered. In addition, an explanation of the spiritual and cultural needs of older people is provided by the use of case studies. An outline of skills development for spiritual care as a preparation for meeting older people's spiritual needs is included. Finally, the nurse's role in preparing the older person and their family for death is highlighted. Throughout the chapter various activities are provided for readers to appraise their thoughts related to spirituality, particularly in relation to older people.

SPIRITUALITY

Today's society is a secular one in which it would appear that each generation has successfully tried to build a way of life and morality as if there were no God or spiritual transcendent. In such a secular world, the preoccupation tends to be on material and tangible things that are immediately available. Concern for the spiritual aspects of person, things that are sacred and eternal, is likely to receive less attention in a world dominated by technological advances and expectations of immediate results. However, religion is still active and well for many people and there is evidence to suggest that even in most secular countries, there is a revival in the spiritual side of life (Reid, 1992). The spiritual dimensions of individuals' lives can be significant; spirituality is expressed in a variety of forms and some individuals find that their religion acts as a medium for expressing it. Human life is governed by social, psychological, physical and spiritual influences.

SPIRITUALITY AND RELIGION

Before proceeding any further with this discussion, it is necessary to examine the differences between spirituality and religion. The concepts of spirituality and religion that emerged when an ideas storming session was carried out are shown in Table 8.1.

Some people draw only small differences between the meaning of 'religion' and 'spirituality', but most people identify many significant differences as noted in Table 8.1. The word religion tends to create images in our minds of external things like buildings, religious officials and public rituals such as baptisms, weddings, or funerals. Indeed, for some people these are the times when they come in contact with something to do with religion, with or without a deeper religious significance. In contrast, 'spirituality' is usually much more abstract, including areas such as the meaning of life, love, humanity, inner peace, tranquillity, meditation, a relationship, individuality, personal worth and so on. These are discussed later within this chapter.

Spirituality is seen as a subjective dimension, implicit in nature, inward and to do with feelings and experiences, a personal entity, and a form of journey. On the other hand, religion is seen as a concrete dimension that is explicit and outward, related to objective things like institutions. For some people religion is a mode of transport for their spiritual journey.

TABLE 8.1	*Religion/spirituality*
Religion	**Spirituality**
God	Beliefs affecting one's life
Church	and how it relates to others
Cathedrals	Something not necessarily religious
Temples	Purpose and meaning of life
Mosques	A source of strength
Doctrines	At peace with oneself
Fanatics	Inner peace
Beliefs	A feeling of security
Church hierarchy	Love and to be loved
Clergy	Self-esteem
Prayer/worship	Inner self
Spiritual leaders	Inner strength
Prophets	Searching
Holy books	Coping
Rituals	Hope
The Cross	Trusting relationship
A way of life	
Baptism	
Weddings	
Funerals	
Songs	
Conflicts	
Rules	

What is spirituality?

From the above discussion one can surmise that spirituality is a multi-dimensional word that defies simple definition. The word spirituality is used widely in the caring context, but despite its common usage there would not appear to be a single authorative definition of it, although a variety of explanations are offered in the emerging literature on this subject.

The Oxford Concise Dictionary (OUP, 1990) defines the word spiritual as:

1. Concerning the spirit as opposed to matter,
2. Concerned with sacred or religious things; holy; divine; inspired (the spiritual life; spiritual songs),
3. (of the mind, etc.) refined, sensitivity, not concerned with material,
4. (of a relationship, etc.) concerned with the soul or spirit etc., not with external reality.

Dictionary definitions are useful when used in the appropriate context, but less valuable when used in isolation. However, Murray and Zentner (1989) offer workable definitions of spirituality and religion (Box 8.1).

BOX 8.1	*Definitions of spirituality and religion (Murray and Zentner, 1989)*

Spirituality

Spirituality is a quality that goes beyond religious affiliation, that strives for inspiration, reverence, awe, meaning and purpose, even in those who do not believe in any God. The spiritual dimension tries to be in harmony with the universe, strives for answers about the infinite, and comes into focus when the person faces emotional stress, physical illness or death (p. 259).

The above definition is relevant to nursing because it is almost comprehensive enough to offer a workable understanding of the spiritual dimension. It is also practical enough to apply to secular and religious contexts related to caregiving relationships. This definition enables us to appreciate that not only believers but non-believers also have spiritual needs. In contrast, Murray and Zentner define religion as follows.

Religion

A belief in a supernatural or divine force that has power over the universe and commands worship and obedience; a system of beliefs; a comprehensive code of ethics or philosophy; a set of practices that are followed; a church affiliation; the conscious pursuit of any object the person holds as supreme (p. 259).

SPIRITUALITY AS A UNIVERSAL DIMENSION

Spirituality can be described as a universal phenomenon in that the capacity for spirituality belongs to all of us. Even the non-religious person, as depicted in Murray and Zentner's definition of spirituality, sometimes exhibits something of the serenity and inward peace which are especially characteristic of those who tend to be religious.

The spiritual dimension motivates us to make sense of the meaningless world we are born into. Indeed, Macquarie (1972) claims that the spiritual person is one who has made sense of the meaningless world and has learned to be at home in the universe by deriving a certain serenity and inward peace. It is implied from this that people in their endeavour to make sense of their world have developed this extra dimension, that is, spirituality. As part of the search for meaning, some people try to find answers to the irrational and meaningless world through religious faiths. This includes spirituality as embracing spiritual life and its activities such as prayer, worship and whatever practices are associated with its development.

According to Macquarie (1972) our motivation to seek meaning and purpose renders us as distinct beings and sets us apart from other physical organisms. In other words, we as individuals, are made up of the body, mind and spirit. In regard to this Macquarie writes:

> We do not relate to other people as if they were only objects that we could see and hear and touch or even as if they were simply living organisms from which reactions could be evoked. We relate to them as persons, and we talk about them or talk to them in a language appropriate to persons. What makes the difference between a person and an animal is not itself something that is to be seen. It is the inevitable 'extra dimension' ... and as we attribute to other beings as well. It is this range of experience that is distinctive of the human being and that we call 'spirit' (p. 46).

The existential view is that an individual becomes a spiritual person when one has made sense of this meaningless world and has learned to be at home in the universe by deriving certain serenity and inward peace. In other words, people in their endeavour to make sense of their world have developed this extra dimension, that is, spirituality. Macquarie's (1972) position on spirituality strengthens the assertion in nursing that spirituality is a holistic notion (Narayanasamy, 1991).

Spirituality as a holistic notion

Spirituality prevails as a holistic notion in healthcare in the sense that an individual is made up of the body, mind and spirit, and that these components are interconnected and interdependent (Stallwood, 1981; Carson, 1989; Shelly and Fish, 1988). The word 'holism' was first used by Jan Christian Smuts (1926), a South African philosopher and politician, in the early part of the century. Holism relates to the study of whole organism or whole system, its spelling derived from the Greek word *holos* meaning 'whole'. In applying it to the western healthcare context, it may be seen as an approach that incorporates the inter-relationships between all aspects of bodily functions and psycho-social functions in a sort of multifaceted approach to the human being.

Holism in both senses means that there is now a drift from the ideas proposed by Descartes who claimed that, in order to study the body as a machine, it could be broken down into its component parts (Bradshaw, 1994).

If holism is accepted in terms of the above perspectives, then it can be suggested that there is a need to study the whole being, and the manner in which the body, mind and spirit interact.

In developing spirituality as a holistic notion in nursing, Stallwood (1981) illustrates its holistic features in her conceptual model of the nature of a person. Unlike Cartesian dualism, Stallwood (1981) explains, in the classical tradition, that an individual as an integrated whole is made up of the body, mind (psycho-social) and spirit, and that these components are dynamically woven together, one part affecting and being affected by the other parts. Figure 8.1 depicts an adaptation of a model developed by Stallwood (1981) as an illustration of a person's wholeness. The person is, and functions as, a dynamic whole. This is depicted in the model by the broken lines and arrows. The body influences, and is influenced by, the psycho-social dimension of the person expressed itself through the body, the biological dimension. The spirit expresses itself through the total being – the psycho-social and biological dimensions.

Unlike Stallwood, Gorham (1989) developed a five-component person model. This model portrays a person as being made up of five of different aspects – the mental, the physical, the social, the emotional, and the spiritual – the interactions are so closely related that they are almost inseparable. The spiritual dimension is the most difficult one to recognize. The interactions of these five components are illustrated in Figure 8.2.

The two models of spirituality presented above appear to demonstrate the holistic nature of this concept.

Further evidence exists in the nursing literature that spirituality is seen as an all-embracing dimension. In developing the holistic notion of health, some theorists have described spirituality as a sacred journey (Mische, 1982); the essence or live principle of a person (Collinton, 1981); the experience of the radical truth of things (Legere, 1984); a belief that relates a person to the world (Soeken and Carson, 1987); giving meaning and purpose in life (Legere, 1984); a life relationship or a sense of connection with mystery, Higher Power, God or Universe (Granstrom, 1985).

So far, we have seen spirituality a universal dimension from a holistic per-spective; however, Hay (1987, 1994) implies that this view is not comprehensive

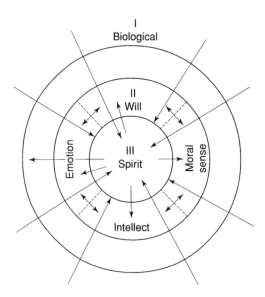

Figure 8.1   Holistic model of the nature of a person.

enough. He asserts that present holistic approach does not include the biological basis of spirituality. By this default of the biological roots of spirituality, any definition of it is not comprehensive enough and therefore cannot be truly holistic in nature.

There is emerging evidence from research studies (Hay, 1987, 1994; Hardy, 1979) to suggest that spirituality is an innate biological dimension which frequently emerges during personal crises. Hay and Hardy, both biologists, view spirituality in the sense of spiritual awareness, i.e. the numinous and mystical states. Using the evolutionary theory, they postulate that spiritual awareness is an innate thing and that it is a universal and everlasting phenomenon because of its survival value. In the light of their research findings related to people's

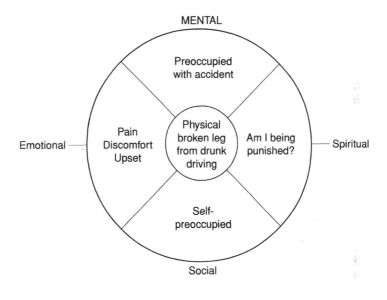

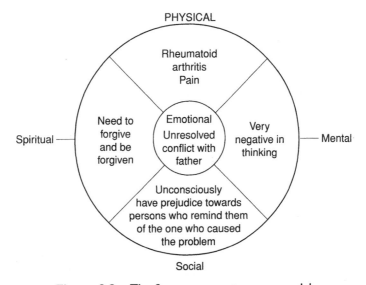

Figure 8.2   The five-component person model.

experience of spiritual awareness they postulate that this has been necessary for the survival of the human species through the natural process of evolution.

Although Hay and Hardy use the concept of spirituality interchangeably with religion, their studies have generated interesting findings. National surveys (Hardy, 1966; Hay, 1987) show a trend that about half of the British adult population would claim they are spiritually or religiously aware from time to time. Further studies (Hay, 1994) boost this figure to about two thirds when there is the opportunity to build trust, that is, when respondents feel confident to trust others to reveal their personal and private experiences. This was borne out by the pilot phase of one study where patients' trust in the interviewer prompted them to reveal intimate details about their spirituality and spiritual concerns (Narayanasamy, 1995).

All of the experiences outlined above are forms of spirituality; that is, being aware of oneself in a holistic relationship with the rest of reality, which in religious experience implies an awareness of God. This spiritual experience is presented in the literature as 'mystical states' (James, 1902; Stace, 1960) and 'numinous' (Otto, 1950).

Hay (1987) suggests that the evidence from comparative religions is that literally anything or any occasion can be associated with a sudden moment of religious awareness or 'herophany'. Records exist of such moments 'during childbirth, at the point of death, during sexual intercourse, at a meal, during fasting, in a Cathedral, on a rubbish dump, on a mountain top, in a slum, in association with a particular plan, stone, fish, mammal, bird and so on ad infinitum' (Hay, 1987, p. 207). In this respect, there is basis in Laski's (1961) suggestion that there are special 'triggers' for experiencing spiritual awareness that is mystical in nature. However, it appears that the British culture does tend to teach us to associate transcendental experience with particular occasions and place.

Interestingly enough, research by Hay (1987) has consistently suggested that people who claimed to have undergone spiritual experience(s) appear to be:

- Calmer and stable
- Finding meaning in their lives
- Concerned with issues of social justice
- Tolerant of others
- Less materialistic
- Less status conscious
- Less likely than others to be racially prejudiced

Spirituality as a culturally universal phenomenon

We are all capable of experiencing spiritual awareness, regardless of our cultural background. However, the way we experience this may differ according to our cultural orientation. Many of us, although capable of experiencing spiritual awareness, tend to shut it out because of social, cultural and psychological conditioning. Some of the explanations for this conditioning process are given below.

In secular societies, the material aspects of life are given greater priority and all our efforts are placed on achieving material wealth to improve the economic position and status (Carson, 1989; Hay, 1987; Narayanasamy, 1991).

However, a very large number of people do experience spiritual awareness in a secular society such as Britain: many feel uneasy when they find themselves to hold an opinion or belief that radically differs from that of the people around them. One way of coping with spiritual experience is to repress it out of consciousness altogether, because it conflicts too violently with our social and moral convictions.

In certain cultures that have a welcoming attitude towards the spiritual aspects of the human consciousness, the following may happen: someone brought up in a western Christian tradition may be enabled to develop this spiritual awareness to maturity. In other words, a more spiritual way of life through religious guidance, public rituals like attendances at church services, or private meditation may enable such an individual to lay open to the divine. Conversely, if one is brought up, for example in the Hindu tradition, it is believed that one can reach the ultimate reality through personal devotion (Bakti) to God (Brahman).

STAGES OF HUMAN DEVELOPMENT AND SPIRITUALITY

Certain spiritual needs feature at different times during an individual's development and growth. It is important to bear in mind that life may not develop in a logical and organized way, as individuals, depending upon their individual capacity, develop in their own individual way. The capacity to develop spiritually is universal in the human species (Hay, 1987). It is argued that because spirituality is an innate dimension due to its biological roots, as discussed earlier, its growth is accelerated from conception. For example, there is also evidence to suggest that the 'oceanic' type of mystical state experienced in mental health crisis has its origins in the internal environment of the mother's womb (Horton, 1973). Indeed, Horton hypothesizes that some people attempt to prevent suicide by inducing this kind of spiritual experience, that is, to evoke the 'oceanic [mystical] experience'. Through this 'oceanic experience' one derives the comfort, safety, serenity, and security once experienced in the mother's womb.

A discussion of the stages of human growth and development follows in order to demonstrate the spiritual journey that older people had undertaken. This includes infancy, childhood, adolescence, young adulthood, middle years and old age.

During infancy, trust is a major spiritual need, and during childhood individuals learn to understand concepts about religion from their parents and people close to them. A child could react with fear sometimes as a response to spiritual needs. Such fear may include sudden movements, loud voices, loss of support, pain, apprehension about strangers or strange objects, heights, or anticipated unpleasant situations. Unmet needs for love and close security may manifest as those fears and meeting the infant's need for basic trust has an impact on spiritual development.

Childhood is a developmental period when one learns to understand religious concepts from parents and other people in his/her environment. Inquisitiveness may prevail when the child may ask questions about basic issues of life, for example, 'What is God?', 'Why doesn't Thomas have a Christmas tree?' and 'Why did granny go to Heaven?'.

The need for love and security is an important feature of spirituality in childhood. This sets the foundation for the development of a trusting relationship and indeed the basis for healthy relationships at later stages of life. We learn and internalize beliefs and values from people we trust during our childhood. The child is likely to imitate his/her parent's faith, and some of his/her concepts of faith may also be based on fantasy.

In childhood one learns moral values, that is, what is 'good' or 'bad' from parents and other significant people. During crisis, say the death of a member of family, the child often has a great difficulty with verbal expression of his/her spiritual concerns. The child does not understand that death is universal, inevitable and irreversible.

In adolescence the search for meaning and value may feature as a part of one's spirituality. People around the individual are useful sources of help and support during this development. The adolescent may experience confusion and act in conflicting ways if this individual is not adequately supported to seek meaning and purpose during this crucial period of development. During adolescence, peer groups act as a useful source of strength and support. Therefore, a stable and supportive environment is necessary for the adolescent's need for the search for meaning and value as part of their spiritual development.

During young adulthood one seeks for trust, love, hope and forgiveness. At this stage of development there may be an experience of tension, expectation and spiritual struggle. It is also a transitional period in which restructuring of religious, moral and ethical values may take place. So this may be the period where reorientation and growth in the spiritual realm takes shape.

In middle years, the questioning of life precipitated by the death of parents or peers, children leaving home, plans for retirement, or an awareness of one's failings may feature. According to Narayanasamy (1991) the four common features of spirituality in middle age are:

■ The need for meaning and purpose in life
■ The need to be forgiven
■ The need to receive love
■ The need for hope and creativity

In old age many take a stock of one's life's successes and failures together with a renewal of religious faith and spiritual beliefs. This is particularly evident within the area of self-esteem and self-actualization. Many older people experience a more positive self-concept (self-esteem and self-image) as a result of feelings of accomplishment and worth (self-actualization). Consequently, many may find great social and spiritual fulfilment in having some kind of religious affiliation. For example, Christian religious ceremonies such as marriages, baptism and burials may become significant. Religious expressions and rituals may be fulfilled by attendance at the church or place of worship. Church or religious affiliation promotes feelings of hope and purpose to life for many older people.

SPIRITUALITY AND CULTURE

The ways in which older people express their spirituality may be based upon their cultural roots or upbringing, this may be reflected in their religious orientations. As pointed out earlier, believers find that their religions are important media for expressing their spirituality. Older people reflect the cultural variations of their society in the way that they practice their religions. Within a multi-cultural society, this can lead to difficulties whereby an older person's spiritual needs are in conflict or inappropriately addressed as a result of the majority culture. This will be further explored by addressing a number of different cultures and approaches to the area.

Western spirituality

In the western tradition, that is in Christianity and Judaism, spirituality is viewed as a theistic notion from the classical theological perspective. The theological perspective is relevant to any anthropological debate, particularly, in discerning a spiritual dimension of humanity as a basis for nursing. Theology has traditionally been defined as knowledge of God, in other words, it was used for the disciplined study which treats God, His nature, His attributes and His relations with the universe and people. Christian theology is embedded in a belief that God reveals Himself in nature and history and human affairs (Brown, 1992; Bradshaw, 1994). Theism, that is, belief in God, and monotheism, that is, belief in one God, are the generic terms for Christians' view of God.

Using a classical theological paradigm, Bradshaw (1994) presupposes revelation focused on the disclosure of God in the person of Christ. In developing the theological argument, Bradshaw (1994) asserts that the place of man and woman (humanity) in the creation is as the image of God. Man and woman are unique and their nature is a unity. They are not a dualistic composition of physical body and spiritual soul, but an entity in which the body finds expression in the whole. Stoll (1989), cited in Carson (1989), illustrates the spiritual nature of a person in this respect as:

> ... an animating, intangible principle that gives life to the physical organism ... [it] integrates and transcends all other dimension of person ... The literal breath of life (p. 6).

In the theological context, spirituality also represents prayer, worship and a range of other practices that are associated with the development of spiritual life.

The well-established holistic notion of a person as being made up of the body, mind and spirit was shattered by Descartes (Williams, 1981; Bradshaw, 1994). Descartes' philosophy challenged classical position on spirituality and proposed that an individual should be perceived as consisting of only reality, that is, mind. Everything else is secondary, and therefore more illusory in nature. Pietroni (1984) attributes the overemphasis of the physical within medicial and nursing care to Descartes, who split off other aspects of the person and allowed them to become irrelevant. This was the inevitable outcome of Descartes' notion of the body as a machine comprising several systems and the belief that if one of these systems fails, it can be fixed irrespective of the individual's spiritual and psychological needs.

We will return later in the chapter to the discussion of the spiritual needs of clients who follow Christianity and Judaism. Next, we will turn our attention to people who do not claim to belong to any of the traditions discussed earlier, that is, humanists.

Humanists

It would be useful to note that a significant number of people in the western culture do not claim to adhere to any of the spiritualities described earlier. Between 25% and 30% of people in Britain today do not have a religion (Narayanasamy, 1991); some are simply silent on the issues of spirituality or claim to be humanists.

Humanists do not believe in God or heaven, but give credence to the power of science, reason and human experience to make sense of life's complicated puzzle. Presently, those who claim to be humanists, or scientific humanists, who subscribe to such journals as *The Humanist* (USA) or *New Humanist* (Britain) are all or almost all avowedly atheist or at least agnostics. They hold the premise that we should use the human qualities of understanding, caring and cooperation to help each other and to make life better for fellow human beings.

Although humanists do not claim to believe in God or a transcendent being they can be just as spiritual as any others. Just like individuals who claim to be religious, humanists engage in the universal search for meaning and purpose, in other words, search for answers to the great puzzles of life: 'Why am I here?', 'What is life all about?', 'What is the universe?' etc. Some humanists look to the facts which people have found out for themselves through experience and by exploring the world scientifically.

Eastern spirituality

Eastern spirituality has its origins in Asia. Asia, with its vast geographical expanse, has been a breeding ground for a rich cultural diversity in languages, customs, ethnic groupings, religious traditions and diverse economic levels. This rich mixture of cultural traditions has produced a variety of spiritual orientations or varieties of spiritualities. These being:

- **Asian Islamic spirituality,** found in Pakistan, Afghanistan, South East Asia and India
- **Asian Buddhism** with different spiritual orientations, found in Theravada, Thailand and Mahayana, Japan
- **Asian Christian spirituality,** also found in India

There are significant differences in the spiritual and intellectual life of Asian peoples. The two great and most ancient civilizations of Asia, India and China, reflect sharp cultural contrasts. India lays its emphasis on the universals, underplays specific particulars and finds creativity in the act of negation. On the other hand, China appreciates concreteness, particulars and practicality. Such clear cultural variations will be evident in the spiritual orientation of older people originating from or having roots in any of these countries.

However, in spite of the differences, there is a common base of Asian spirituality. This becomes evident when it is compared with western spirituality. Relatively speaking, Asian spirituality is concerned with undifferentiated totality before creation. Hence, the pantheistic view that all things are part of one creation. While, in western spirituality a sharp distinction is drawn between the Creator God and His creations, the notion of dualism originates from this. In general, the fundamental contrast between western and Asian spiritualities is that Asian spirituality is cosmological while western spirituality is eschatological (transcendent). Kosuke Koyama (1983) describes this eloquently:

While the cosmological spirituality proclaims that my help comes from heaven and earth, eschatological spirituality would say 'my help comes from the Lord who made heaven and earth' (p. 30).

African spirituality

It is important to also mention African spirituality as it has some differences to the already mentioned western and eastern spirituality (meaning Asian spirituality). Africa, apart from its own cultural traditions, shows plurality in its spirituality. It is a vast continent with a diversity of culture and religions, contributed by native Africans, Africans of western and Arab origins, to name a few. Thus, Africa shows plurality when it comes to spirituality, namely Christianity and Islam. However, some older people of Afro-Caribbean origins or traditions may express spiritual beliefs based on Rastafarianism which has its origins in Africa (Ethiopia, to be precise).

BOX 8.2   *Spiritual needs of older people*

The following are offered for your consideration:

The search for meaning and purpose

- Finding meaning and purpose in life
- Finding meaning and purpose in illness and suffering
- Searching and seeking motivation as to why and how to live

Love and harmonious relationships

- A universal need, especially love that is unconditional (no strings attached to it)
- Relationships with people, living harmoniously with people and their surroundings
- Deriving inner peace and security from love and harmonious relationships

Forgiveness

- Guilt is a universal human phenomenon that needs to be ridden by forgiveness
- Believers may seek forgiveness through their faith/religion; however, non-believers may not have such opportunities but still need to find the means to be forgiven

Hope and strength

- Sources, religious or spiritual, that give hope and strength to go on living, face challenges of life

Trust

- Emotional and physical security
- Stable environment and living gives security and peace

Personal beliefs and values

- Life principles and values
- Religious and cultural beliefs
- Humanistic needs

SPIRITUAL AND RELIGIOUS NEEDS

Acknowledging the spiritual needs outlined above, some value may still be ascribed to identifying the universal spiritual needs of older people (Box 8.2). These, however, must be considered in the light of the individual's personal belief systems.

RELIGIOUS AND CULTURAL BELIEFS

Previously suggested religious and cultural beliefs may be strong motivating influences upon older people and how they live their lives. The next section of this chapter will consider these issues in the context of delivering nursing care using case studies and activities to explore relevant issues.

Christianity

Most healthcare practitioners will be familiar with Christianity in some form or another. It is the largest and most universal religion, with more than one billion believers, and is based on the belief that Jesus Christ is the son of God.

Beliefs of Christianity are explained within the Old and New Testament books of the Holy Scriptures. These include belief in God, Jesus Christ, the Holy Spirit, Sin, Redemption, Salvation, and Retribution or a final accounting with God at the end of life.

For further details, readers are advised to consult sources given in the further reading list at the end of this chapter.

Mrs Elsie Hunter, a physically dependent woman aged 88 years, has been dressed and sat in a chair at the side of her bed. She asks the nurse if she can go out of the ward to walk to the chapel as she wants to pray there. The nurse knows that Elsie is a Christian, but takes no action because the lady is in danger of falling if allowed to walk unaccompanied.

■ What issues may influence the nurse in not acting upon the information given?
■ What might be the effect upon Mrs Hunter if she is not able to go to the chapel and pray?
■ What needs to happen to allow her to do this?

You may have considered the lack of importance the nurse placed upon spiritual and religious needs, particularly when compared to the perceived risk of further injury as a result of a fall. By taking such an approach, you may have reflected on the feeling of isolation and lack of self-esteem that Mrs Hunter may feel from not being able to pray. When thinking about what needs to happen to allow Mrs Hunter to pray, you may have thought about additional places/ways in which she may pray or you may have considered exploring her situation within a risk management framework, to help with the decision-making process.

Judaism

Judaism is the faith of the Jewish people, numbering around 300,000 followers in Britain. Actual numbers are difficult to gauge as there is a lack of consensus about how to determine 'who is a Jew'. Traditionally, whoever is born to a Jewish mother is considered to be a Jew. However, there are also thousands of 'secular' Jews who show no affiliation towards the religion in any outward form.

In modern Judaism there are three main divisions: Orthodox, Conservative and Reform. Reform Judaism is more liberal than the other two divisions in its beliefs and practices. Orthodox Judaism is the stricter of the two, and adherents hold the belief that God gave the law and that this should be followed precisely as written. Certain beliefs are shared by all Jews:

- God is the one and only God
- He is holy, sacred, and separate from the world and people
- By his word he creates, rules, and judges the world and people, and speaks to Israel and people
- He will bring history to fulfilment, in the messianic age

The theory and practice of Jewish ethics include:

- The moral law comes from God; as such it is absolute, universal, revealed, and human
- The law consists in the Commandments of God which are interpreted by the Rabbi, to be studied and followed by all, as a blessing for them and for the world

Synagogues are Jewish centres of worship, education and socializing. Worship in the synagogue takes the form of prayers and readings, especially from the Torah. The Torah contains five books of the Bible and is considered to be the most important of Jewish sacred writings. The worship is often led by a rabbi or a singing leader called a 'cantor'.

The Jewish home is valued as more important than the synagogue for ensuring the continuing of the Jewish faith. Followers of this faith eat only food that has been prepared in accordance with God's law to make it 'Kosher' (fit). Meat and milk products must never be eaten at the same time or prepared with the same utensils and many foods, including pork and shellfish, are forbidden by the Torah.

TABLE 8.2	Major Jewish festivals
Rosh Hashanah	A festival for the Jewish New Year which falls in September or October
Yom Kippur	Also called *The Day of Atonement*, this festival comes ten days after Jewish New Year. The most sacred day in the Jewish calendar, it is spent in prayer, fasting and asking God's forgiveness for wrongdoings
Passover	Or *Pesack*; falls in March or April and signifies the night when the Israelite children were saved or 'passed over' by the Angel of Death when plague threatened them before their escape from slavery in Egypt
Seder	The most important ceremony in which some of the food and drink has a special meaning
Hanukkah	The Festival of Lights which falls in November or December. A candlestick with nine branches is used

Mr Joseph Goldstein, an Orthodox Jew aged 80 years, is dependent upon insulin and has been admitted to hospital with unstable diabetes eight days after the Jewish New Year. His family have informed the ward staff that he is a strict observer of his religion and not to give him porcine based insulin. Plan care for Mr Goldstein that aims to meet his spiritual needs, particularly as he will be in hospital during the festival of Yom Kippur.

Problem/need	Goal	Care plan

The Sabbath

The Sabbath (*Shabbat* in Hebrew) is the Jewish holy day, which begins at sunset on Friday and lasts until nightfall on Saturday. It is a day for rest and contemplation.

Table 8.2 shows the major Jewish festivals.

Rastafarianism

Rastafarianism, a recent religion, was founded in the 1930s and is strongest in Jamaica but has spread to other Afro-Caribbean communities, particularly in the USA and Europe. When Ras (Prince) Tafari was enthroned in Ethiopia in the 1930s as Emperor Haile Selassie, he was hailed as the black messiah who had been predicted to arrive in Africa.

Rastafarians accept some of the teachings of the Bible as it is the tradition of Ethiopia, basing their belief that God took human form first as Christ, then as Ras Tafari. Rastafarians draw similarities with that of the Israelites in that they liken the fate of all black people in the west to that of the Israelites within the Old Testament and believe that Rastafarians will not be free unless they return to Africa. This is interpreted by many Rastafarians as a spiritual state of mind rather than the actual place.

John Isaac, a 68-year-old man, states that he is Rastafarian when his nursing assessment is carried out. He further declares that he is a follower of his faith and eventually wants to return to Africa, where he feels his spiritual roots are.

How can the nurse help John to achieve his spiritual goal of being at one with his spiritual roots?

Islam

Muslims are followers of Islam and two million of them live in Britain. Most muslims were born in the UK, although their families may have come from Turkey, Somalia, West Africa, South Asia (mainly, Pakistan and India). In the UK most people of Pakistani origin, and some with Indian descent are Muslims. Some British people have converted to the Muslim faith.

More than a fifth of the world's population practise Islam. There are muslim communities in more than 120 countries, the largest being in Indonesia.

Islam originated in the Middle East at the beginning of the seventh century by Prophet Muhammad. Muslims believe in one God, Allah, and Muhammad, His prophet provides the key to Muslim beliefs. Muslim means 'peaceful submission to God's will'. The beliefs and way of life of muslims, Islam, is laid down in the Qur`an (Koran) as well as the life and teaching of the Prophet Muhammad.

There is a great deal of similarity in the practices and beliefs of all Muslims; however, some differences exist in the interpretations and explanation of Qur`an by the main (two) sects in Islam – the Sunni and Shi`ah believers (McAvoy and Donaldson, 1990). Sunni Muslims adhere to the traditions of the early elected 'khalifahs', or leaders, who were obedient to the example and teaching of Muhammad. On the other hand, Shi`ah Muslims follow descendants of Muhammad, with extra beliefs and customs. Today, a large of number of Shi`ahs is found mainly in Iran and Iraq. In Britain and the rest of world, most Muslims are Sunni.

To Muslims, the five central pillars of belief are important. These show how their beliefs should be put into action in daily life (see Table 8.3).

Many older Muslims visit the mosque and this is an important feature of their lives. It is a place for individual and communal prayer as well as a facility for study and for the discussion of community matters. On Fridays all Muslims attend the congregational prayer (jumma) at midday.

TABLE 8.3	*The five pillars of Islam*
The Shabadah	The declaration of one's faith, which is repeated several times a day. 'There is no God but Allah and Muhammad is His Messenger'
Salat	This is the formal prayer, recited five times daily: at home, mosque or place of work. This prayer is carried out in Arabic at dawn, just after mid-afternoon, just after sunset and after dark. The prayers may be recited in any clean place and extra prayers may be observed at any time. Muslims carry out ritualistic washing and take off their shoes before prayer, for cleanliness
Sawn	Muslims should fast during the daylight hours in the month of Ramadan, health permitting. Fasting focuses the minds of Muslims to be conscious of Allah and reminds them of the poor and hungry. It brings them to the same level as the poor, thus fostering the notion of equality. Ramadan is the time for intense studying of the Qu`ran and for practising self-discipline and charity
Zakat	A Muslim's obligation, if it can be afforded. At least 2.5% of one's untouched wealth is given annually for the wealth of the community: to support the mosque, charities and others in need
Haji	Or *Makkah*, the pilgrimage of Mecca. This should be made once in a lifetime, if possible to visit Ka`bah

Muslim dress

Modesty in dress is expected of men and women. Women normally cover their head, arms and legs. Some Muslim women may observe strict dress code, that is, cover their faces too when outside the home. Of course, dress rules are interpreted differently in different places and by different people.

Muslim diet

In Islam all meat must be halal (permitted), which means it has to have been prepared in a certain way. Pork and pork-based products are forbidden because muslims believe these are unclean. Alcohol is strictly forbidden because it clouds people's minds and leads them to forget their duties to Allah, such as prayer.

Amina Abdul, aged 80, a Muslim woman with a learning disability, lives in a 'group home' where 24-hour support is available. The care staff have been giving Amina bacon sandwiches which she appears to enjoy.

What are the relevant issues in this situation and how may it be resolved to the satisfaction of Amina's family?

When considering this case, you may have identified some of the following issues. Who gave Amina the first sandwich? What is the level of awareness of staff regarding Amina's cultural and spiritual needs? How much importance have staff placed upon Amina's personal choice, and to what extent does this conflict with other important issues relating to her cultural needs and her family's feelings?

Hinduism

Older people of Indian origins or ancestry are likely to be Hindus, although some may follow other faiths. Approximately 360,000 of the world's 700 million Hindus live in Britain. Many of British Hindu families have not migrated directly from India, but from East Africa or, in some cases, from other parts of the world including Trinidad and Fiji.

It is estimated that about 70% of Britain's Hindu community originate from the western Indian state of Gujarat. Their customs, their dialect, as well as their food, their festivals (Table 8.4) and styles of worship, reflect this. Cultural variations in their practices related to their religions among Hindus are common. These differ according to their ancestral region, their caste (social grouping) and the gurus (or spiritual teachers) whose path they follow.

The second-largest group of Britain's Hindus, an estimated 15%, have their roots in Punjab, a state divided between India and Pakistan in 1947. There are also smaller Hindu communities in Britain which originate from other Indian states such as West Bengal, Maharashtra and Tamil Nadu.

Hindus believe in one God, but one which can be worshipped in many forms, the important ones being Brahma (the Creator), Vishnu (the Preserver), and Shiva (the Destroyer). Hindus hold beliefs about non-violence and reincarnation.

TABLE 8.4	*Important Hindu festivals*	
Holi		At the end of March, this is a spring festival of Krishna. It represents the gaiety and fun of Krishna in his youth. It is common for Hindu children to throw coloured powder and water at each other
New Year		Mid April
Diwali		Mid October – the Festival of Lights

Reincarnation is the cycle of birth and rebirth. It is based on the notion that individuals are responsible for their actions in each life, and undergo a cycle of rebirth until their lifestyles rise above their previous lives and unite them with God. Current lifestyles of Hindus are predestined according to the behaviour in the last life.

Religion is a way of life for many Hindus and one that is constant and pervades all aspects of their lives. The Hindu sacred book is the Bhagavad-Gita. The Ramayana and Mahabhrata are the two great epics in Hinduism (in recent years the latter was shown on British television as a long-running serial).

Many Hindus worship at shrines in their homes, in front of various pictures of incarnations of the Deities, where incense is burnt. There is no standard form of worship in Hinduism. Some Hindus meditate, some pray; some combine meditation, prayer and physical exercises, as in Hatha-Yoga.

Hindu attitudes towards various life events tend to be based along the following lines:

- **Birth** – The older relative may require the mother of a newborn baby to rest for 40 days
- **Abortion/family planning** – Hindu women feel that they have a duty to produce a son. Needs of the family are more important than those of society. May be against abortion
- **Diet** – the cow is a sacred animal and is never eaten. Many Hindus are vegetarians
- **Death** – Hindu priests may be needed to perform certain rituals and blessings. Nursing staff can wash the body. Cremation is usual. The eldest son is responsible for funeral arrangements
- **Other** – The Hindu faith is centred on the transmigration of the soul with indefinite reincarnation. As a soul moves from body to body it hopes to become purer and purer until it reaches God

Mr Ram Das, a 75-year-old Hindu, is transferred to a medical ward following treatment at the coronary care unit. He is found to be distressed and upset whenever he has been visited by his family.

A nurse found that he had requested his sons to bring a statue of Shiva, his personal Deity, but they had refused because of the fear that the ward staff would object to their father praying to it. It was found that Mr Ram Das likes to listen to religious songs and music.

Outline a care plan for Mr Ram Das that aims to meet his spiritual needs. Insert Problem/Need, Goal Care, Plan Box.

How can the religious and spiritual needs of Mr Ram Das be integrated?

Sikhism

Sikhism was founded by Guru Nanak in India; it is younger than Hinduism and is based on the teachings of ten Gurus. Sikhism is based on one God, with great importance given to worship to, and to a personal relationship with, God. Its faith is a combination of elements of both Hindu and Muslim beliefs, but tends to be more flexible. The followers of Sikhism, known as Sikhs, believe in reincarnation but reject the notion of caste on the grounds that all people are equal. Many worship in a Gurdwara – a Sikh temple (place of Guru). The Holy Book is the Guru Granth Sahab, a collection of the writings of the ten Gurus.

'Taking Amrit' is special devotion in Sikhism. Sikhs who undertake this are known as 'Amrit Dari'. They promise to wear the five signs of Sikhism (see Table 8.5), carry on special prayers, not eat meat, and attend the Gurdwara every day.

TABLE 8.5	*The five signs significant to Sikhism (5Ks)*	
Kara	A metal bangle which is usually not removed, worn by men and women (sign of eternity)	
Kesh and Keski	Uncut hair and turban	
Kangha	The comb (sign of cleanliness). Used to secure long hair under a turban	
Kirpan	A small symbolic dagger (sign of strength)	
Kacchehra	A sacred undergarment (pair of shorts). Symbol of action and goodness	

Other important considerations are:

- **Birth** – similar to Hindu
- **Abortion/family planning** – often same problems about contraception and abortion apply as to Hindus
- **Transfusion** – generally accepted
- **Diet** – beef forbidden. May be vegetarian
- **Death** – five traditional symbolic marks should be worn (not to be removed). No objection to hospital staff handling the body

Mr Jaginder Singh, a Sikh, aged 78, is admitted to a continuing care setting in a state of confusion, disorientation and aggressiveness. The nurse discovers that he carries a small dagger and removes it to give to his wife because of his mental state. However, his wife, who has some difficulty with the English language, manages to insist that the dagger should not be removed, but does not offer any explanation for this because of communication difficulties.

What spiritual issues are important for Mr Singh?

SKILLS DEVELOPMENT FOR SPIRITUAL CARE

As well as an awareness of knowledge about spiritual needs, a nurse needs to develop skills of self-awareness, communication (such as listening), trust building, giving hope, and acting as a catalyst for clients' spiritual needs (Narayanasamy, 1991, 1996). Only an outline of these skills development is given in this section. The details relating to aspects of self-awareness and communication are given elsewhere in this book.

Self-awareness

Self-awareness can be elaborated as an acknowledgement of our own:

- Values, attitudes, prejudices, beliefs, assumptions and feelings
- Personal motives and needs and the extent to which these are being met
- Degree of attention to others
- Genuineness and investment of self, and how those above might have an effect on others, i.e. the intentional and unconscious use of self

Communication skills

- Active listening without being judgemental
- Showing genuineness and unconditional acceptance of clients
- Creating the right climate for clients to express spiritual thoughts and feelings

Trust building

- Showing genuine concern and giving attention to clients enhances trust and promotes a sense of security
- Being reliable and keeping promises made to clients to adhering to care plans and carrying them out promptly

Giving hope

- Showing humility and humour
- Enabling clients to maximize their potential, worth and talents
- Working out with clients to reaffirm their faith, if required; this gives them hope and strength
- Enabling them to uplift their good memories

Being a catalyst for clients' spiritual growth

- Share and learn about each other's spirituality
- Give attention to clients along the points identified earlier – these will enable spiritual growth for both

THE NURSE'S ROLE IN PREPARING THE OLDER PERSON AND THEIR FAMILY FOR DEATH

As some older people are near the end of their life it would seem appropriate here to cover aspects related to their spiritual needs and care. There is evidence to support spirituality as a significant human experience during death (Reed, 1987; Narayanasamy, 1995, 1996). In some instances a sense of spirituality acts as a resource when one is facing death. Spiritual well-being and indeed a positive mental health state is°related to low death fear, low discomfort, decreased loneliness, emotional adjustment and positive death perspectives among people who are facing death (Gibbs and Achterberg-Lawlis, 1978; Miller, 1985; O'Brien, 1982; Narayanasamy, 1995, 1996).

The older person facing death is likely to have the following spiritual needs: forgiveness and reconciliation, prayer and/or religious services, spiritual assistance at death, and peace.

Forgiveness and reconciliation

There may be the feeling of unaccomplished relationship in that the dying older person may not have been granted forgiveness. The client may seek ways and means of achieving reconciliation. This may reflect as wanting forgiveness and reconciliation with their God. The client may also need to forgive and be reconciled with others.

Prayer and religious services

Prayer, as indicated earlier, can be a source of comfort and strength. Religious services in Christian context such as receiving sacraments, or blessing of departures, can all be very comforting to the client and their family.

Spiritual assistance at death

The presence of a significant person, such as a doctor, nurse or chaplain at the bedside of a dying client can be a very comforting spiritual assistance to the client. This is an invaluable gift that can be given to a dying client and their family.

Peace

Peace and tranquillity can be achieved through expression of one's spirituality.

SUMMARY AND CONCLUSION

Despite the elusive dimension and nature of spirituality, a number of definitions have been explored within this chapter. For many of us spirituality comes into focus when we are facing stress often induced by a variety of factors, including illness. Spirituality refers to a broader dimension which is sometimes beyond the realm of any explanation but is very much an important part of our daily lives.

Spirituality features as a significant dimension in many older people's lives. Therefore, its significance as part of their personal growth and development is highlighted in this chapter. The positive effects of spirituality in maintaining one's self-esteem and mental health emerged in the discussion. The relationship between culture and spirituality was highlighted with a brief introduction to some of the western and eastern spiritual beliefs and practices. This chapter also drew attention to the needs of humanists, which may well be neglected as a result of our lack of understanding.

An outline of skills related to spiritual care was given in order to help readers to develop these whilst practising care. Further attention was drawn to the needs of older people and their families whilst facing death as an important aspect of one's spiritual journey.

FURTHER READING

Bradshaw, A. (1994) *Lighting the Lamp: the Spiritual Dimension of Nursing Care*. Scutari Press, London.
An in-depth treatment of spirituality is offered in this book from a variety of perspectives. Although the author writes in favour of the classical theological traditions some of the assertions are almost justified in the context of caring.

Carson, V.B. (1989) *Spiritual Dimensions of Nursing Practice*. W.B. Saunders, London.
The concept of spirituality is adequately treated in chapter one of the above book.

Department of Health (1996) *Directory of Ethnic Minority Initiatives*. HMSO, London.
Readers will find that this directory contains catalogues of the initiatives that have been funded by the Department of Health since 1988. It covers resources such as leaflets, as well as other larger initiatives such as research and projects. The directory is particularly useful when readers wish to find addresses and telephone numbers of leading organizations related to minority ethnic group initiatives.

Narayanasamy, A. (1991) *Spiritual Care: a Practical Guide for Nurses*. Quay, Lancaster.
This book makes a good introductory reading to the subject of spirituality and care. Various self-directed exercises are found in this book.

Shelly J.A. and Fish, S. (1988) *Spiritual Care: the Nurse's Role*. Inter Varsity Press, Illinois.
Although written from a Christian perspective readers will find useful sections which explore the concept of spirituality. Chapters one to three are particularly useful and assist the reader to 'grasp' the concept of spirituality. The book also includes a workbook section which contains individual exercises for developing spiritual awareness.

Sampson, C. (1984) *The Neglected Ethic: Religious and Culture Factors in the Care of Patients*. McGraw-Hill, London.
This provides useful information on approaches to cultural factors in a caring context. Readers will find sufficient material in this book to increase their awareness of some of the cultural and religious aspects of care.

The following also make useful further reading:

Fellows, W.J. (1979) *Religions: East and West*. Holt, Rinehart & Winston, London.
Keeley, R. (ed.) (1992) *An Introduction to the Christian Faith*. Lynx Communication, Oxford.
Lion Handbook (1982) *The World's Religions*. Lion, Oxford.
McGilloway, O. and Myco, F. (1985) *Nursing and Spiritual Care*. Harper & Row, London.
Parrinder, G. *Asian Religions*. Sheldon Press, London.
Wakefield, G. (1983) *A Dictionary of Christian Spirituality*. SCM, London.

REFERENCES

Bradshaw, A. (1994) *Lighting the Lamp: the Spiritual Dimension of Nursing Care*. Scutari Press, London.

Brown, C. (1992) Relating philosophy and theology. In *An introduction to the Christian Faith*. Keeley, R. (ed.) Lynx Communication, Oxford.

Carson, V.B. (1989) *Spiritual Dimension of Nursing Practice*. W.B. Saunders, London.

Collinton, N. (1981) The spiritual dimension of nursing. In *Clinical Nursing*, Belland, E. and Passos, J.Y. (eds). Macmillan, New York.

Gibbs, H.W. and Achterberg-Lawlis, J. (1978) Spiritual values and death anxiety: Implications for Counselling with terminal cancer patients. *Journal of Counselling Psychology*, **25**, 263–269.

Gorham, M. (1989) Spirituality and problems solving with seniors. *Perspective* **13**(3), 13–16.

Granstrom, S.L. (1985) Spiritual nursing care for oncology patients. *Topics in Clinical Nursing* **7**(1), 39–45.

Hardy, A. (1966) *The Divine Flame*. Collins, London.

Hardy, A. (1979) *The Spiritual Nature of Man*. Clarendon Press, Oxford.

Hay, D. (1987) *Exploring Inner Space: Scientist and Religious Experience*. Mowbray, London.

Hay, D. (1994) The biology of God: What is the current status of Hardy's Hypothesis? *International Journal for the Psychology of Religion*, **4**(1), 1–23.

Horton, P.C. (1973) The mystical experience as a suicide prevention. *American Journal of Psychiatry*, **30**, 294–296.

James, W. (1902) *The Varieties of Religious Experience*. The Fontana Library, New York.

Koyama, K. (1983) No handle on the cross. Cited in Wakefield, C.S. (ed.) (1989) *A Dictionary of Christian Spirituality*. SCM Press, London.

Laski, M. (1961) *Ecstasy*. The Cresset Press, London.

Legere, T. (1984) A spirituality for today. *Studies in Formative Spirituality*, **5**(3), 375–385.

Macquarie, J. (1972) *Paths in Spirituality*. SCM, London.

McAvoy, B.R. and Donaldson, L.J. (1990) *Health Care for Asians*. Oxford University Press, Oxford.

Miller, J.F. Assessment of loneliness and spiritual well-being in chronic ill adults and health adults. *Journal of Professional Nursing*, **1**(79) 6–10.

Mische, P. (1982) 'Toward a global spirituality' in the *Whole Earth Papers*, Mische, P. (ed.) Global Education Association, East Grange, NJ, No 16.

Murray, R. and Zentner, J.P. (1989) *Nursing Concepts for Health Promotion*. Prentice Hall, Englewood Cliffs, NJ.

Narayanasamy, A. (1991) *Spiritual Care: a Practical Guide for Nurses*. Quay, Lancaster.

Narayanasamy, A. (1995) Research in brief: Spiritual care of chronically ill patients. *Journal of Clinical Nursing*, **4**, 397–400.

Narayanasamy, A. (1996) Spiritual care of chronically ill patients. *British Journal of Nursing*, **5**(7), 411–416.

O'Brien, M.E. (1982) Religious faith and adjustment to long term hemodialysis. *Journal of Religion and Health*, **21**, 68–180.

Otto, R. (1950) *The Idea of the Holy*. Oxford University Press, London.

OUP (1990) *The Concise Oxford Dictionary*. Oxford University Press, London.

Pietroni, P. (1984) Holistic medicine: New map, old territory. *British Journal of Holistic Medicine*, **1**, 3–13.

Reed, P. (1987) Religiousness among terminally ill and healthy adults. *Research in Nursing and Health*, **10**(5), 335–344.

Reed, P. (1992) An emerging paradigm for the investigation of spirituality. *Research in Nursing and Health*, **15**, 349–357.

Reid, G. (1992) The spiritual dimension. In *Introduction to the Christian Faith*, Keeley, R. (ed.), pp. 18–22. Lynx Communication, Oxford.

Shelly, A.L. and Fish, S. (1988) *Spiritual care: The nurse's role*. Inter Varsity Press, Illinois.

Smuts, J.C. (1926) *Holism and Evolution,* Macmillan, New York.

Soeken, K.L. and Carson, V.J. (1987) Responding to the spiritual needs of the chronically ill. *Nursing Clinics of North America*, **22**(3), 603–611.

Stace, W.T. (1960) *Mysticism and Philosophy.* Lippincott, London.

Stallwood, J. (1981) Spiritual dimensions of nursing practice. In *Clinical Nursing*, Belland, I.L. and Passos, J.Y. (eds). Macmillan, New York.

Stoll, R.G. (1979) Guidelines for spiritual assessment. *American Journal of Nursing,* **79**, 1574–1577.

Stoll, R.G. (1991) The essence of spirituality. In *Spiritual Dimension of Nursing Practice*, Carson, V.B. (ed.). W.B. Saunders, London, pp. 4–28.

Williams, J. (1981) Life after death. *Epworth Review*, January (8), 29–34.

INTRODUCTION

The National Health Service and Community Care Act (NHSCCA) (HMSO, 1990) reinforces the need for multiprofessional collaboration in care delivery. This has resulted in the need for nurses to develop opportunities to network with colleagues from other professions and services. Networking and the value of strong networks is not, however, solely related to the professional domain. The emphasis within the NHSCCA upon providing services within the community has created an increased need for nurses to consider the social networks of the clients with whom they work. This is reinforced within the Act when considering the role communities are expected to take in the support of individuals with health and social care needs. A second reason for all nurses to consider the concept of social networks is the potential for this area to either enhance or detract from a person's health and the quality of their lives.

From the perspective of those older people with mental health needs and/or a learning disability, it is important to consider the additional impact of repeated or lifelong involvement with institutional care upon the development of their personal networks and consequently upon their health. Within learning disabilities, additional issues which support the need for nurses to consider the value and importance of relationships and social networks can be seen in the principles outlined in the concept of 'ordinary living'.

◀3

The fundamental principles discussed within 'ordinary living' mirror those outlined within the NHSCCA (HMSO, 1990). This shift towards community care has resulted in the increase in residential provision for many client groups, including older adults. In many instances such provision is seen as preferable to large institutions by both clients, their carers and professionals. However, Kinsella (1993) suggests that many of these smaller homes are miniature versions of the institutional environments from which clients have been discharged. Thompson (1994) argues that such environments are often characterized by a lack of valued contact with members of the local community and an over-emphasis upon professional support. Therefore in order to counteract the institutional culture, nurses will need to enable clients to develop meaningful relationships in other situations. The skills of maintaining existing external relationships will be of paramount importance in care delivery.

With regard to a non-disabled older person accessing healthcare provision, there are a number of important issues when considering the nature of an individual's network. These include the network changes that occur due to admission to hospital, which may result in an inability for the individual or their friends to maintain contact. Secondly, the increased involvement of professional health care staff may alter a person's social network. All the above need to be considered when planning with an older person to meet their care needs. These areas will also be of importance when developing an individual's discharge plan.

It is the intention of this chapter to consider what constitutes a social network and the ways in which different people define this complex concept. This exploration will include discussion and activities relating to the key characteristics and properties of networks in the context of older people. Consideration will also be given to the ways in which networks change over time and how growing older can and does impact upon this area. Finally, practical examples will be given to assist nurses to work in this area with people they are providing care for.

DEFINING SOCIAL NETWORKS

In order to enable nurses to use the concept of personal networks within practice, it is useful to outline what is meant by the term social network. Bott (1957) identifies networks as all or some of the social units with whom an individual is in contact. This work defines a social unit as being any individual or group of people. Within this, Bott is suggesting that a social network is all those people or groups of people that an individual has contact with during the course of their everyday lives. A network can range from those people you see on a daily basis

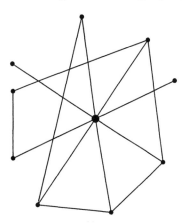

● Person at the centre of the network

● Contacts – friends, family, etc.
   Interactions between individuals

Figure 9.1　Representation of a person's network.

such as children or spouse to people you may see infrequently and who offer you services, such as accountants, bank manager or estate agent.

Barnes (1954) suggests that it is possible to represent your network pictorially. This would take the form of a series of points, some of which are connected by lines. The points are the people and the lines are those individuals that communicate with each other (see Figure 9.1). In this definition Barnes is alluding to the inter-relatedness of networks. Central to this is the way in which different people's networks can and do overlap with one another. Individuals move from being the focal point of their own network to being a component part of many other people's networks. In principle a social network can be seen as fundamental to a person's existence and is directly related to their health and well-being and overall quality of life.

CHARACTERISTICS AND PROPERTIES OF NETWORKS

Atkinson and Williams (1990) identify the key components of networks as family, friends, neighbours and acquaintances, people with common interests and finally, service providers and professionals.

Family

The family is generally regarded as the major influence in people's lives and is perceived as being of central importance to many people in the maintenance of their own personal health and well-being. Parents, children and siblings are often seen as the primary kin of individuals, though care must be exercised when considering clients from different backgrounds. This is relevant where the nurse is from a culture in which nuclear families are common. The nurse's personal experience of nuclear families, can, on occasions result in insufficient attention being given, during both assessment and care planning, to the different dynamics that exist within the extended family, or within single-parent and single-sex families. Within many cultures the closest family members live in reasonable proximity to one another. Within these relationships, the kinship bond is generally enduring in its nature, with a long-term commitment and unconditional positive regard often implicit within it.

Both the nuclear and the extended family situations may call for particular effort to actively involve the relevant people in their relative's life. When attempting to involve family members in the care of a relative it is essential to achieve a careful balance between the expressed needs of both parties. This is important as the needs or wants of the individual concerned will not always match those of their family.

List some of the areas in which your needs and wants have been similar to those of your family and occasions when they have been different.

What similar situations are you able to identify from your practice experience?

How is your nursing practice affected in situations where the client and their family have different expectations?

Friends

As with families, friends may provide support, physical care and companion-ship. Richardson and Ritchie (1993) identify three major characteristics of friendship. These are intimacy, company and practical help. Intimacy is described as the deepest level of friendship. Intimate friends are those with whom you share private experiences and emotions. Richardson and Ritchie (1993) suggest that regular contact, either direct or otherwise is not essential to the maintenance of these relationships. Interactions are based upon the feeling of value and that some sort of a bond has been established between the individuals involved. The resulting relationship relies very heavily upon trust, loyalty and the expectation of some longer-term reciprocal involvement.

Company is that element of friendship that is concerned with having people around, individuals with whom you are comfortable to share time. This is identified as different to intimacy in that company provides a sense of society and sociability. Its very existence provides those involved with the opportunity to engage in an active social life.

Practical help is an aspect of friendship that is not often overtly acknowledged. It may consist of a variety of means of assistance including small services, advice, or help with details of ordinary living. Allan (1983) and Wilmott (1986) also identify key aspects of friendships, many of which will be discussed later in this chapter. These aspects include:

- Affection and attachment
- Personal choice
- Same gender
- Equality
- Reciprocity
- Exchange
- Equivalent social position
- Sharing of interests
- Caring about rather than caring for

Neighbours and acquaintances

Building neighbourhood relationships and friendships is a different process but can be seen as important to feeling, and being part of a community. Though neighbours are easily identified and defined it is much more difficult to identify the characteristics of a positive neighbouring relationship (Bulmer, 1986). Neighbourhood relationships are generally casual and not very intimate, being based upon a friendly distance designed to maintain a healthy respect for the privacy of those individuals involved. On this basis, neighbours are generally more suited to providing small acts of kindness and support in crises situations rather than longer-term ongoing support. However, there are many examples of neighbours providing ongoing crucial support for older people within their community.

Consider how many times you see your neighbours and what sort of a relationship you have. What factors influence how often you see them?

Neighbourhood relationships can be affected by a number of factors. These include age, individuals' stage in the life cycle, gender, social class, mobility, personal history and ethnic background. When considering an individual's needs, either in relation to developing this aspect of a network or maintaining one already in existence, it is essential to have some understanding of these issues.

Acquaintances, as with neighbours, are frequently based within the immediate geographical area in which a person lives. Acquaintances may be related to an individual's work setting; they are casual contacts characterized by face-to-face interaction and mutual recognition. Nevertheless, acquaintances are able to provide individuals with access to a range of ideas and information, potential new friends and partners, involvement within a local area or group and an extension to the social circles within which an individual operates (Atkinson and Williams, 1990).

People with common interests

People with common interests can be seen as the initial starting point for those people with which an individual is able to develop a more intimate and reciprocal relationship. In order to facilitate such relationships it is useful for nurses to consider the places in which the client will meet people with similar interests. It is important to focus upon the potential of individual situations to facilitate interaction. It is possible to differentiate between socially integrated and socially isolating activities. In this context, places such as work, and membership of churches, self-help groups or other organizations and clubs, can be seen as socially integrated activities. Conversely, those pastimes such as watching television, reading, going to the cinema and theatre and shopping can be identified as socially isolating.

Identify how many of your own leisure activities can be described as socially isolating.

Now carry out the same activity for an older person with whom you work.

Consider the living environment of the care setting in which you work. Does this promote social integration or social isolation?

People within the work setting often have common interests by the very nature of the encounter. Work-based relationships consist of day-to-day and face-to-face involvement in which people spend some small but significant time interacting. For many older people these relationships, which may have been built up over a significant period of time, often disappear through the process of retirement and bereavement, thus leaving a potential gap in their network that may have knock-on effects to their health and the successful adjustment to retirement. As such, therefore it is an important area for nurses to discuss with clients and when necessary to act upon the information acquired.

Service providers and professionals

Victor (1994) identifies that as people age they increasingly require input from a variety of external sources, in particular health and social care services. As a consequence, older people are often perceived as consuming the majority of the available welfare resources (Wells and Freer, 1988). This increase in the number of health and social care professionals involved within an older person's life can result in a shift from a position of control over their everyday activities to one where they are perceived as dependent. Synonymous with this is the belief that older people are unable to manage their activities of living independently. Ultimately this can lead to an imbalance between those people interacting with the older person because they are paid to do so, and those who are involved because they value the individual.

A potential difficulty that may arise within the nurse–client relationship as a consequence of dependence is that one party may act out of duty and obligation to the other. Implicit within any such relationship is the issue of who is perceived as having the 'power'. Due to the very nature of any caring relationship there is always some imbalance of power; this can lead to the older person becoming dependent, and therefore, vulnerable. The potential within such circumstances is the exposure of the older person to situations of exploitation, neglect and abuse.

Consider:

■ Your own contact with professionals
■ A client's contact with professionals

In these contacts, who controls the focus and balance of the relationships?

You may have identified that your own personal contact with health professionals relates in the main, to the work situation. Additional contacts are on an infrequent basis, they are often instigated by yourself and you tend to have some control over the nature and length of the interaction. A client's situation may produce a very different picture. For example, there may be a predominance of professional contacts which take place on an ongoing basis. Within these relationships the control may well be with the professional, such as a district nurse who chooses the time of a home visit.

PROPERTIES OF SOCIAL NETWORKS

Having explored the characteristics or component parts of a network it is now possible to consider each of these areas in the context of the properties. The properties of a social network can be identified as size, intensity, density, multiplexity, durability, reciprocity, symmetry and clustering (Atkinson and Williams, 1990).

The size or range of a network refers to the number of people with whom the client has contact. Wenger (1991) identifies that active social networks consist of anything between 16–50 people, but that most people receive help or support from a minority of close individuals. However, in previous research Wenger (1984) found that older people usually have between 5–7 people in their social network.

Analysis of any network over time can identify the ways in which an individual's social contacts change with regard to range and size. The strength that is attributable to any specific relationship is defined as its intensity. The 'density' of a network refers to the frequency with which individuals within the social circle contact each other independently of the person at the centre of the network. A network which has a large number of people who communicate regularly with the central person and with each other is referred to as a high-density network. Wellman (1981) states that high-density support networks have been shown to be well-integrated, solidary groupings. Such networks are generally small and are likely to provide strong emotional support (Craven and Wellman, 1973). The support network of an older person is likely to be high-density since the majority of its members will live in close proximity to the person at the centre (Wenger, 1991).

Conversely, low-density networks are large, more fragmented and heterogeneous (Wellman, 1981). Members of such networks may be better able to secure help. Craven and Wellman (1981) state these networks may provide better access to resources; however, such relationships may be less reliable. d'Abbs (1982) suggests small, dense networks appear to hinder the flow of knowledge and that members of close-knit dense networks are less likely to seek help from formal sources (McKinley, 1973).

The number and types of exchanges that occur within a network and between the client and their contacts is defined by the term 'multiplexity'. Wenger (1991) uses the term linkages to describe this concept. She suggests that multiple linkages are stronger and likely to be of a reciprocal nature. For older people support networks tend to have a core of highly multiplex relationships, for example, a daughter may provide emotional as well as practical support. In addition, the older person may have a periphery of uniplex relationships, for example, a neighbour who collects their pension but provides no other physical or emotional support. Wenger (1991) identifies that, in western cultures, ties tend to be asymmetrical, with one partner benefiting more than another. All such ties are potential sources of support and vary in intensity. Wellman (1981) suggest that in general, the stronger the tie the more likely it is to become a source of support, and the closer the relationship the more likely that one of the partners will be able to ask for support. In the professional domain the types of exchanges will be very different from those which naturally occur in ordinary life simply as a result of the purpose underpinning any healthcare interventions. In addition, the difference in the power relationship between a nurse and the client will alter the nature of any exchange. This balance or imbalance of the power between two people, within the context of networks, is referred to as 'symmetry'.

The degree of stability that exists between the client and those individuals with whom they have contact is termed 'durability'. This may or may not be influenced by time or expectations of continuity, such as those that exist in families. Within the concept of social networks, 'clustering' refers to the gathering together of cliques, or groups of people. This is particularly relevant for nurses if it results in an imbalance within any one of the component parts of a network.

The way in which the above characteristics and properties of a network integrate allows nurses and other healthcare professionals to categorize that person's network. This can be achieved using the framework identified by Wenger (1991).

Types of network

In her study, Wenger identified five distinctive types of networks. These range from what is described as a local integrated support network to a more private and restricted support network, depending upon the interplay between the properties already discussed.

- **Local integrated support network.** This includes close relationships with local family friends and neighbours and is usually based upon how long someone has lived within the community and how active they have been within it
- **Local self-contained support network.** Such networks typically have infrequent contact, if any, with local kin and tend to rely mainly upon neighbours. Community involvement is low key
- **Wider community-focused support network.** This includes distant kin, many friends, some neighbours and is characterized by a high level of community activity and involvement
- **Family-dependent support network.** This has its primary focus on close local family ties with few peripheral friends or neighbours. These are often based upon a shared household or close proximity to an adult child
- **Private restricted support network.** This network is characterized by an absence of local kin, other than spouse and limited contact with the local community. No local friends and superficial contact with neighbours

This work is important for nurses in that it provides a framework by which they can predict the nature and amount of professional support that an individual may require. It allows the nurse to explore, with the client and their family, other areas where support may be needed in order to develop a package of care that is individually based and meets the needs and expectations of the older person, their family and friends.

THE IMPACT OF AGEING UPON NETWORKS

Networks are affected by numerous aspects of a person's life; examples include a person's gender, marital status, social class and health status. Mugford and Kendig (1986) and Wellman (1981) suggest that women have larger networks than men, more friends and more multiplex ties. While the networks of both men and women in adulthood and older age tend to be family orientated, older women's networks are more likely to have bonds or ties outside the family (Corin, 1982).

d'Abbs (1982) states that social class affects networks as a result of issues with financial resources. Amongst middle-class people there is evidence of extensive mutual aid and financial help and an increased likelihood of them being affected by the migration of their offspring. However, such people are less constrained by distance as they have greater access to transport and communication networks. Warren (1981) identifies that middle-class people develop relationships more quickly, are less likely to turn to family, and are more inclined to seek help from friends.

Mugford and Kendig (1986) state that working-class older people have small social networks which are kin dominated. Such networks tend to have intense ties with neighbours. Individuals at the centre of these networks tend to be more seriously affected before seeking help, especially if it is outside the family.

The transition from what is seen as a productive working adult into retirement from the official workforce can be seen to have a dramatic effect upon an individual's social network. The sense of purpose and well-being that an individual gains from the everyday contact with work colleagues is an obvious loss when work patterns change. This loss of contact with people at work not only affects the size of a person's network, but also has the potential to impact upon its intensity, durability, multiplexity and symmetry.

The potential impact of retirement upon the intensity of relationships can be twofold. Firstly, those work relationships that continue to exist become less intense through reduced frequency and the loss of common purpose. Secondly, the reduction in intensity of these relationships can lead to re-focusing upon the family relationships, which in turn alters the durability of an individual's network. The individual's perception of these changes is dependent upon their personal beliefs and value system.

Parents can be seen to be the central focus of a child and adolescent's social network. During this time they, and other close family members, provide stability and security for their offspring. During the late teens/early twenties, the focus typically changes to include an individual's own partner, and ultimately their own children. At this point in time, parents may appear secondary within their children's network. With further life changes some individuals may see alterations in the dynamics of their network. Children may take on an increasingly significant role in their parents' lives, therefore strengthening the multiplexity and symmetry of that relationship.

In addition, the effect of the loss of spouse, family and friends through bereavement has a specific impact upon an individual's personal network. Bereavement can significantly reduce the size and durability of a person's social contacts. This may be particularly significant if the person who has died was the centre of much of the couple's joint network. In this situation the person left behind may find themselves returning to smaller less-resilient contacts with friends and family as a result of the loss of the contact with their partner's network. In addition, an individual who has lost their partner may have more and different contact with their offspring, which in turn can affect the reciprocal nature of those relationships. Wenger (1984) identifies that in widowhood, men's networks shrink, whilst women's tend to remain stable. For men this may mean that their networks become more polarized and focus more significantly upon their child, thus leading to opportunities to further strengthen their

Using the five characteristics of social networks identify the members of your own social network.

How does your current network differ from your network when you were 16?

How would your network be affected by a change in workplace, long-term illness or unemployment?

Thinking into the future, how may it have changed by the time you are 75? (You may find it helpful to think of an older person you know to complete this section).

With respect to the above activity, it is possible to consider the changes you may have identified in the context of losses and gains to an individual's network, both within their family and external to their filial ties.

relationship with their offspring. From the women's perspective the stability that Wenger (1984) identifies may provide a significant support mechanism during times of need.

QUALITY OF LIFE

Garbarino (1986) suggests that a network which includes close, reciprocal and intimate relationships is one that is rich and supportive. It is important to acknowledge that the size of a network does not always indicate quality. For some individuals a small close-knit network may be sufficient and more conducive to achieving happiness and contentment, particularly when the large network offers the opportunity for numerous interactions, in many places, but little or no attachment and commitment. Conversely, for others it may be necessary and appropriate to have contact with a greater number of people.

Irrespective of the size or range of a network it is important to consider the impact that a strong network is able to have upon a person's mental health and their quality of life. Within most models of health there is an implicit belief that the amount of social contact any individual has with others has implications for their health. This is important with regard to that individual's psychological and mental health. The effects of poor-quality networks can be seen to be social isolation, loneliness and stress. Work by Townsend (1973) and Tunstall (1966) identify that loneliness and isolation from the outside world are particular problems for older people who have a disability. It may be that the experience of being cut off from other people may cause that individual to experience the symptoms of stress and other health-related problems. This is relevant to mental health, where social isolation may result in a person becoming disorientated and insecure in their environment.

Victor (1994) argues that the concept of social isolation is problematic as it consists of both objective and subjective components. Early studies such as Townsend (1973) relied heavily upon the use of numerical data, for example the number of contacts and visits that an older person had within a defined period. On a more subjective level, social isolation relates to perceptions of loneliness and isolation and concerns the response of older people to the quality of their social contacts.

Jerrome (1982) suggests that certain social groups are more vulnerable to loneliness than others. In respect of older people we tend to consider widows, childless people, the never married and those who live alone, as at risk. In fact, this is not necessarily the case; Jerrome (1981) and Gubrium (1975) state that people who have never married are less vulnerable as they have developed strategies for establishing and maintaining social contacts. Wenger (1984) found that the most lonely person is as likely to be married as unattached. Acute loneliness is often a feature of the lives of women who have concentrated their emotional resources in marriage and find themselves in widowhood with a lack of friends (Jerrome, 1983).

Social isolation can also be seen to exist in what Goffman (1961) described as the 'total institution', in which individuals live, work and play within the same physical environment. Atkinson and Williams (1990) suggest that segregation is not conducive to a good quality of life. This scenario can be reflected in some hospitals, group homes and nursing homes where people requiring long-term continuing care reside. The negative aspects of such care provision is widely acknowledged within the literature, for example, Norton *et al.* (1962) identified that in such circumstances people became institutionalized. This results in a variety of symptoms, which include confusion regarding date, time and place, shuffling gait and withdrawing from social contact with others. This process of withdrawal often results in a deterioration in all aspects of an individual's social network and ultimately their health and hence their quality of life.

When considering older people with a learning disability or long-term mental health needs, many of the above factors remain pertinent. It is also important to note the different life experiences of these client groups and opportunities through which people have developed their social networks. For many of these individuals their social contacts have been controlled both by families and professional carers. In many instances this has resulted in networks that are either mediated through another person, such as a parent, or that are focused purely within the institutional settings. People who have spent many years in hospitals are unlikely to have an extensive network of their own to utilize.

Atkinson and Williams (1990) suggest that an individual's network can provide an indicator of a person's social identity. An individual's social network becomes the essence of who they are, and one can expect that their network will change throughout their life cycle. The transition into older personhood is important in relation to the inherent changes within this and its impact upon the individual's social identity. For many older people these changes are reinforced as a consequence of the ageing process, particularly difficulties that can occur with mobility, visual/hearing ability and also many other outcomes of the normal process of ageing.

The way in which society perceives older people may also have an effect upon a person's social identity. Of particular relevance are the attitudes that society holds about older people. The belief that an older person is unable to live an independent quality lifestyle is absorbed not only by society as a whole but also by the older person themselves.

THE NURSE'S ROLE IN DEVELOPING SOCIAL NETWORKS

Traditionally, the development and maintenance of social networks has not been seen as part of healthcare provision and consequently not part of the normal role of the nurse. It is hoped that the issues addressed within this chapter challenge this assumption. An individual who has a supportive and integrated network will have an increased sense of their value and self-worth in a way that has positive repercussions for their health, well-being and quality of life.

The role of the nurse within the arena of social networks has three important aspects. These are firstly, the face-to-face nurse–client interaction, the development and maintenance of contacts that are external to the caring situation, and finally, the supportive function that underpins this area.

Nurse–client interaction

It is within this arena that nurses are able to offer a significant contribution to both the health of the individual and also their quality of life. Within this is the perception that closeness with another human being is a positive experience. This closeness and positive human experience is espoused as the central focus of many of the theories related to nursing, with an emphasis upon the importance of communication and relationship building.

Practical nursing interventions that may be of value within this include the use of communication skills such as listening to clients, providing space and time for clients to explore their feelings and emotions, effective questioning skills, and appropriate self-disclosure in order to support the development of trust within the relationship. These skills can be used in order not only to build relationships between the nurse and the client, but also to facilitate the client in building and

➤10–13 maintaining relationships with others.

Developing and maintaining external contacts

The previous section focused predominantly on the responsibilities of the nurse within their relationship with the client. As already outlined, an additional responsibility of the nurse is that of the relationships that exist within the mainstream of an individual's life. In order to address this area the nurse needs to work with the client in order to assess their existing network. This can be achieved by using both the key characteristics and properties of networks that are identified within this chapter. Practical ways of achieving this will be considered through using a systematic approach. The elements of assessment, planning, implementation and evaluation will be utilized.

Assessment

Assessment of a person's social network is obviously a component part of a much more comprehensive approach to the nursing care of the individual. Such an assessment effectively complements the biographical approach to assessment as defined by Brost and Johnson (1982).

The purpose of assessing a person's social network is to identify both the strengths and limitations of their network. The nurse and client need to ascertain what the present situation is with regard to that individual's network. It must be remembered that this process will only ever reveal a snapshot of information; it does not indicate either past or future networks. This information may, however, still be required in some circumstances. In such cases the nurse needs to work with that client to provide a retrospective picture, or negotiate with them their future network developments. It is the latter situation that provides the focus of many nursing interventions in this area.

Returning to the provision of a snapshot of a personal network, the purpose of assessment is to identify who is part of that individual's life. This should be compiled as a simple list of names with whom that person has contact. Such a method would not, however, produce qualitative information upon which the nurse could base care. In order to improve the quality of the information acquired it is useful to categorize it based upon the criteria identified within the properties and characteristics of networks. This will provide information in relation to those contacts that a person has which are strong in nature, those which are experiencing some degree of stress or pressure and have the potential to breakdown, and lastly those areas where gaps exist. All this data can be compiled to produce a map of the person's current network.

This may provide the following types of information for the nurse: that the person has contact with a similar number of contacts/people within both their family and their neighbours and acquaintances, few contacts they regard as friends, little involvement with people with common interests, and an abnormally large number of people within the professional and service provider area. Taking the category of friends and utilizing the information identified within the section looking at the properties of networks, the following assessment data may be compiled.

The range of people within this section is small in number; however, all the individuals within this network, know and contact one another independently of the central person (density). The relationships within this category are all long-standing friendships which provide emotional support and practical help when needed (durability and reciprocity). Finally, within the area of friendship it is possible to identify a subtle difference in the balance of power between a person at the centre of the network and their friends. In the context of care delivery, it can be seen that though the actual number of friends is small, the nature of these relationships is enduring. The possible areas requiring nursing intervention are the maintenance of these friendships and attention to the imbalance of power within them.

Planning

Having identified the areas upon which nursing interventions should focus, the planning of care to meet those needs will, in reality, result in an accumulation of many areas of knowledge. Of paramount importance within this knowledge of the client is their wants, needs and preferences. For example a person who has few friends but wishes to increase their contacts in this area, will need to consider what their areas of interest are and possibly utilize these to initiate contacts which may ultimately develop into friendships. If such assessment identifies dancing as an area of interest, this will necessitate different nursing interventions to an individual who enjoys rambling or clock making.

It is important to consider the competence of the person in a number of areas, for instance the stated interest, ability to develop and maintain friendships and communication skills. The outcomes of assessment in these and other similar areas will also determine the required competence of the nurse in implementation of the planned care.

Implementation

Within the skills of developing and maintaining networks is the need to support both the client in this process and also the person they wish to develop a relationship with. This is important in the early stages of relationships where the potential exists for one person to become 'overdependent' leading to an imbalance within the relationship which may ultimately result in either undue stress or a breakdown of that relationship. It is easy to see the sensitive nature of any attempt to build networks for other people. It is essential that nurses consider this process carefully, particularly in the context of the UKCC Code of Conduct (UKCC, 1992) and Guidelines for Professional Practice (UKCC, 1996).

Support can be seen as an integral part of any healthy relationship. In this context 'support' is defined as 'being there' for an individual. Equally, it may entail doing something for someone, for example, helping an individual wash and style their hair. More often, however, it means working alongside a person and ensuring that they retain a sense of autonomy. Support may operate at different levels, it may mean participating in social 'chit-chat' with someone, or talking in a more meaningful way, based upon a caring two-way relationship. The relationship may operate on a more intense basis where people actively seek to support one another, particularly in times of difficulty. Where such relationships occur between relatives and over a longer period of time, these relationships often take an overt caring focus. In this way support begins to look very much like informal caring (Atkinson and Williams, 1990).

Evaluation

The prime focus of evaluation is the extent to which the individual's social network has been either maintained or developed in keeping with the person's wishes. Data relating to this can be produced by systematically revisiting the network mapping process. This new snapshot can then be compared with the previous information. This process should identify any area of change within the individual's network; this can then be compared with the goal statements within the person's care plan and be utilized as the focus of interviews to gain qualitative data regarding client satisfaction with the outcomes of that plan.

➤15

CONCLUSION

In this chapter we have explored the fundamental importance of social networks to the health and well-being of older people. In doing this we have explored the concept of networks and established that this includes all contacts a person experiences. This chapter provides information regarding the characteristics and properties of networks, supported, where appropriate, with actual examples. These have been used to give constructive examples of how nurses can develop and maintain the networks of people to whom they provide care. Finally, this chapter explores the role of social networks in the context of social identity, health and the quality of an individual's life. Each is of fundamental importance to the delivery of high-quality nursing care and as such makes this area of work essential to all nurses working with older people.

FURTHER READING

Richardson, A. and Ritchie, J. (1993) *Developing Friendships: Enabling People with Learning Difficulties to Make and Maintain Friends.* Policy Studies Institute, London.
This is a useful and practical text, focusing upon ways of developing friendships. Though specifically related to people with learning disabilities, there are some valuable insights for other areas of nursing to use in practice.

Trevillion, S. (1992) *Caring in the Community: a Networking Approach to Community Partnerships.* Longman, London.
This text has a very strong basis in social work and community care. However, it does provide a very interesting perspective upon network therapy.

Wenger, G.C. (1991) Support networks in old age: constructing a typology. In *Growing Old in the Twentieth Century*, Jefferys, M. (ed.). Routledge, London. *This chapter describes many of the key features of networks in the context of older people. It identifies five different types of networks and provides a synopsis of her research into networks and older people.*

REFERENCES

d'Abbs, P. (1982) *Social Support Networks: a Critical review of Models and Findings.* Monograph No 1, Institute of Family Studies, Melbourne.

Allan, G. (1983) Informal networks of care: Issues raised by Barclay. *British Journal of Social Work*, 13, 417–433.

Atkinson, D. and Williams, P. (1990) *Networks.* Open University Press, Milton Keynes.

Barnes, J.A. (1954) Class and committees in a Norwegian Island Parish. *Human Relations*, 7, 39–58.

Bott, E. (1957) *Family and Social Networks.* Tavistock, London.

Brost, M. and Johnson, T. (1982) *Getting to Know You.* Wisconsin Coalition for Advocacy, Madison, WI.

Bulmer, M. (1986) *Neighbours. The Work of Philip Abrams.* Cambridge University Press, Cambridge.

Corin, E. (1982) Elderly people's social strategies for survival: a dynamic use of social networks analysis. *Canada's Mental Health*, 30(3), 7–12.

Craven, P. and Wellman, B. (1973) The network city. *Sociological Inquiry*, 43(3–4), 57-88.

Garbarino, J. (1986) Where does social support fit into optimism, human development and preventing dysfunction? *British Journal of Social Work*, 16(supp), 23–37.

Goffman, E. (1961) *Asylum.* Penguin, London.

Gubrium, J.F. (1975) Being single in old age. *Ageing and Human Development*, 6, 29–41.

HMSO (1990) *The National Health Service and Community Care Act.* HMSO, London.

Jerrome, D. (1982). The significance of friendship for women in later life. *Ageing and Society*, 1, 175–197.

Jerrome, D. (1983) Lonely women in a friendship club. *British Journal of Guidance and Counselling*, 11(1), 10–20.

Kinsella, P. (1993) *Group Homes.* National Development Team, Manchester.

McKinlay, J. (1973) Social networks, lay consultation and help seeking behaviour. *Social Forces*, 51, 275–292.

Mugford, S. and Kendig, H. (1986) Social relations: networks and ties. In *Ageing and Families; a Social Network Perspective*, Kendig, H. (ed.) Allen and Unwin, Sydney.

Norton, D., Mclaren, R. and Exton-Smith, A.N. (1962) *An Investigation of Geriatric Nursing Problems in Hospital.* Churchill Livingstone, Edinburgh.

Richardson, A. and Ritchie, J. (1993) *Developing Friendships: Enabling People with Learning Difficulties to Make and Maintain Friends.* Policy Studies Institute, London.

Thompson, J. (1994) Social networks. *MHNA Journal,* June, 15–18.

Townsend, P. (1973) *The Social Minority.* Allen Lane, London.

Tunstall, J. (1966) *Old and Alone.* Routledge and Kegan Paul, London.

Victor, C. (1994) *Old Age in Modern Society*, 2nd edn. Chapman & Hall, London.

Warren, D.I. (1981) *Helping Networks: How People Cope with Problems in the Urban Community.* University of Notre Dame, Indiana.

Wellman, B. (1981) Applying network analysis to the study of support. In *Social Networks and Social Support*, Gottlieb, G.H. (ed.). Sage Publications, Beverley Hills, CA.

Wells, N. and Freer, C. (eds) (1988) *The Ageing Population: Burden or Challenge.* Macmillan Press, London.

Wenger, G.C. (1984) *The Supportive Network: Coping with Old Age.* Allen & Unwin, London.

Wenger, G.C. (1991) Support networks in old age: Constructing a typology. In *Growing Old in the Twentieth Century*. Jefferys, M. (ed.). Routledge, London.

Wilmott, P. (1986) *Social Networks, Informal Care and Public Policy*. Policy Studies Institute, London.

UKCC (1992) *Code of Professional Conduct*. UKCC, London.

UKCC (1996) *Guidelines for Professional Practice*. UKCC, London.

3 THERAPEUTIC INTERVENTIONS

This section explores some of the therapeutic interventions currently utilized in specialist areas of nursing practice. The first chapter addresses communication in the context of nursing older people. Other areas covered include touch as therapy, exploring sensory stimulation, stress and relaxation. In the exploration of these interventions consideration is given as to how they can contribute to the development of the nurse–client relationship.

10 Enabling positive communication

Brenda Maslen

INTRODUCTION

Most people think they know what communication is about. Some naively think that as they are good 'talkers', they are good at communication. However, think of our anatomy, and notice that we have two ears and only one mouth; a good rule of thumb about communicating effectively might be to listen twice as much as you speak!

We are all exposed daily to many forms of communication, such as hoardings, television, radio, newspapers, telephones, magazines – the list is almost endless. Something as simple as traffic lights which we see daily have an important communication function – as anyone will know after trying to negotiate a junction when the lights have not been working!

Communication is a fundamental aspect of any relationship and this is true for the relationships developed and utilized in a caring partnership. Virtually any text related to care will contain information regarding the skills of effective communication. However, William Reid, the health ombudsman, amongst others has highlighted that dissatisfaction with how information and support are communicated is inherent in most complaints about the health service. It seems that communication can, and still does go wrong (Wilson Report: DoH, 1994).

If you look at the key concepts you will see that this is not a chapter that you will merely read, but a focus for various experiences which will be unique to you and which will create a connection between theory and practice. These experiences will be built around a genuine case study which, through the use of activities, reflection, think points, questions and your own experience, you will easily be able to contextualize to your own particular sphere of practice.

Perhaps a pragmatic outlook is required to some extent which takes the view that 'If it works – it's good', but this need not detract from the theoretical underpinnings of many of your everyday activities. Some of the material will already be part of your own communication system and will connect to information you already have in your mind. This is a process called extra-integration, where what you already understand will link with new skills being learned. Because we are all human beings and many of the exercises will require you to look at your own feelings, thoughts and attitudes, there are often no 'right' answers. The answers to most of the topics being explored are not simple, but lie in how you feel about what you are doing and how, for instance, others react towards you. However, from time to time if there is a specific answer this will be given, and there will also be suggestions as to what you may discover as a result of the activities undertaken.

SOCIOLOGICAL PERSPECTIVE

You will have read previously in this book the social and theoretical concepts associated with ageing, and this brief perspective simply aims to contextualize this to communication. For example, the media often influence what we think; what we read in the papers, see on television or listen to on radio can and does modify our views – a fact that is crucial to the advertising executive!

Government departments are perhaps as guilty as anyone else when, either in opposition or in office they mention policy which targets the old, sick and infirm, suggesting that there is a correlation between the three. Whilst the incidence of sickness and infirmity is higher in older adults, it is not universally so. This may appear to be pedantic, but it serves to emphasize how beliefs, prejudices, and stereotypes are formed or modified. For example, what kind of message is being given by the Ministry of Transport road sign, sited near residential homes for older people, which depicts two bowed figures with walking sticks (Figure 10.1)? That this sign is the same as that relating to people with disabilities insinuates that older age is a disability and it is a warning sign generally associated with hazards of one sort or another.

It is not only the media which influences our value bases. These are laid down in our childhood and reflect, to some extent, the views held by significant people in our lives. If, therefore, we see older people held in high esteem, consulted for their vast experience, and generally made a focus of the family and society in which they live, then we are more likely to see them as valuable members of that particular group.

If, on the other hand, we are exposed to beliefs which see people in their fifties

Think for a moment of any time that your ideas have been changed, your thoughts stimulated or your feelings affected by something you have seen or heard in the media. How powerful an influence do you think this is?

If you come to the conclusion that these are very powerful channels of communication, then ask yourself what implications there might be in the fact that off-the-cuff, seemingly innocuous, apparently funny comments are made about older adults. For example, it raises quite a laugh when a 58-year-old contestant on a quiz show 'confesses' to being a member of a veteran cricket team – and the host suggests he might be out ZBW – Zimmer-frame before wicket. The more insidious message is – 58 is old; old people have difficulty in mobilizing; this is amusing. None of these facts, of course, is generally correct.

Figure 10.1   Department of Transport sign.

as 'over the hill' and denigrate older people as useless, slow, senseless lumps of baggage waiting to die, then we may internalize and even share some of those opinions. Attitudes thus formed are often difficult to change as they include an emotive element, and whereas intellectually we recognize the worth or otherwise of our value base and behaviour, it is an enduring state.

There are numerous references in common parlance to 'old gits' or 'old duffers', 'silly old sods' and the like, often used as terms of endearment. There is also that common negative misnomer 'dirty old man' conjuring up visions of the grubby mac being thrown open to the distress of onlookers. The statistics reveal that it is young men who are most often convicted of indecent exposure – but this all adds up to a negative perspective with the common factor being the use of the word 'old'. Nurses, or other carers are obviously part of society as a whole, and are exposed to these negative influences.

It would seem that the older adult in the western world gets a raw deal from society in general, and that this is likely to be exacerbated when the necessity for some sort of caring intervention is needed. No doubt we would claim that this does not apply to us – but genuine self-examination might indicate differently.

Think about your own responses when you approach an older adult or when you are working in a caring situation with older people. Have you been influenced in any way by what has been said to you, or what you have read or seen in the media? If so, how do you think this has affected your behaviour – and what do you think you could do about it?

I am reminded of a group of registered nurses with whom I was working as an educational facilitator. When discussing her onerous workload, one senior sister said that things were made more difficult because 'they got all the "grot" on her ward'. When pressed as to the meaning of this, she sheepishly admitted that 'grot' referred to geriatric patients. She maintained, however, that this was merely a word and that it did not affect the way in which the staff worked. What do you think?

THE THEORY OF COMMUNICATION

There are lots of definitions of communication and in considering these, and choosing, it is important that a working definition is utilized. Consider the following, selected from literally thousands which are available. Communication is:

the exchange of information between people (Groenman *et al.*, 1992)

all the processes, verbal and non-verbal, conscious or unconscious by which one mind may affect another (Blattner, 1981)

social interaction through messages
about creating shared meaning and understanding (Weinstein, 1992)

In the definition by Weinstein (1992) the word 'interaction' focuses on a vital ingredient: the opportunity of feedback, without which there is no real communication. So, checking back, asking for clarification, feed back one's own interpretations and understanding – only then are we truly communicating. The alternative is a monologue.

The interaction involves three elements: the use of language (our prime, but not sole means of communicating with one another) our behaviour, and other symbols (e.g. status symbols). The 'message' is what we are trying to convey, and what we inadvertently convey.

In addition to numerous definitions, communication has its own jargon words. It has been said that successful communication is not possible without (Hurst, 1991):

- Understanding
- Common ground
- Perception
- Awareness
- Self-confidence
- Clarity

and it may be in these areas where communication breakdown can occur.

For the purposes of this chapter it might be useful, although not typical of theoretical texts, to use a working definition which encompasses some of the fundamental definitional aspects. Perhaps it will be enough to say that communication is a two-way process which follows the principles outlined in the classical diagrammatic representation shown in Figure 10.2.

If we consider the following illustration, we may begin to understand how breakdowns in communication may occur:

A boy from a working-class background was asked to describe a net. He replied: 'A lot er oiles tied togeder wi' string' (A lot of holes tied together with string).

Dr Samuel Johnson's definition in his *Dictionary* is:
Anything reticulated or decussated at equal distances with interstices between the intersections (cited in Bernstein, 1970).

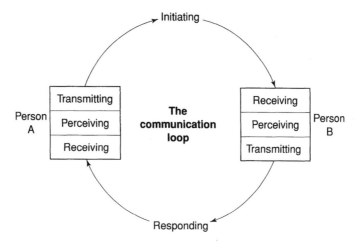

Figure 10.2   The communication process. (Reproduced from *Social and Behavioural Sciences for Nurses*. Groenman, Slevin and Buckenham (1992) Campion Press Ltd, Edinburgh).

There is no intention to look very deeply at communication theory, for as has already been mentioned, this has been done extensively by other authors. However, the previous illustration of the use of a restricted and an elaborated code might be pertinent and then those who wish to delve further into the intricacies of this highly complex, well-documented but often ill-practised phenomenon may care to consult the reading list at the end of this chapter.

PHYSIOLOGICAL IMPLICATIONS

Biological changes that affect communication gradually occur with the ageing process. Esberger and Hughes (1989) suggest that there is a marked decrease of the senses involved with communication after the late mid-adult years, between the ages of 55 and 60, and Ostro (1989) specifies the following changes. Vision is affected by changes in the crystalline lens, decreasing the ability of the eye to focus on near objects, whilst the rigidity of the iris causes an increasing inability to accommodate the amount of light let into the eye. The tympanic membrane gradually becomes less effective in transmission of sound, and wax may build up in the ear and the ability to taste and smell may be significantly affected. The alteration to the dermal layer of the skin may reduce tactile sensations which

►12   may cause problems with the perception of pain or pressure.

The gradual onset of these changes usually allows the individual to adapt to them and maintain communication, but it is important when caring for the older adult to be aware of these changes and ensure your own communication skills are adjusted to reduce the difficulty the client might experience. This should, of course, be done in a sensitive and meaningful way – we have all seen, unfortunately, the person who shouts at the top of their voice when 'communicating' with older people.

Specific conditions may have a more significant effect. Perhaps the most apparent elements of this are the neurological and sensory changes which affect the ability both to receive information (for example read, hear conversations)

I am very short sighted, a problem which is corrected by spectacles; on occasions when I have had to remove my glasses I have felt my confidence plummet, and sometimes I have felt quite frightened. When someone speaks to me I have been known to say (and this usually prompts amusement) 'Hang on a minute while I get my glasses, I can't hear what you are saying'. I have not got a built-in hearing aid, but sight is very important when listening, and this illustrates the inter-relationship between verbal and non-verbal communication.

and to transmit information (for example speak and write). Acuity of vision and hearing are obviously fundamental to the communication process, but what is not as immediately apparent is the fear, anger, or hostility which may be provoked by the absence of good hearing and clear vision.

Physical conditions such as a cerebrovascular accident can create a communication barrier, as can other neurological changes such as organic brain syndrome or aphasia, but it is important to check out other physiological and environmental factors whilst assessing the client's ability. Sometimes new spectacles (or even clean spectacles!), syringing the ears, a hearing aid or simply better lighting might be enough to make all the difference.

This detail, however, concentrates on the physical aspects of communication, and it might be important to consider the meaning behind what we say to each other as illustrated in the case study which follows (from Groenman *et al.*, 1992) which may be played out in any number of homes:

CASE STUDY   **Elsie and James Archer**

Six o'clock in the evening. James is sitting in the living room with his feet up on the table. He pretends to be reading the newspaper. His wife Elsie is in the kitchen. The cooker extractor hood is whirring, she is cooking.

She thinks: he's just come home and he's sitting in the living room. Why doesn't he help, and then we could both sit down together? She says, 'Are you comfortable?'

He thinks: I've just come home, I've had a hard day, why doesn't she come and sit down with me, so we can tell each other what sort of day we've had, and then we can cook and eat together afterwards. He shouts to the kitchen, 'Will it take much longer?' The cooker hood continues to whir.

Think about the scenario you have just read. What is happening here? Can you identify with this and perhaps think of a relationship between client and nurse which gave rise to mutual misunderstandings because meanings were unclear?

Meanings are often badly packaged in words, so that we may not find the meaning through the words. In this case only if you know the underlying thoughts of the couple do you begin to understand what they mean. We often react to what we think the other person means. It is quite likely that the woman in the example thinks: 'If he carries on doing this, I shall walk out tomorrow, I'm fed up with being treated like his servant'. If, however, she was to say something like that to her husband, he would be flabbergasted. He would not understand where this reaction came from. This is reflected in the statement in the following:

> You may think you understood what I said, but I'm not sure what you understood was actually what I said.

With regard to the relationships formed with clients, that we should love them may be viewed as a dangerous concept, since love has various connotations, some of which are rightly seen as having no place in a professional relationship. However, if we look upon it in association with the work of Simone Weil (1952) it concerns an openness to the reality of one's own self and through this a receptiveness to the reality of the other person. There is here an appreciation of the self as one exists in the world, and an intentional going out to the other as a person, a willingness to experience and accept the other with all their goodnesses and badnesses, strengths and weaknesses, well-being and non-well-being. Perhaps this is the least that we can do for those who enter into our sphere of care.

The case study which follows allows you to explore through real-life situations the various facets of communication skills and does so in a way which will be meaningful when applied to your own practice. It is essentially a story, but it is a story which requires you to read into and around the actual facts recorded and adopt some of the feelings which it will provoke. From time to time you will be directed to leave the study in order to allow the consideration of theoretical concepts and their application to your own experiences.

CASE STUDY

Elsie was 69 years old when her husband died suddenly of a heart attack. Theirs had been a long and happy marriage and she could still remember him saying to her 40 years before 'Tha's nowt t' worry about lass, I'll tak care o' thee' – and he had.

She was desperately shocked on hearing about his death from a very anxious chap from the bowling club, where he had gone just a couple of hours before, and sent immediately for her daughter Lena. Lena had been the light of her father's eye, and she was as distressed as Elsie. There followed the rush and bustle of the funeral arrangements, and it all seemed rather like a dream to Elsie, or a nightmare from which she struggled to awaken.

When Lena returned home to re-join her husband in running their successful business, Elsie felt bereft and alone in her small bungalow. True, she knew how to cook and shop and clean, but, as Fred had said, money was a man's business and she was not to worry her pretty little head about it. He had laughed as he said it, and she could still see those crinkles which appeared at the corner of his eyes and feel the protective warmth of his arm around her.

So she managed for a little while on the money she had, and she had not felt able to tell Lena, or friends about the fact that she didn't even know how to write or cash a cheque. Another thing was, she couldn't put petrol in the car in these new fangled serve-yourself outlets. Fred had always done this, and although Elsie was proud of her ability to drive, she seldom did. Fred had always taken her everywhere and somehow, she didn't really know why, her confidence seemed to have deserted her.

Time passed, and people she met appeared to be avoiding the one topic which occupied her every waking thought – Fred. Waking thoughts got ever longer, for she found she could not sleep in the once warm haven of her double bed, and she took to roaming the house late into the night. Lena, of course, telephoned her on a regular basis, given that she was so busy with the shop, and appeared to think her mother should be getting on alright. She often ended their conversations by saying to Elsie 'Come on Mam, where's the Dunkirk spirit'? to which Elsie replied 'It's still there' and after replacing the receiver turned her tearful attention to trying to find it.

When the bills came she put them behind the clock on the mantlepiece, their usual place, and wondered about paying them, thought of getting in touch with the bank manager, but again her confidence deserted her when she heard the reply from the switchboard. After all what would they think of her, a grown woman, not knowing what to do. Anyway she could cope, she didn't eat much, no one left to cook for, and so when the gas was cut off she managed on sandwiches and bits and pieces from the local shop. After all, she and Fred had survived the war – and all Hitler had thrown at them!

She plucked up courage to see the family doctor, a kindly man, who offered her sleeping tablets and anti-depressants, but she had never been one much for taking tablets, and what good would they do anyway?

She became ever more forgetful and withdrawn, and when Lena finally realized the situation, not being able to get through on the phone, she said something had to be done.

Perhaps that was why this nice young man, who said he was a social worker (but Elsie doubted it, he looked more like a schoolboy) was taking her to hospital. She didn't think she should be going there, wasting doctors' precious time, but she had to agree that something had to be done.

When they pulled up outside the imposing looking building and made their way to the ward along what seemed like endless corridors which convinced Elsie that, should she be required to, she would never find her way out again, she was surprised to see that everyone was wearing ordinary clothing rather than nightwear. The nurse who greeted her, in a very kind way, was also not wearing a uniform and this seemed very strange. Sandy, the admitting nurse, looked at this shrunken frail-looking woman, and recalled her recent discussion with a colleague when they had been informed of the admission. The 'confused old biddy' of their conversation was standing here in front of her. With a sigh, she directed Elsie to a chair, and proceeded to talk with the social worker about the situation. Not able to cope, was the phrase which sprang to mind, and whilst they discussed the merits, or otherwise, of her being there, Elsie took stock of this very strange place.

ENVIRONMENTAL INFLUENCES

Consider the influence the environment has on communication. It has long been accepted that the environment has an effect on social behaviour and how we interact with others, for all social behaviour takes place in a physical setting. Sometimes settings have been deliberately arranged, for example by positioning desks and chairs, and sometimes the physical arrangements are a leftover of previous encounters and have 'unconsciously' been arranged by the people who most use the setting.

The presence or absence of a desk can have a significant effect on whether a patient is at ease or not when visiting a doctor. Argyle (1967) found that only 10% of patients were perceived to be at ease when the doctor's desk was present and the doctor sat behind it. This figure increased to 55% when the desk was absent.

Think of your working environment. Can you identify fittings and furnishings which may either enhance communication or make this more difficult? Pursue these thoughts as you do the following activity.

There is the following furniture in a room:

- One desk
- Two easy chairs (of equal height)
- Four upright chairs (of equal height)
- One coffee table
- One bookcase full of books

Think about the best way to arrange the furniture to take account of the following situations:

1. An interview for a job (with a panel of three)
2. An informal discussion with a colleague on a joint project
3. A meeting between yourself, as a manager, and an employee of lower status, who is to be reprimanded
4. A meeting between yourself as a manager and an employee who has asked to see you about a personal problem

How would you arrange the furniture – and why?

The following examples are offered.

For the panel job interview (Figure 10.3), because the chairs are all of equal height this would indicate equality amongst all parties, but the desk would act to a certain extent as a barrier, and a confrontation situation may exist between the central interviewer and the interviewee. This, however, may be intentional on the part of the person setting up the interview in order to assess the interviewee's reaction to this situation.

A more informal set up would be to place the four upright chairs equidistant around the coffee table.

For an informal discussion with a colleague (Figure 10.4) perhaps the best set up might be the two easy chairs close to each other by the coffee table with the other furniture moved out of the way. This is called the co-operative position. It also allows both parties to look at any written material. By placing the chairs on the same side of the table this would indicate working together.

Whilst reprimanding a person (Figure 10.5) the usual position adopted would be the competitive–defensive position. This position is taken by people who are either competing with each other or if one is reprimanding the other. It can also establish that a superior or subordinate role exists when it is used in the manager's office.

Finally, for the counselling situation, you may decide to have the furniture as shown in Figure 10.6. This corner position allows unlimited eye-contact and the opportunity to use gestures and observe the gestures of the other person. The corner of the desk provides a partial barrier should one person begin to feel threatened, and this position avoids a territorial division on the top of the table (Pease, 1981).

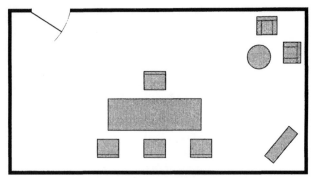

Figure 10.3   Panel job interview.

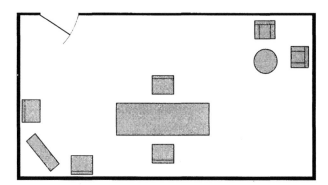

Figure 10.4   Informal discussion with colleague.

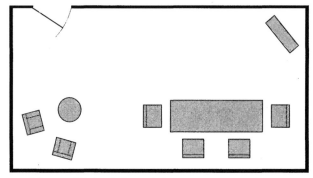

Figure 10.5   Reprimanding: establishing senior/subordinate position.

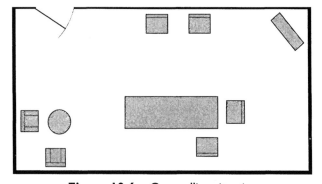

Figure 10.6   Counselling situation.

Think back to the case study; what kind of environment might Elsie have found herself in? It was in fact a small office, with a desk behind which sat the nurse, with the social worker at the side of the desk and Elsie in an upright chair against the wall. How might this have made her feel? Using what we have just done, how could this have been a different and more positive experience?

Returning to the case study:

CASE STUDY

Elsie ventured to ask where she was to sleep and the nurse said 'hang on a minute, pet, and I'll take you down there'. She seemed nice and Elsie did not want to do anything which would cause a problem, so she hung on for about an hour.

Re-read the preceding paragraph, and identify any aspects of it which you find problematical. Are there implications in the language used, and what of those minutes which turn into an hour – how might this be perceived by Elsie?

CASE STUDY

Finally, the conversation between the nurse and the social worker was brought to an end by a hasty summons for the social worker to be elsewhere, and Elsie was conducted to a room, off another anonymous – and she thought grey – corridor. There were four single low divan beds and four lockers, and not much else as far as she could see. The nurse took Elsie's overnight bag (all she had brought, for she wouldn't be staying long), and after removing her things from it, the nurse said she would put it away for safe-keeping. Elsie felt doubly sad as the tapestry bag which she and Fred had chosen in Malta on their first overseas holiday disappeared in the nurse's hands, and she looked around the rather sparse, cold, small space which had been allotted to her.

PERSONAL TERRITORY

This territorial ownership applies more especially to those who do actually own a building (e.g. their own home), but some personal territory issues are more transient than this, for example your space in a communal office, your locker in the changing room, a room you have booked in a hotel for a holiday, or a table booked in a restaurant.

What do you regard as your own personal territory?

Perhaps it is your own room at home, or your garden or the office you have at work. Imagine for a moment that you have your own office at work and one day you discover someone sitting in your chair, at your desk, looking at your papers. How would this make you feel?

I thought that I was really aware of my own behaviour and that I fully respected the rights of the clients with whom I worked. I always knocked on doors – but – I then entered without waiting for an invitation to do so. The token gesture of a tap on the door was merely window dressing – I entered anyway because I felt I had the right to do so on my ward. Perhaps you can relate to this and even extend it to other activities.

Contextualize what you have considered and apply it to your sphere of practice. Is the furniture arranged so that it encourages interaction or not? If not, how could it have been improved. Compare these findings with what you observe in social venues. Are there differences between physical settings outside care settings and those inside?

You may well conclude that, whereas many venues actively arrange the environment to encourage interaction, as in the case of small booths in restaurants, care area settings very much tend to do the opposite. Have you ever been into anyone's home and found the furniture arranged completely around the walls? I would hazard a guess that you have not.

Now try the following.

Look at the arrangement of furniture in the area in which you are working and note how it is used by occupants both from a territorial and an interactive point of view. Do this for a period of one week. What are your conclusions?

Try rearranging the furniture to improve interaction and observe for a similar period of time the resultant changes. Did increased interaction occur? Did the new arrangement 'stay in place'? If not, who moved it, clients or staff?

If increased interaction did occur, what implications might this have for you in your working life. If it did not occur, or if the furniture was restored to its usual arrangement, why might this have happened and what can you do about it?

It may be that people feel uncomfortable with things which are new and different, particularly in long-stay areas of care where sometimes things have remained as they are for a very long time.

Reflect upon your answers to the activities where you identified your own personal territory, and the instances given regarding 'ownership' of a particular space. Then answer the following:

Do we always allow clients this type of territorial privilege? Do we allow them to feel that their bed space, chair, part of the sitting room – is theirs? Or do we sometimes actively try to prevent this ('There are no personal chairs here', or 'I can't see your name on that chair')? If it seems important to us, do we make assumptions that it is not important to them?

Ownership of various items of furniture or particular spaces may provide a crumb of comfort in an otherwise alien world – and perhaps we should recognize this. This might particularly apply to the environment in which Elsie found herself.

CASE STUDY

They, the staff that is, and there appeared to lots of them, talked with Elsie and asked her questions about how she had come to be here. She responded in the way she thought would be helpful to them, and did not want to confess all her shortcomings about managing. A doctor, whom she had never seen before, reiterated lots of these questions and Elsie occasionally did not bother to answer. She could not understand, either, what was wrong with Lena, who appeared angry at the situation and who abandoned her mother by returning home, with, however, promises to keep in touch.

NON-VERBAL COMMUNICATION

This section concentrates on non-verbal communication (NVC), not because there is no recognition of the importance of verbal communication, but because NVC is an area of expertise which people often neglect. It is also less overtly under concious control. So what is NVC? Ekman and Oster (1979) defined it as:

> any movement or position of the face or body, chiefly perceived through the visual sense organs, occasionally supplemented by auditory and tactual sensations.

It is made up of many parts, some of which are conscious enhancements of what we are saying, others which are unconscious and may not match, in emotion, the spoken word. An example of a conscious NVC is something which is known as an 'emblem' and is almost universally accepted. One such emblem would be pointing with the index finger to indicate something. Others might be waving; thumbs up or down; shoulder shrug; fist shaking; and many more.

Affect displays are merely facial expressions, but they can say a lot to us. Someone who is anxious is likely to have a furrowed brow, wide open eyes and may be biting their nails – so without a word being spoken you perceive an emotional state.

Just briefly stop and think of other facial expressions, perhaps with some small additions, like a particular hat or hairstyle or clothing – can you envisage this and deduce information from what you see?

Do verbal and non-verbal messages always match?

Reflect back to a time when someone was telling you something with their words, but their non-verbal signs were opposite to what they were saying. For example, a person saying he is not anxious, but wringing his hands, sweating, worried expression, fidgeting. Which type of communication did you take most note of at the time?

Now imagine what non-verbal signs might have been displayed by Elsie in her current situation, and the importance that these were read and recognized by the staff.

CASE STUDY

A woman in one of the other beds appeared friendly and tried to establish contact with Elsie. When Elsie told her she was 'Just in for a short while until she "got her bearings" after her husband's death' the other woman, who was apparently called Maud snorted with laughter and said 'Aren't we all!' in a way which made Elsie uncomfortable, although she could not exactly say why.

It was a few days before she realized that she was in a psychiatric hospital, which explained the strange arrangement of getting up each day early, getting dressed and eating in a kind of cafeteria, where there seemed to be an assortment of other 'patients' and some of them men. There were men too on her ward, and it seemed strange to see them passing what she thought of as her bedroom. On one day, she missed the midday meal entirely, having not been successful at finding the dining room, and when she mentioned this to a member of the catering staff who was just clearing away the remnants of lunch she was told 'You'll have to be quicker next time'. She began to wonder if there would be a next time, as she had no appetite. Her bungalow and its now overgrown garden – once Fred's pride and joy – beckoned unremittingly and she asked to go home.

There are several channels of NVC. Proxemics – already considered from a physical point of view – is the way we use space including touch distance and positioning, whereas personal space in a western culture varies according to the interaction taking place and the person involved (Figure 10.7):

- Intimate zone – we allow lovers, parents, spouses, children and close friends into this space (the clear area in Figure 10.7 is the close intimate zone and can only be entered during physical contact)
- Personal zone – we stand at this distance at office parties, social functions and friendly gatherings
- Social zone – we stand this distance from strangers (the doorstep caller, the decorator, local shopkeeper and people we do not know very well)
- Public zone – we use this distance when we address a large group of people

Thinking of Elsie's situation, and this information regarding personal space, how might she have felt about being in close proximity with 'strangers'?

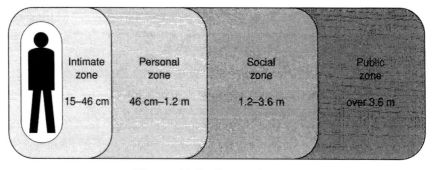

Figure 10.7   Personal space.

There are, of course, situations when we are in very close contact with strangers, for example in a crowded lift. Next time you are in this situation note your own behaviour and that of others.

You may be able, by this observation, to discover the 'unwritten' rules in such a situation. These rules usually include:

1. You are not permitted to speak to anyone, often including the person you know
2. You must avoid eye contact with others at all times
3. You are to maintain a 'poker face' – no emotion is permitted to be displayed
4. If you have a book or newspaper you must appear to be deeply engrossed in it
5. The bigger the crowd the less body movement you are permitted to make
6. In lifts you are compelled to watch the floor numbers above your head

It could be reasonably assumed that Elsie is very worried about her situation. How might this affect her uptake of information given to her?

In order that you might approach some understanding of this, try the following. Imagine you are very worried about things, you could imagine you are being admitted to hospital – or some other situation which you would find anxiety-provoking – and there are lots of thoughts whirling around in your mind.

Make a tape recording of these 'worry thoughts' – a constant drone of 'What if this or that happened?', 'Is everything alright at home?', 'Will the cat/dog/kids be alright?' and anything else you might like to add.

Now with the co-operation of a friend, put on headphones which will relay to you the 'worry thoughts' and ask the friend to read some information to you – it could be something as simple as the TV programmes for that evening. Do this exercise for about two or three minutes and then try to recall and repeat what your friend has been saying to you. How much of the information has actually been received and remembered by you? Is it less than you would normally be able to recall?

Now this is an activity which you have devised and therefore its impact will be reduced. But use the information you have gleaned to apply to Elsie's situation. It should help you to understand why sometimes our information is apparently not understood.

PERSONAL PROPERTY AND FREEDOM OF MOVEMENT

CASE STUDY   When Elsie asked to go home it was explained, very clearly to her, that this was not a good idea. After all she had demonstrated that she could not cope and they were trying their best to get her better, but she didn't seem to be helping them at all. She felt quite angry and betrayed by this, and demanded her bag back to pack. She knew they couldn't make her stay, even though this hospital seemed a world away from the one where she had had Lena – her only other experience of hospitalization.

When she realized that the bag was not going to be forthcoming, she became tearful and then angrily accused the staff of stealing it. They said they were not going to have any of that kind of talk and that an entry would be made in her notes and she was making false accusations, even further evidence, if any were needed, that she did not know what she was doing.

Nurses obviously violate personal space boundaries on a regular basis, but how could the distress this might cause be minimized?

You have considered personal space and the invisible 'bubble' around us all. Refer back to the text and activities on environmental territories and our need to 'own' the spaces we occupy and link this to the concept of personalizing space.

When a person enters any sort of caring environment how important is it to them that they are aware of the space which is theirs, and that they are able to personalize that space? How may they personalize that space?

Are we always able to accept this need and allow the person to display their individuality in this way? Or do we occasionally, in our pursuit of tidiness and order, preclude this expression? What happened to Elsie's tapestry bag? How much might this seemingly innocuous activity have meant?

Leaving proxemics, we move on to kinesics, movements, gestures and expressions, which are popularly known as body language and include gaze, posture, and even to some extent the way we dress.

Look at the representations of posture in Figure 10.8. See if the message of each is clear to you. Are you able from this very limited information to make some sort of assessment of what the figure is thinking or feeling?

Some may be more difficult to identify than others, and indeed some may have a dual meaning. Is the central bottom figure cheering in triumph or shaking their fists in rage? However, no form of non-verbal communication should be taken in isolation and these postural messages need to be considered in the context of other observed phenomena.

What might Elsie's posture be? How might this have been read? How might this have been mis-read?

It might have been shoulders hunched, arms hanging by sides, head bowed, eyes lowered, gait slow. This type of postural picture may indicate that someone is decidedly unhappy and can also be seen in those who have been in an institution for a number of years and who have lost the ability to make choices and significantly influence their own lives.

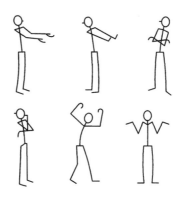

Figure 10.8   Some postures with clear meanings. (Reproduced from Pease, K. (1974) *Communication without Words*. Vernon Scott Associates).

THE IMPORTANCE OF PRIVACY

CASE STUDY   Time passed in a kind of limbo. Things did not improve. The meagre belongings she had brought needed increasing, and she was asked if her daughter would be visiting and bring her more things. She said she was sure she would be, unaware that this was increasingly more unlikely. In the end the nice social worker appeared with some things from her house. If she had been more 'on form' she would have asked how he had got them, but by now she didn't care.

Always a neat and tidy person, she began to neglect her appearance, and the staff, to give them their due, did help her by taking her into the bath on a regular basis. It seemed funny having someone with you in this most private of places, and sometimes they even had to wash her. Elsie castigated herself, what was she thinking about letting strangers wash her as if she was a baby – why sometimes even a man – yes there were male nurses here, they would even come in the bathroom for keys or some such nonsense on occasions. She felt very embarrassed by this, it appeared to be 'the norm', but she had great difficulty in figuring out what the rules were here. When she caught sight of herself in the mirror she thought Marjory, down at the hairdressers, would have had a fit if she could have seen her hair, she had always done it so nicely for her.

There are perhaps two issues to be addressed here. With regard to the invasion in the bathroom – reflect on the material we have used with regard to personal space, own sense of identity, and try to empathize with the feelings associated with someone actually seeing us in a situation which is normally totally private.

When you are in a public lavatory, and the lock is broken – what position do you usually adopt? Do you stretch out a leg or arm to its ultimate in order to prevent someone entering? Do you practice bodily contortions which have never been seen before in order that you might at least prevent the door opening WIDE? If so, and this is a common response, you should have no difficulty in relating to Elsie's feelings.

What about clothing? What about the change from neat, tidy, clean, well turned-out to dishevelled, somewhat dirty? Does this have a message for us, and how should we respond?

Judgements are often made about people filling certain roles as to their personality traits. Take nurses for example: nurses are kind, caring, dedicated – they are also apparently female, young, attractive, and prone to wearing stockings (black) and suspenders! This is one example of a stereotype. If you went to see a bank manager, would you be surprised if you were confronted by someone with an orange mohican haircut, a large stud in his nose, jeans, braces and Doc Marten boots? I think perhaps you would. For we all make, and have been socialized into making, judgements according to role and external accoutrements such as clothing.

How important do you think it is to be aware of our own sterotypes and recognize their influence upon our behaviour? What might be a stereotype of some older people? However positive, outward appearances need to monitored in order to ensure we are aware when someone's habits change significantly. This often is a sign that all is far from well.

Sometimes we are caught out. I remember a rather bombastic sister on an acute ward being faced with a rather scruffy middle-aged gent some half an hour after visiting time was over. After a cursory glance – over the top of her glasses – she informed him that visiting was over in no uncertain terms – and returned to her writing. The 'visitor' then informed her bowed head that he was Mr Jones, a consultant surgeon, who had been called to visit one of the clients. He apologized for his dress, but explained that he had just been working on his boat when called. As you can imagine, this provoked a very different response.

On a more serious note, it is important that we do not allow our prejudices to cause us to make assumptions about people, merely by their outward appearance.

CASE STUDY There was some talk of treatment, by electric shock, which seemed a funny sort of treatment to Elsie. 'You don't want to stand for it', said Maud. Elsie started laughing softly to herself when she thought she didn't have the strength to sit for it, never mind stand for it. If only they would just listen a bit more – if she could get up the courage to tell them – and help her to sort out finances, simple things which had lain in Fred's domain, and if only Lena seemed more understanding. She agreed to the treatment, and in her short conversations with various transient fellow clients heard stories about it both good and bad. Apparently it had 'Done Marge over the way the world of good, made a new woman of her' while Ernie said ominously it was like being 'Plugged into the National grid'.

She knew by now she could not leave, as some forms had been filled in by the nice young man; Lena was somehow involved and a very important consultant. It was all explained very carefully, something to do with an Act of Parliament, but to her it felt very much like being imprisoned. The nurse agreed, that 'Yes it was like this, but it was for her own good so she should try and comply with what they wanted her to do'. The staff were OK, they did their best in often trying circumstances, but nobody seemed to have the time or inclination to talk with her and when they did it appeared to her that they were making impossible demands. She missed the contact of others, not just Fred, and longed for someone to just hold her hand, or put their arms around her. She thought it was perhaps her own fault that nobody did.

TOUCH

➤ 11   Touch is the earliest and most primitive form of communication. It has been described as a basic human need which becomes important during gestation and continues to remain a fundamental component of communication throughout life. It is a potent means of non-verbal communication and can convey a myriad of positive and negative messages between people (le May, 1986).

Human touch can be a great comfort in times of distress and can serve to emphasize a verbal message. There are, however, people who like to be touched and those who find it uncomfortable, so it is important for care workers to be aware of not only the client's feelings about this, but their own as well.

Think about yourself and how often you touch others during the everyday course of your life. Are you a person who likes to touch and be touched? Make yourself aware of your own touch behaviour.

Not only do we need to be aware of what we are unconsciously telling clients when we touch them, but it is worth considering how we can use touch consciously, to communicate with clients who have a greater need than normal for touch.

Most research on touch has been conducted on clients who are suffering from a physical condition, and has shown that if expressive touch is used (as opposed to merely mechanical touch to carry out some procedure) then recovery rates are improved and the clients report feeling better in themselves.

In a situation where a person is expressing either physical or emotional distress – and you reach out to touch him – what non-verbal signs would indicate whether he would welcome the touch?

The way in which testing of touch works is as follows:

- Carer feels empathy and reaches out to touch client
- Positive response can be identified in facial expression, eye contact and no sign of limb withdrawal (withdrawal would be literal, a distinct movement away, gaze averted)
- Carer touches client and maintains touch
- Client continues to accept touch

Make a note of observations you could use to help you become aware of the limits and benefits of touch in your work setting. Select a few clients and hold a small discussion, either individually or as a group, to ask them what their feelings are about touch.

If we take the plight of clients on long-stay wards, we will see that they are often denied through circumstances and loss of family contacts, many forms of touch. Rubin (1963) noted in situations where clients were under intense personal stress, feeling isolated and vulnerable, no other method of communication compared in immediacy to the comforting and quieting effects of touch.

Contact within a social context is mainly limited to the hands. Intimate relationships are characterized by touching, but in our society, friends and acquaintances are usually very inhibited in using touch as a means of communication.

The touch mentioned here is not the phenomenon known as therapeutic touch – merely touch as a means of communication. Another very important facet of non-verbal communication is eye contact, something which Elsie was trying to establish in her situation.

CASE STUDY

On occasional good days, she tried to discuss this, but it now took her so long to say anything and the staff appeared to have a great deal of paperwork to do and often did not even look up, except initially when she approached. Sometimes her concerns were swept away by statements such as 'Well we mustn't be negative must we?' – it seemed to her, in her more lucid moments, she had plenty to be negative about.

Reflect on any occasions when you have been trying to say something to someone and they have, for instance, kept on writing without looking up. How did this make you feel?

If you are unable to identify such a situation, perhaps you could set up a role-play to enact the scenario with a colleague. Make it as realistic as possible and note your feelings when you are the person trying to speak. You might well conclude that what you were saying was of so little import that it did not even merit recognition. This might have grave implications for your self-esteem.

Have you ever been 'guilty' of doing such a thing? Bear this in mind next time you are busy and a client, a colleague or a relative wants to talk.

We have expectations about eye behaviour and perhaps only become aware of these expectations when we meet nervous, very shy or mentally disturbed individuals who do not demonstrate usual eye behaviour.

The pattern of eye behaviour acts as punctuation and in this way the conversational turns are passed around like a ball.

There is a well-known saying that 'It's not what you say – it's the way that you say it', and this is where the non-verbal skill of paralanguage comes in. This is the tone, volume and inflexion of your voice. The words spoken may be quite innocuous but the way in which they are spoken will demonstrate the feeling behind the words.

Reflect on the implications of this for those who may not fully be able to follow the conversation and may miss their chance at 'catching the ball', for example those who are blind. How might you need to adjust your own communications to accommodate this?

Observe a group of people talking and see if you can identify the role that eye contact plays in punctuating conversation. Then observe a group of people who are not in a familiar environment – for example clients in a care setting – and note whether eye contact is used to facilitate interaction or appropriately used as punctuation.

Compare these two activities. What was the difference – if any? If you have discovered any differences, why might this group of people be behaving differently and how could you use your skills to remedy this?

If you have discovered this or any other anomalies in client/client or client/staff communication, what problems might this pose to therapeutic interaction – and how might these be remedied or reduced? What message may have been unintentionally sent to Elsie when the member of staff did not look up from the task in hand?

It might be that simply by practising appropriate eye contact, and other non-verbal activities, you will increase therapeutic interaction – at least between yourself and those you interact with – but there may be some strategy you could devise to help clients interact with each other.

Take the following words or phrases and try saying them out loud, with a colleague for feed-back if you wish, in two different ways so that the meaning is altered.

1. You look lovely in that dress
2. Stop that
3. Go away
4. Come with me
5. Isn't this a lovely day for a picnic?

What different meanings did the words adopt?

Take, for example, the last sentence. If this is said on a sunny day with a smile, perhaps rubbing hands and a 'lilt' in the voice, it has one meaning. If it's pouring with rain and it is said with a glum expression and a sarcastic emphasis, then the meaning is entirely opposite – but – the words are exactly the same.

The nuances and the subtle different emphases we place on words, both intentionally or unintentionally can affect how the message is received.

MEANINGFUL ACTIVITY

CASE STUDY   There appeared to be nothing to do here. Right enough, some people came and took Elsie to activities, but she could not seem to relate to the other people there. She knew she had been good at many things and had taken care of and dealt with all the things associated in caring for her husband and daughter, but she had to agree she didn't seem too good at anything else. Fearing failure, she didn't even try. She saw it as a kind of victory when they didn't send her there anymore.

Activity theory, as a sociological approach to ageing, postulates that life satisfaction in later years occurs when individuals maintain an optimal level of social activity. Less active older persons were found to be less successful in coping with the demands of everyday life (Watson, 1982).

It is important that clients should have a choice of activities in which to participate and three types of activity are described in Lemon *et al.*'s (1972) theory. Informal activities such as those of a social nature and involving relatives, friends, and neighbours; formal activities such as social interactions in voluntary organizations and the church; solitary activities such as hobbies, handicrafts and playing a musical instrument.

Very often the television is the chosen mode of distraction, turned on by a member of staff, and subsequently left on. This kind of activity, although of some limited worth is essentially an isolating activity.

EPILOGUE

CASE STUDY

Elsie knew she shouldn't have stopped eating and drinking, but the food seemed to choke her. She lost track of time, and when transfer was mentioned to a long-stay hospital, she remembered it by name as being the place the patients said was where they sent 'no hopers' and the place the staff said, unfortunately in her hearing although not to her specifically, where they sent people who wouldn't conform.

Seven months after admission, Elsie got into what seemed like the same car, with the same nice young social worker and was transferred to a long-stay facility some four miles away.

During the next three years she had various treatments, many setbacks, lost her home, but on one day, which she would never forget, a nurse, with whom she had talked extensively, argued a case for Elsie to be placed in a sheltered house with another patient. Not many people were for it, but by some miracle (she later thought) she got the place.

This was the turning point. Elsie again had someone to care for – even if it was not her beloved Fred – and part of the transfer scheme was to work with patients on aspects of social living, including financial management. In her better moments Elsie thought this was quite amusing as she now had so little money to manage as she was on the basic benefits – but gradually out of the nightmare came little glimmers of hope.

This story has a happy ending. Elsie, now aged 79, lives in sheltered accommodation in the community. She is a spry, neat, determined woman, who against all the odds, survived. She has been reconciled with her daughter, who appeared to abandon her in her time of most need, and goes occasionally to visit her three grandchildren. She still misses Fred, and cannot remember the full extent of her time in the hospital. Her favourite nurse, the one who got her out, as she likes to put it, is now retired herself, and visits Elsie on the basis of true friendship every week.

CONCLUSION

In conclusion, the core skills of communication and relationship building are essential fundamental skills for nurses. From analyzing Elsie's experience it is obvious that failure to listen to clients and hear what they are really saying, rather than what we, as nurses, think they are saying, can have an enormous impact on the outcomes of care. In this way, communication breakdown is not simply the 'fault' of the older person who may not be able to clearly articulate, or are in a strange environment. Nurses need to take responsibility for their part in the way in which any communication evolves, including in those situations which do not work. The nurse is responsible for their abilities to not only send messages, but also to receive them. The more difficulties the older person has in communication the greater the nurse's skill in interpreting and receiving messages needs to be.

FURTHER READING

Argyle, M. (1983) *The Psychology of Interpersonal Behaviour*. Methuen, London. (1988) *Bodily Communication*. Penguin, Harmondsworth.
Good source books on communication in general.

Bebb, R. (1987) Care to talk? *Nursing Times*, 16 September, 83(37), 40–41.
Explores the diminishing, but still present, belief that talking to clients is a lower priority than functional tasks and the guilt feelings this prompts, particularly in student nurses.

Berne, E. (1968) *Games People Play*. Penguin, Harmondsworth.
Popularized with move towards personal growth and understanding; likely to clarify roles and motives both personal and professional.

Faulkner, A. (1984) Communication. In *Recent Advances in Nursing*. Churchill Livingstone, Edinburgh.
This series of publications gathers together research-based papers providing an authoritative perspective on a subject of current interest.

Gaze, H. (1990) Making time to talk. *Nursing Times*, 86(13), 38–39.
This article suggests that nurses need to be more aware of the therapeutic value of allowing patients to express their fears in a hospital environment.

Kagan, C., Evans, J. and Kay, B. (1986) *Manual of Interpersonal Skills for Nurses*. Harper & Row, New York.
This book adopts an experiential approach and is a mix of activities and well-packaged theory. The discussion issues provide useful prompts for further exploration.

Morris, D. (1981) *Manwatching*. Triad, St Albans.
Now a classic in the public domain. Readable, interesting and revealing.

Pease, K. (1974) *Communication without Words*. Vernon Scott Associates, Boston.
Clearly identifies the role and impact of non-verbal communication. With very good illustrations, this book is effective in relating this area of skill across a broad range of situations.

Stockwell, F. (1971) *The Unpopular Patient*. RCN, London.
Not about communication as such, but highlighted within the text is how appropriate and inappropriate communication skills leave patients in no doubt as to how they are perceived.

Williams, J. (1991) Meaningful dialogue. *Nursing Times*, 23 January, 87(4), 52–53.
Explores the nurse's contribution to communication with confused older people.

REFERENCES

Argyle, M. (1967) *The Psychology of Interpersonal Behaviour*. Methuen, London.

Bernstein, B. (1973) *Class, Codes and Control*. Routledge and Kegan Paul, London.

Blattner, B. (1981) *Holistic Nursing*. Englewood Cliffs, NJ.

Department of Health (1994) Being heard: the report of a review committee on NHS complaints procedures.

Ekman, P. and Oster, H. (1979) Facial expressions of emotion. *Annual Review of Psychology*, 30, 527–554.

Esberger, K.K. and Hughes, S.T. (eds) (1989) *Nursing Care of the Aged*. Appleton & Lange, Norwalk, CT.

Hurst, B. (1991) *The Handbook of Communication Skills*. Kogan Page, London.

Groenman, N.H., Slevin, O. D'A. and Buckenham, M.A. (1992) *Social and Behavioural Sciences for Nurses*. Campion Press, Edinburgh.

le May (1986) The human connection. *Nursing Times*, 19 November.

Lemon, B.W., Bengston, V.L. and Peterson, J.A. (1972) An exploration of the activity theory of aging: activity types and life satisfaction among in-movers to a retirement community. *Journal of Gerontology*, 27(4), 511–523.

Ostro, M. (1989) Care of the elderly person. In *Nursing Practice and Health Care*. Hinchliff, S.M., Norman, S.E. and Schober, J.E. (eds). Edward Arnold, London.

Pease, K. (1981) *Communication Without Words*, 2nd edn. Vernon Scott Associates, Boston.

Rubin R. (1963) Maternal Touch, *Nursing Outlook*, 11, 828.

Watson, W.H. (1982) *Aging and Social Behaviour*. Wadsworth, Monterey CA.

Weil, S. (1952) *Gravity and Grace*, Routledge & Kegan Paul, London.

Weinstein, K. (1992) Managing communication. In *Handbook of Management Skills*, 2nd edn, Stewart, D.M. (ed.). Gower, London.

11 Touch as therapy

Gill Johnson and Alan White

INTRODUCTION

> The human need for touch . . . does not lessen as we grow, develop and age. Rather the need for touch on all levels increases with age and wisdom (Fanslow, 1990, p. 542).

The role and value of touch is an integral part of nursing practice. It encompasses a range of interventions from the fundamental, everyday contact with clients to the more specialized and specific use of touch that is the use massage in practice. The concepts of 'touch as therapy' and 'therapeutic touch' are interpreted, for the purpose of this chapter, as any touching act which is of benefit to a client. This is considered in the context of cultural and gender issues. In addition, the concepts of caring and comforting in relation to touch are explored. The skill of massage and its appropriate integration into nursing practice is examined and its use is placed with the context of the Code of Professional Conduct (UKCC, 1992). This chapter aims to challenge your perceptions and assumptions by asking you to reflect upon your practice, your knowledge and your attitudes in relation to the use of touch.

Touch is a central component of human existence; age is no barrier to this, indeed the need for touch may increase as we grow older. Consequently, as nurses, we need to consider the use of touch in our care of older clients. There has been a growing interest in, and literature on, the use of touch in caring environments in support of this. Some of this has focused on touching in general, whilst others have concentrated on more specific issues around touch, including its links to care, comfort, age, culture and gender (Sanderson *et al.*, 1991; Ernst and Shaw, 1980; Krieger, 1979; Fraser and Ross-Kerr, 1993; Montagu, 1986). The need for touch to aid growth and development physically, psychologically and socially at all ages, is recognized by Montagu (1986). The tactile senses in the skin are represented by a large area in the brain. Montagu (1986) uses this evidence to emphasize the need for physical contact and tactile stimulation to enhance and promote holistic health and well-being. Lack of appropriate touch in childhood can have implications throughout the lifespan resulting in potential problems such as aggression, depression, social withdrawal and challenging behaviours (Sanderson *et al.*, 1991). This emphasizes the importance of recognizing the older client as being at one point on a developmental continuum that began in infancy, the effects of this being reflected in their responses and desire for touch in older age.

To help you focus on the idea of touch, observe an interaction between two people. Watch their touching behaviours. How did this make you feel? Did the touch convey any messages? Were these congruent with what was being said? Were there any factors that helped or hindered this interaction?

Perhaps it is the first time you have ever consciously considered the use of touch. It may have alerted you to why this medium of communication needs to be used with care as the messages touch is able to convey can be very powerful. It may be assumed that people who enter the nursing profession value physical contact and are comfortable touching others – this may not always be the case. You will, therefore, be asked throughout this chapter to reflect on personal and professional experiences that may affect how you feel and behave in situations involving touch.

Consider for a moment how you feel about being touched. Are you comfortable touching others and being touched? What messages do you intentionally or unintentionally send or receive?

◄10   The concepts of communication and interaction may be seen to be central to the use and meanings attributed to touch. From this it can be seen that having communication and interaction as a central and vital component of the nurse–client relationship may be more complex than first thought. However, this emphasizes the need for a deeper understanding of the complexities surrounding the use of touch in client care.

THE NATURE OF NURSING

This chapter is attempting to address the concept of touch from the perspective of the older person – this therefore necessitates an understanding of nursing which has this client focus as its primary consideration. It has already been alluded to that there is no such thing as a standard person, either nurse or client, and therefore it may not be possible, or indeed desirable or appropriate, to create a clinical protocol for the use of touch in practice settings. The nurse must have a thorough appreciation of what touch may mean to the client and also the potential benefits and harm that can occur through its use. This is important if touch is to be used, in both planned for and spontaneous care events in a therapeutic and effective manner. It is also necessary to consider that whereas it is appropriate and possible that a client may not wish to be touched, it cannot be seen as permissible to have a nurse who will generally avoid physical contact with clients.

The beliefs and values held about nursing and people will affect how care needs are identified, prioritized and managed.

What do you believe about nursing? What do you think are the important components of effective care?

Chinn and Kramer (1995) suggest that the nature of nursing is based around a helping process which has its primary focus on interpersonal relationships between a nurse and another individual. Touch as a potential facet of this relationship has already been highlighted when recognizing the use of touch in communication and interactions. Nursing can subsequently be seen as centrally pivoted around this concept of an interpersonal process.

The nature of this process will vary. The client may not wish to have anything more than a functional relationship with the nurse. It may, however be appropriate to develop deeper therapeutic relationships with the client. Whichever the case, touch used with consideration and thought can play a therapeutic role.

CARING

The nature of the relationship between nurse and client and the attitudes, knowledge and skills that go towards its development may also be linked to the notion of nursing as a caring profession. The Report of the Committee on Nursing chaired by Briggs (HMSO, 1972) made a powerful statement when they referred to nursing and midwifery as the major caring professions. This report predates the large volume of literature that has emanated from the United States on the concept of caring and must be seen as foresighted and worthy of some consideration.

 Consider for a moment what you consider to be the necessary skills, knowledge and attributes for a nurse in today's care settings

This report (HMSO, 1972) identifies nursing as encompassing kindness, responsibility, skill, intelligence, and sensitivity, with clients and the public, judging caring in qualitative ways via the perceived quality of the care received. It also recognizes nursing's integrative function not just in the co-ordination of care in hospital and in the community but also in terms of understanding and responding to a person's physical, social and psychological needs. This report, although not as well argued as some nursing theories, does portray some of the ideas that should be directing the nurse at the end of the 20th century.

The writings of Briggs (HMSO, 1972) do not, however, lead us into the true complexities of what it means to care. The *Oxford English Dictionary* (1989) suggests that the origin of the word care is from the Anglo-Saxon *carian*, meaning to 'trouble oneself'. As the meaning is investigated further this, in essence, is what is required. To care is as much about having a deep commitment as it is having a sound knowledge base. The values and beliefs of the nurse are as important as the skills. A commitment to the individual as well as to the client group at large would seem essential to the genuine and effective development of a caring relationship.

These issues are reflected by Lawler (1991), Savage (1995) and Morrison (1994), all of whom identify the deep and profound way the relationship and interactions between nurse and client affect care. Savage (1995) identifies how nurses in her study sample felt the need to get close to people in both physical and emotional ways in order to be effective carers.

However, Lawler (1991) indicates that nurses central involvement with the body as an 'object' requires the nurse to develop strategies to recognize the 'lived body', the body as experienced by living people. This involvement with 'the body' often takes place at a time when clients are facing feelings, described by Morrison (1994) as 'crushing vulnerability'.

Stevens Barnum (1994) develops these ideas by identifying three meanings for the word care: care of, care about and careful. The first can be seen as having the practical skills to nurse. The second relates more to the attitudinal or emotional involvement with the client. The third meaning relates to the caution or precision in carrying out the practice of nursing. These three definitions should not be seen as mutually exclusive. When nursing older adults the 'care about' is as important as the practice and precision of the skills of care. When considering touch, the messages that may be sent and how they are interpreted may reflect the nurse's attitude towards the client regardless of the functional task being performed. Ersser (1991) reinforces this point in his study on the therapeutic nature of nursing, where it found that clients interpret the therapeutic actions of the nurse in both expressive and technical ways. In other words it was perceived by clients that the 'how' of doing the caring emphasized the nurse's value judgements as to the worthiness of the client.

Watson (1988) argues that caring is the essence of nursing. Nursing is viewed from both a philosophical and practical perspective with an emphasis on the importance of seeing the individual in a holistic and humanistic capacity whilst also keeping the science of the body in balance. Caring is seen as a transpersonal, intersubjective, mutual exchange between the nurse and client. There is a need for the nurse to know themselves so that their own part in the relationship can be recognized. Leininger (1981, 1991) holds similar views on caring, but, coming from an anthropological background has rooted her views in the cultural domain. The emergent transcultural theory of nursing focuses the nurse on to the need to recognize and be responsive to the cultural variations that exist between groups and individuals. The cultural influences on perception of care, that is, what is acceptable and appropriate, also require consideration when initiating or returning a touching act. These aspects will be more fully developed later.

When reflecting on the role of touch, care and the older client, Watson's and Leininger's theories highlight the need to consider the nature of the relationship. This includes beliefs about initiating touch, past experiences and their influences on touching behaviours as well as the mutuality and power relationships that may affect the interactions and types of touch used.

The need to consider the notion of care and its relationships to touch would seem to centre on the use of touch in a practical and functional sense. It can also be a way of sending affective and accepting messages and developing relationships with clients. All these factors depend on the nurse's beliefs about values about nursing, people in general and specifically older people, the nature of care, and the relevance of touch.

The relevance of caring to nursing is beginning to take shape. Nursing has as its central point the notion of an interpersonal process (Chinn and Kramer, 1995). Therefore the theory that drives nursing must have the interpersonal dimension firmly embedded within it. We have also seen that nursing can be about dealing with people in a very intimate and deep manner, therefore another aspect of our theory must be to guide us in relation to our values and beliefs.

The expression of care and its links to the form of the relationship developed between people is the subject of a study by Morse *et al.* (1992). This study suggests that in order to fully take into account the person who needs care, the nurse has to focus on the clients response to the care delivered. Morse *et al.* (1992) also identified other levels of engagement which moved from this fully attuned, connected sense to a detached self-focused manner in which care was delivered with no notice being taken of the emotional impact on the client. When the nurse becomes engaged with the client's emotions, genuine reflexive responses are elicited which are identified as: pity, sympathy, consolation, commiseration, compassion and reflexive reassurance. These responses, exhibited in a variety of interpersonal ways, including touch, when used in an immediate and genuine way provided the client with a deep sense of comfort.

Comfort

Comfort is the most important nursing action in the provision of nursing care for the sick. Whereas caring provides the motivation for the nurse to nurse and to provide maintenance, restorative and preventative actions to promote health, comforting is the major instrument for care in the clinical setting (Morse, 1983).

Kolcaba and Kolcaba (1991) analyzed the concept of comfort and identified six meanings that are in use:

- A sense of relief from discomfort and/or of the state of comfort
- The state of ease and peaceful contentment
- Relief from discomfort
- Whatever makes life easy or pleasurable
- Strengthening; encouragement, incitement, aid, succour, support, countenance
- Physical refreshment or sustenance, refreshing or invigorating influence

They identify from this that three technical senses of comfort can be identified:

- The state sense – in which the state of being comfortable is experienced
- The relief sense – in which an uncomfortable state is relieved
- The renewal sense – in which the person is strengthened and invigorated

The implications that can be drawn from this suggest that a client may require different therapeutic strategies to help them achieve a state of being comfortable. This requires an assessment of the client's current state and the creation of a plan which will meet the individual client's requirements. Hamilton (1989) suggests the following framework, which is able to assess the client's ability to feel comfortable and which can be used by the nurse to guide care planning:

- Disease process
- Self-esteem
- Positioning
- Approach and attitude to the staff and hospital life

Touch may be seen to play a role in this plan, either as a specific intervention, such as massage, or as part of other comfort strategies such as repositioning or the light touch of a supportive hand. The framework also emphasizes the multi-dimensional nature of comfort, in which touch may play a part. This multi-dimensional nature is emphasized in Hamilton's (1989) observation that older adults view their relationships, their environment and their feelings equally as important as the physical components of comfort.

THERAPEUTIC USE OF TOUCH

To touch says 'I care',
Being touched means 'I exist and I am worthy of care'
(Ernst and Shaw, 1980, p. 193)

Estabrooks and Morse (1992) claim that touch as a means of providing comfort has been neglected in nursing theory, although Bottorff (1991) cites several studies where caring, comfort and touch have been linked.

 Do you think that touch is an integral part of providing care and comfort to your clients? What has made you think in this way?

Historically, touch has formed part of nursing (Robb, 1910), although Wright (1995) suggests that in some areas its use may have become lost or marginalized. Henderson (1966) reflects on the mechanistic, procedure-orientated aspects of her nurse training and identifies how this approach limited and invalidated efforts to enhance the art of nursing. Perhaps you can identify with Henderson and can recognize areas within your own training, education or experience where value has been placed on learning procedures or doing tasks rather than nursing people. More recently, Benner (1984) has identified that the nursing domain does extend to providing healing and helping roles and relationships, some of which include: 'Providing comfort and communication through touch' and 'Presencing', which is defined as being with a patient (p. 50). Duke (1992) reiterates this and states, 'Caring is to listen, to touch and reach out to others' (p. 40).

It may be no surprise that in a study by Barnette (1972) it was found that nurses touch people more than any other healthcare workers. This study identified that older people, the acutely ill or people with psychotic disorders were touched least. These findings are also supported in other studies by Goodykoontz (1979), Watson (1975), Aguilera (1967) and Tobiason (1981). These studies emphasize the problems that may exist around the use of touch for certain client groups. This awareness is important if nurses are being charged, to 'devise a more personal approach to care . . . to enhance the therapeutic role of the nurse' (Wright, 1995, p. 16).

Wright (1995) considers that using touch in therapeutic ways may be one way in which this can be achieved. Therapy, therapeutic, care and comfort therefore seem to be linked and appear to create a range of opportunities for use in nursing practice.

DEFINING TOUCH

There is a need to more fully explore the nature of touch, its definition, meanings and uses, to clarify its potential for appropriate use in nursing older clients.

Consider for a moment how you would define the word 'touch'. What features does your definition have?

Watson (1975) defines touch as an intentional physical contact between two or more people. You may think that this meaning is rather limited and that it does not take into account the complexities that constitute an understanding of the word 'touch'. Several other writers (Wright, 1995; Montagu, 1986; Weber, 1990; Weiss, 1986) recognize that touch can encompass not just physical but also emotional, social and spiritual aspects. They recognize that these dimensions interlink and that at all these levels touch can be a powerful means of contact and communication.

Consider for a moment whether you think it is possible to touch someone without making physical contact. Can someone's behaviour touch another emotionally?

The idea of touching someone other than physically is seen in Benner's (1984) and Ersser's (1991) idea of 'presencing' or 'being with' a person and is also examined by Paulen (1984), who suggests that nursing may also be about touching the spirit of another human being.

Work done by Krieger (1979) extends the boundaries of touch in nursing in her work on therapeutic touch. This form of touch includes the transfer of energy and feelings between individuals without making physical contact.

Some of these issues are highlighted in the following quote from a client who had been visited by the district nurse to have a leg ulcer dressed. The nurse had taken a birthday card for the lady who was celebrating her eighty-second birthday.

> You're always so kind and take good care of my leg.
> I didn't even know you knew it was my birthday.
> Thank you, I'm very touched.

Fanslow (1990) reminds us that for older people:

Physical, psychological, and emotional touches are all essential for the proper establishment of internal sources of security, self image, trust and interdependence (Fanslow, 1990, p. 543).

TYPES OF TOUCH

How and why we touch can communicate many messages, may take many forms and may be used unconsciously or consciously for a variety of reasons.

Consider two situations in which you have touched a client. What was the reason for the touch? Were there differences in the type of touch used?

You may have identified:

- Doing things for clients, for example, performing a task
- Conveying a message
- Comforting
- Greeting someone
- Gaining information about a client's skin condition or temperature
- Validating them as a person and recognizing their presence

Differences may have included:

- Linked with a physical task
- To give emotional support
- To protect yourself or the client
- To stimulate or relax muscles
- To gain information rather than convey a message

Tutton (1991) cites several studies where the types, amount and style of touch nurses use have been identified. These styles are also reflected in studies by Burnside (1981) and Sims (1986), Morse (1983), Estabrooks (1989), Watson (1975) and Weber (1990). These types of touch include:

- Task, functional, instrumental or procedural touch (Sims, 1986; Watson, 1975). This links to Benner's (1984) domain of 'doing to or for a person'
- Comforting or caring touch (Morse, 1983)
- Expressive, systematic and therapeutic touch (Sims 1986, Watson 1975)
- Protective touch – a form that may be used by nurses or clients to control or provide a distance between another person (Estabrooks, 1989)

From your previous reflections on experience you may be able to identify aspects of these types of touch in your interactions with clients. It is interesting to note that in a study by McCann and McKenna (1993), most of the observed interactions in continuing care settings for older adults were instrumental in nature, the focus being on tasks and 'doing for another'. Although this suggests that one type was prominent it does not identify if other messages or meanings were being conveyed during the interaction which could turn a potentially routinized and mechanistic procedure into a therapeutic event.

Think back to a task you have recently undertaken with a client, perhaps helping them to move, adjusting their clothing or assisting them with their hygiene needs.

Is there a difference between handling someone and touching them?

When considering the different types of touch and touching styles it is important to recognize that they can be used together and not, necessarily in isolation. When we perform tasks we can also gain information, express emotion or feelings and convey messages that may or may not be associated with care and comfort. The type of touch we use, the message received or conveyed as well as the initial reason for the touch requires careful and reflective thought to ensure we act in a therapeutic rather than mechanistic fashion. The way that these different forms of touch can be integrated is illustrated by the following example.

CASE STUDY

A nursing student had been caring for an older gentleman with learning disabilities for several weeks. This client was profoundly physically and mentally disabled and required a great deal of intimate physical care. This necessitated the use of instrumental touch. Towards the end of the placement the student realized that although she had frequently touched this client he had never touched her purposefully nor had there been any cues from him that he knew or recognized her. She felt as if the relationship was uneven and that she knew the client better than he knew her. The next time she worked with this gentleman she deliberately let him touch her face and hair. He responded by stroking her hair and lightly touching her face. Almost imperceptibly, the student felt the relationship had become more recognized, balanced, and equal.

Hollinger (1980) identifies that the type of touch used by the nurse when first meeting the client is a major determinant in the development of a trusting nurse–client relationship. The initiation of this contact also requires thought. The social status of the participants may influence how the touch is perceived. Burnside (1981) and Watson (1975) indicate that the touch initiator is often seen culturally and socially as the most powerful member of the relationship. This knowledge is relevant at any point in the nurse–client relationship; however, at an early stage when the nurse and client are meeting as strangers (Peplau, 1952) the initiation of touch could subtly define the power relationships within the care environment. The student in the above example recognized the implications of power relationships in her care of the client and used this knowledge to purposefully plan care to try and redress some of the imbalance. It also emphasizes the need to reflect on personal value systems to ensure touch is used in a client-sensitive way.

An in-depth awareness of the following statements and their inter-relationship indicates the importance of the personal beliefs in the context of touch.

I have my own views of touch, I have a cultural heritage and a personal value system. I have prejudices and I bring myself into each encounter. I perceive you and you perceive me. A result of this is that everything the nurse does is value laden. The style of dress, posture, speech, and touch conveys messages which may affect the client. Likewise, the client's style of dress, posture, speech and touch conveys messages which affect the nurse. This has two implications: one is that my beliefs and values will affect how I see you and therefore may affect the care I give you. Secondly, the client's values and beliefs will affect how they respond to me as a person and the care offered.

Morrison (1994, p. 127) highlights this in relation to the idea of mutuality, and how difficult it is to achieve the goal of the mutual relationship in which there is true acceptance of the other to create true companionship due to the very nature of the professional relationship. However, to use Buber's (1958) I-thou I-it concept it is possible to see how the nurse can reduce the client to the level of an object (it) to be nursed and also how the client can reduce the notion of the nurse to an 'it' giving institutional care as opposed to a person delivering client centred care.

THE CONTEXT OF TOUCH

Touch also needs to be seen within the social context in which it takes place. Nurses and other carers have privileged access to clients' bodies in a way that would not be usual in society at large. This, often intimate, access may also occur at the beginning of a relationship. Societal norms need to be considered in any discussion on touch to ensure the touching is acceptable and therapeutic and not invasive or demeaning.

Consider the two body outlines in Figure 11.1.

Indicate on the two figures where you would touch a person:

- Socially
- In your role as a nurse

What factors affected your choice?

You may have considered issues such as:

- Gender
- Culture
- Relationships
- Environment
- Context

- Age
- Status
- Past experiences
- Physical appearance
- Behaviour of the person

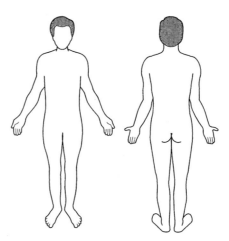

Figure 11.1   Body outlines (front and back).

This idea of body accessibility was investigated by Jourard (1966) who identified some of the above factors as particularly relevant when considering touch in a social context. Similarly, Bottorff (1991) recognized that the context in which touch takes place can fundamentally alter the meaning attached to the interaction. This work has since been partly substantiated by Lawler (1991) in her study on how nurses deal with the contact they have with the human body. In a study by Watson (1975) it was seen that touching was a selective process. Factors found to affect a person's touching behaviour included the parts of the body being touched, the gender and social status of the people involved, plus the physical appearance of the person to be touched. Physical stigma, deformities or frailties were found to produce varying responses from staff including positive and negative behaviours.

It needs to be recognized that nursing actions are governed by both intuitive and rational thought processes (Benner, 1984; Watson, 1988). Touch may be intuitively initiated by either the nurse or client in response to a perceived need or may be used purposefully and deliberately as the result of a planned sequence of events. It may also be used without regard to its effects or reasons for use. It would seem essential for therapeutic nursing to ensure that any touch is based on knowledge and skills gained from reflective practice and relevant reading.

The importance of this is supported by studies which identify that touch can have a therapeutic effect for both client and nurse (Seaman, 1982; Rowlands, 1984; Preston, 1973; Fraser and Ross-Kerr, 1993). Anecdotal evidence and case study approaches also indicate the value of touch when nursing older clients (Fascione, 1995; Passant, 1990; Sanderson *et al.*, 1991). However, Bottorff (1991) cautions that some of the literature may be biased, emphasizing the positive nature of touch without consideration of the influencing factors in the data collection. Bottorff (1991) identifies some of these constraints as:

- The sample population used was biased towards clients who would benefit from touch rather than those who would be harmed
- Researchers tended to use sampling techniques and data collection methods that only looked for positive outcomes
- Studies where client feedback was required suggested clients may have been constrained by the presence of the 'toucher'

Despite these timely reminders of the need to use touch in a considered and thoughtful way, touch used in a therapeutic way is seen as offering certain advantages.

 Consider for a moment your practice and the ways in which touch may enhance the care that clients receive.

The following list provides some of the advantages taken from a variety of sources (Fascione, 1995; Passant, 1990; Fraser and Ross-Kerr, 1993). These studies suggest touch can have therapeutic benefit by:

- Minimizing the effects of institutionalization
- Acting as a humanizer in an otherwise impersonal system
- Enhancing and increasing communication and interaction

- Decreasing sensory deprivation
- Reducing feelings of isolation and vulnerability
- Relieving stress and anxiety and helping to balance moods
- Promoting engagement
- Modifying behaviour
- Guiding and supporting
- Alleviating pain

Leininger (1991) also suggests that nurses need to identify the cultural requirements of their client so that the care they receive is congruent with their needs. If this does not occur, then the nurse may be seen to be imposing their own values and beliefs on to the client, which restricts any efficacy the care may have to offer. It is also a feature of the nurse retaining the power in the relationship. De Santis (1994) talks of simultaneous dual ethnocentrism in which:

> nurses are judging and reacting to clients on the basis of their own perceptions of clinical reality and their expectations of patients. Simultaneously, patients are judging nurses according to their beliefs about the health encounter and their expectations of the nurse (p. 708).

The ability to recognize the appropriate use of touch is therefore important. Not all client encounters may be enhanced by touch.

Consider a situation when touching a client may be inappropriate. Was it the type of touch that may be inappropriate rather than no touch?

DeWever (1977) found that some clients in a nursing home, especially men, were uncomfortable with expressive touch (arm around the shoulders) when instigated by the nurse. These findings were supported by McCann and McKenna (1993) who identified that expressive touching of the leg, face and shoulders was often perceived by older clients as uncomfortable. The reasons for this have already been alluded to and include:

- The context in which the touch took place
- The socialization and cultural expectations of the client
- A feeling of being dominated or patronized by the nurse
- The gender of the nurse, which may have sexual connotations

Ernst and Shaw (1980) cite sources that suggest touching clients may be countertherapeutic due to its sexual connotations. Psychoanalytic theory is used to justify claims that touch may be taboo with some clients. However, other sources are cited to argue that touching can have a powerful emotional and therapeutic effect. Situations may also occur when touching a client may precipitate a violent or inappropriate response (Farell and Gray, 1992). In these circumstances the nurse needs to be skilled in recognizing cues which suggest touch would be inappropriate and counterproductive.

CASE STUDY   Clare, a young staff nurse, was using the bobath technique to transfer a 78-year-old gentleman from bed to chair. The ward was very busy, client contact time was limited and Clare had only recently met this client. Mr James Nixon was an unmarried gentleman who had suffered a cerebro-vascular accident a week previously. Mr Nixon had a right-sided weakness and very labile emotions. He had previously been a very active man who had a wide circle of friends and an active social life. As Clare moved Mr Nixon he snuggled his face into her neck and stroked her back. Clare felt uncomfortable and completed the move as quickly as possible.

 Consider how you would have dealt with this situation.

The need to recognize the implications of this situation for both the nurse and the client are clear. Clare said she felt like avoiding Mr Nixon, potentially isolating him and labelling him as unpopular. She was confused as to whether the behaviour was as a result of his illness, the need for contact, or whether it represented his normal behaviour. Mr Nixon clearly felt the need for physical contact and due to the ward circumstances was perhaps only being touched when the need for moving arose.

For a wide range of reasons some older clients may have some degree of altered sensory tolerance, changing their perception and acceptance of touch. This does not mean that touching is taboo, indeed these clients may particularly benefit from a planned programme of touch. Preston (1973) and Sanderson *et al.* (1991) indicate that where cognitive functioning is impaired the use of touch via the touching and holding of hands and other non-verbal interaction can increase and/or modify engagement and interaction with others.

The use of touch to promote engagement is also explored by Langland and Panicucci (1982), whose study examines the use of touch alongside other sensory stimuli as a means of enhancing nurse–client interaction. This study is particularly relevant when considered alongside Hollinger's (1980) assertion that with age comes an increasing need to adapt to incoming sensory signals as the ability to recognize and differentiate some stimuli decreases.

The extremities of the body are seen as the exploratory parts of the body and as active organs of perception. These considerations are important and may enable a more therapeutic stance to be adopted with Mr Nixon. Factors which would help in the analysis of the situation could be considered using the following guidelines.

- Location
- Method
- Duration
- Intensity
- Frequency of contact
- Client's and nurse's position
- Recipient's response

This checklist follows Weiss's (1992) and LeMay and Redfern's (1989) work on touch, much of which was done with older clients. It does provide a useful framework against which touch could be planned and may be one way that the care situation with Mr Nixon could be considered.

TOUCH AND THE USE OF MASSAGE

It is not the purpose of this chapter to give you the competencies required to practice massage on clients. It is the intention to give an overview of different types of massage and their potential for use when working with older clients. Further reading and contact addresses for information on courses will be found at the end of the chapter.

Massage is a an ancient form of touch which has its origins in both western and eastern cultures. For some time it has been used in nursing practice as a means of promoting care and comfort, although during the technological revolution of the mid-twentieth century its use became marginalized or omitted from nursing care (Robb, 1910; Wright, 1995). Massage is one of many 'hands on therapies' which are often described as complementary therapies.

It is interesting that many nurses are now considering the use of these therapies to enhance their client care. The holistic approach of complementary therapies emphasizes the interaction and synergism of the body, mind and spirit, a notion that appears in many nursing models and theories (Wise, 1989). The body's ability to heal itself, the 'feel good' factor and the belief that clients should have control, where possible, over their health, are all important features to consider when using complementary therapies. Smith (1993) considers that nurses are now seeking to revive and legitimate the healing and caring potential of nursing via the use of massage and therapeutic touch.

There are several different types of massage. Some focus on specific areas of the body as in reflexology, others on muscle and soft tissues, as in Swedish massage, nerves and muscles, as in neuromuscular massage. Multisensory and interactive massage are identified as being useful for clients with learning disabilities as they have been seen to have therapeutic social, psychological and physical effects (Sanderson *et al.*, 1991). Interactive massage uses a planned sequence of interactions to gently and slowly allow clients to respond and become involved at their own pace. It uses touch as a means of developing a therapeutic relationship with a client. Although this approach was originally developed for use with deaf–blind infants (McInnes and Treffry, 1982), it has potential for use with older clients.

Eight stages are identified through which the client may progress:

- Resists the touch
- Tolerates the touch
- Passively co-operates
- Enjoys
- Responds co-operatively
- Leads
- Imitates
- Initiates

Multisensory massage uses other sensory stimuli alongside massage to provide a rich and varied environment (Sanderson *et al.*, 1991). It can be used with clients who have a variety of sensory impairments to increase their interaction and understanding of their surroundings. Even if you are not skilled in the use

Consider for a moment helping a client with hygiene needs.

It involves instrumental touch and could be seen as just another mechanistic task to be completed. By letting the client dip their hands in the water, feel the temperature and texture of the water, smell and feel the soap, hold the flannel and feel your hands gently touching theirs, what is often seen as an intimate nursing task becomes a therapeutic event.

➤12

of these techniques, some elements may be considered useful in your everyday contact with clients.

Reflexology is a form of massage that is concerned with zones on the hands or feet which reflect specific areas of the body. By stimulating and massaging these areas it is believed that beneficial effects can be achieved ranging from relaxation to the relief of physical symptons such as digestive discomfort and constipation. Two small studies (Thomas, 1989; Taylor, 1995) indicate how reflexology has been used as a means of reducing pain from arthritis, relieving anxiety and increasing interaction in older clients. The report by Taylor (1995) is particularly interesting as it identifies a six-month pilot study entitled 'Health Alternatives for Older People' commissioned by the charity 'Central and Cecil Housing Trust', which studied the use of three 'hands on' therapies in residential homes in London. The recommendations from this initial study are that complementary therapies should be available as a regular part of the care and that care staff should have the opportunity to develop competence in selected 'touch therapies'.

Swedish massage forms the basic technique taught in many initial massage courses. It can be seen as a form of systematic touch – manipulating the soft tissues of the body. This can sound very mechanistic and may appear to involve little expressive touch or relationship building. To ensure the benefits are maximized, the way in which the client is approached, the attitude and interpersonal skills of the nurse, their ability to pick up and interpret 'cues' from the client are important, as are competency in the massage technique being used. Together they can provide a powerful method of showing care and providing comfort.

Several research studies and anecdotal reports attest to the value of massage when caring for older clients (Fraser and Ross-Kerr, 1993; Fascione, 1995; Rowlands, 1984; Passant, 1990). A gentle hand massage (Box 11.1) can produce a feeling of relaxation and well-being and can be a non-threatening use of the massage techniques.

The need to recognize personal accountability for practice is important and to ensure that client safety is maintained. Before using massage the client, where possible, should give informed consent. Some organizations have forms where this can be documented. The care should be documented in the care plan and appropriate evaluation strategies employed. In a situation where the client is not able to give informed consent the potential use of the therapy should be discussed with relatives/friends, other staff and your manager and guidance taken from any available policies or protocols to ensure the needs and safety of the client are maintained (Johnson, 1995).

BOX 11.1	*Giving a simple hand massage*

Ask a colleague to act as a 'guinea pig'.

Remove any rings or watches that may damage the skin. Ensure your hands are clean and dry. Check your partner's hands for any contraindications such as cuts, bruises or rashes. Do not proceed with the massage if these are evident.

If any of the joints are swollen it would depend on the cause of the swelling as to whether massage would be appropriate. Under these circumstances avoid the use of massage until you have undergone appropriate training.

Note the colour, condition and texture of the skin. Extra care should be taken if the skin is thin or friable and the massage technique and pressure used adjusted accordingly.

As a massage medium use a hand cream or an oil such as grapeseed or sweet almond. Check with your partner that they are not allergic to any perfumes or food such as nuts and ensure that the massage medium is suitable for their use.

Support their hand and arm in a relaxed position, if necessary resting it on a cushion or pillow. Protect clothing with a towel.

Warm the cream or oil in your hands then gently spread it over their hand and wrist. Hold their hand in your hand with their palm down.

With your other hand gently stroke their hand starting from just above the wrist and covering the fingers. Complete the movement in the air to the starting point and repeat several times.

Support their hand using both your hands and gently use your thumb pads to make small light circular pressures over the wrist.

Continue these pressure circles between the bones of the hand from the wrist to the base of the fingers. Move across the hand massaging the soft tissues between the bones of the hand.

Now focus on each finger in turn and use your thumb pad to circle around the fingers, below, across and above the knuckle joints.

Support your partner's hand between your hands and turn their hand palm up. Using your thumb pads gently use the pressure circles over the palm of the hand.

Support their hand with your fingers whilst using your whole thumb length to stroke the palm open, starting at the base of the fingers and moving outwards and upwards.

Turn the hand palm down and complete the massage by stroking from wrist to finger ends as at the beginning.

Denote the end of the massage by a gentle squeeze of the hand.

Points to consider

- Some people may only tolerate the initial stroking, especially if they are unused to being touched, feel embarrassed or are feeling ill
- Focus on what you are doing and make the rate of the massage slow and relaxing

- Sharp or sudden movements will be counterproductive
- Maintain contact with the person's hand throughout the massage
- Ask your partner if the pressure is correct: too little and it may tickle; too much may cause damage and be uncomfortable
- If their skin is thin and friable use gentle stroking movements only and ensure you use adequate oil or cream to prevent your movements dragging on the skin

Considerations before using complementary therapies with clients

In your role as a nurse you need to be mindful of the requirements of the United Kingdom Central Council (UKCC). In order to expand your role by offering massage to clients consideration needs to be made of the following:

- Competency to practice
- Informed consent
- Policies of employing authorities
- Co-operation of other colleagues

The UKCC documents which offer guidance for the nurse are:

- The Code of Professional Conduct (UKCC,1992)
- The Scope of Professional Practice (UKCC, 1992)
- Standards for the Administration of Medicines (UKCC, 1992)
- UKCC Guidelines for Professional Practice (UKCC, 1996)

CONCLUSION

The use of touch in a therapeutic way to enhance client well-being and promote care and comfort is, perhaps, more complex than it would at first appear. An individual nurse's beliefs about people and the nature of nursing will influence the importance placed on aspects of care, the way care is organized and provided and the knowledge, skills and attitudes perceived as necessary for the caregiving. The Royal College of Nursing, in *The Value and Skills of Nurses Working with Older People* (RCN, 1993) reiterates the importance of skilled, insightful and knowledgeable nurses in the care of older clients. The considerations and influencing factors around the reasons for touch, the types of touch and moderating influences, such as culture, age, gender and past experiences should alert the nurse to its potential for therapeutic use in practice.

The humanity, power and potential of thoughtful nursing care using appropriate touch should not be underestimated. However, lest we feel that Henderson's (1966) reflections are a thing of the past, they need to be considered alongside Gillan's (1995) warning.

There are now programmes of research dedicated to developing robots able to care for patients (Gillan, 1995, p. 58).

We also need to reflect on McIntosh's letter to the *Nursing Times* (McIntosh, 1995) in which she reaffirms that the unseen, qualitative skills that are needed to care for this client group are not 'basic skills' but that they should be seen as positive, essential and fundamentally important to ensure that nurses and clients grow and develop together.

The knowledge, skills and attitudes required to provide care, comfort and touch as a therapeutic act should not be underestimated. We hope that this chapter has enthused and stimulated you to explore areas more deeply, to reflect on your own practice and to consider acquiring other therapeutic skills. Further reading and a list of useful addresses have been included to enable you to develop your interests.

Nurses are frequently touching the people in their care. This chapter has identified that the touching act has many meanings for people and that the potential benefit of touch can be lost if it is used inappropriately. The goal of this chapter has been to raise some of the issues relating to the use of touch, both positive and negative. The use of touch has been placed within the context of the Health and Safety legislation and the Code of Conduct for Nurses, Midwives and Health Visitors (UKCC, 1996). The chapter has given practical advice on how to approach the use of massage in the clinical context. The main aim of the chapter was to place the use of touch within the current thinking on the nature of caring.

FURTHER READING

Krieger, D. (1979) *The Therapeutic Touch. How to Use Your Hands to Help and Heal.* Prentice Hall, Englewood Cliffs, NJ.
One of the original texts documenting and explaining the use of therapeutic touch – 'a method of using the hands to direct human energies to help and heal' (p. 1.)

Krieger, D. (1981) *Foundations for Holistic Health Nursing Practices. The Renaissance Nurse.* J.B. Lippincott, Philadelphia.
Contains debates about the sources and concept of holism. Cultural influences are examined and their influence on the understanding and provision of holistic care. Chapter 16 by Catherine Salveson, entitled 'Holistic health for elders – nursing and ageing in America today', provides a stimulating account of the holistic approach and the use of touch, within the care of older clients.

Montagu, A. (1986) *Touching – the Human Significance of the Skin*, 3rd edn. Harper & Row, New York.
Much of the book is relevant – in particular Chapter 9, 'Touch and Age'.

Sanderson, H., Harrison, J. and Price, S. (1991) *Aromatherapy and Massage for People with Learning Disabilities.* Hands on Publishing and Training, Shirley Price, Birmingham and Hinckley, Leicestershire.
A practice-based guide to the use of aromatherapy and massage. Although the main focus of the book is on people with learning disabilities many of the techniques would be transferable into other settings.

Wells, R. and Tschudin, V. (eds) (1994) *Wells' Supportive Therapies in Health Care.* Baillière Tindall, London.
The chapter on therapeutic massage provides a comprehensive overview on the origins and use of massage.

USEFUL ADDRESSES

Complementary Therapies Forum,
Royal College of Nursing,
20 Cavendish Street,
London W1M 0AB

The Research Council for Complementary Medicine,
Suite 1
19A Cavendish Square,
London W1M 9AD

REFERENCES

Aguilera, D.C. (1967) Relationships between physical contact and verbal interaction between nurses and patients. *Journal of Psychiatric Nursing*, January/February, 13–17.

Barnette, K. (1972) A survey of the current utilization of touch by health team personnel with hospitalised patients. *International Journal of Nursing Studies*, 9, 195–209.

Benner, P. (1984) *From Novice to Expert: Excellence and Power in Clinical Nursing Practice.* Addison-Wesley Co, Menlo Park, CA.

Bottorff, J.L. (1991) A methodological review and evaluation of research on nurse–patient touch. In *Anthology on Caring*, Chinn, P.L. (ed.). National League for Nursing Press, New York.

Buber, M. (1958) *I and Thou*, 2nd edn. T. & T. Clark, Edinburgh.

Burnside, I.M. (1981) *Nursing and the Aged*, 2nd edn. McGraw-Hill, New York.

Chinn, P.L. and Kramer, M.K. (1995) *Theory and Nursing: a Systematic Approach,* 4th edn. Mosby, St Louis.

De Santis, L. (1994) Making anthropology clinically relevant to nursing care. *Journal of Advanced Nursing*, 20(4), 707–715.

DeWever, M.K. (1977) Nursing home patients' perception of nurses' affective touching. *Journal of Psychology*, 96, 163–171.

Duke, S. and Copp, G. (1992) Hidden nursing. *Nursing Times*, 88(17), 40–42.

Ernst, P. and Shaw, J. (1980) Touching is not taboo. *Geriatric Nursing*, 1(3), 193–195.

Ersser, S. (1991) A search for the therapeutic dimensions of nurse–patient interaction. In *Nursing as Therapy*, McMahon, R. and Pearson, A. (eds). Chapman & Hall, London.

Estabrooks, C.A. (1989) Touch: a nursing strategy in the ICU. *Heart and Lung*, 18, 392–401.

Estabrooks, C.A. and Morse, J.M. (1992) Towards a theory of touch: the touching process and acquiring a touching style. *Journal of Advanced Nursing*, 17, 448–456.

Fanslow, C.A. (1990) Touch and the elderly. In *Touch: the Foundation of Experience*. Barnard, K.E. and Brazleton, T.B. (eds). International Universities Press, Madison.

Farell, G.A. and Gray, C. (1992) *Aggression – a Nurse's Guide to Therapeutic Management.* Scutari Press, London.

Fascione, J. (1995) Healing power of touch. *Elderly Care*, 7(1), 19–21.

Fraser, J. and Ross-Kerr, J. (1993) Psychophysiologic effects of back massage on elderly institutionalised patients. *Journal of Advanced Nursing*, 18(2), 238–245.

Gillan, J. (1995) Human beans. *Nursing Times*, 91(7), 58.

Goodykoontz, L. (1979) Touch: attitudes and practice. *Nursing Forum*, 18(10), 4–17.

Hamilton, J. (1989) Comfort and the hospitalized chronically ill. *Journal of Gerontological Nursing*, 15(4), 28–33.

HMSO (1972) *Report of the Committee on Nursing (the Briggs Report).* Her Majesty's Stationery Office, London, Cmnd 5115.

Henderson, V. (1966) *The Nature of Nursing.* Macmillan, New York.

Hollinger, L. (1980) Perception of touch in the elderly. *Journal of Gerontological Nursing*, 6(12), 741–746.

Johnson, G.R. (1995) Complementary therapies in nursing. Implications for practice using aromatherapy as an example. *Complementary Therapies in Nursing and Midwifery*, 1, 128–132.

Jourard, S.M. (1966) An exploratory study of body accessibility. *British Journal of Social and Clinical Psychology*, 5, 221–231.

Kolcaba, K.Y. & Kolcaba, R.J. (1991) An analysis of the concept of comfort. *Journal of Advanced Nursing*, **16**, 1301–1310.

Krieger, D. (1979) *The Therapeutic Touch: How to Use Your Hands to Help to Heal*. Prentice Hall, Englewood Cliffs, NJ.

Langland, R.M. and Panicucci, C.L. (1982) Effects of touch on communication with elderly confused clients. *Journal of Gerontological Nursing*, **8**(3), 152–155.

Lawler, J. (1991) *Behind the Screens: Nursing, Somology and the Problem of the Body*. Churchill Livingstone, Melbourne.

Leininger, M. (1981) *Caring: an Essential Human Need*. Charles B. Slack, New Jersey.

Leininger, M. (1991) *Cultural Care Diversity and Universality: a Theory of Nursing*. National League for Nursing, New York.

LeMay, A.C. and Redfern, S.J. (1989) Touch and elderly people. In *Directions in Nursing Research: ten years of progress at the University of London*, Wilson Barnett, J. and Robinson, S. (eds). Scutari Press, London.

McCann, K. and McKenna, H.P. (1993) An examination of touch between nurses and elderly patients in a continuing care setting in Northern Ireland. *Journal of Advanced Nursing*, **18**, 838–846.

McInnes, J. and Treffry, J. (1982) *Deaf Blind Infants and Children – a Developmental Guide*. Open University Press, Milton Keynes.

McIntosh, E. (1995) I do not feel wasted in caring for older people (letter). *Nursing Times*, **91**(4), 24.

Montagu, A. (1986) *Touching – the Human Significance of the Skin*, 3rd edn. Harper & Row, New York.

Morse, J.M. (1983) An ethnoscientific analysis of comfort: a preliminary investigation. *Nursing Papers: Perspectives in Nursing*, **15**, 16–19.

Morse, J.M., Bottorf, J., Anderson, G., O'Brien, B. and Solberg, S. (1992) Beyond empathy: expanding expressions of caring. *Journal of Advanced Nursing*, **17**, 809–821.

Morrison, P. (1994) *Understanding Patients*. Baillière Tindall, London.

Oxford English Dictionary (1989) Clarendon Press, Oxford.

Passant, H. (1990) A holistic approach in the ward. *Nursing Times*, **86**(4), 26–28.

Paulen, A. (1984) High touch in a high tech environment. *Cancer Nursing*, 7, 201.

Peplau, H.E. (1952) *Interpersonal Relations in nursing*. Putman & Sons, New York.

Preston, T. (1973) When words fail. *American Journal of Nursing*, 73(12), 2064–2066.

Robb, I.H. (1910) *Nursing: It's Principles and Practice for Hospital and Private use*. J.F. Hartz, Toronto.

Rowlands, D. (1984) Therapeutic touch: it's effects on the depressed elderly. *The Australian Nurse Journal*. 13(11), 45–52.

RCN (1993) *The Value and Skills of Nurses Working with Older People*. The Royal College of Nursing, London .

Sanderson, H., Harrison, J. and Price, S. (1991) *Aromatherapy and Massage for People with Learning Difficulties*. Hands on Publishing & Training, Shirley Price Aromatherapy.

Savage, J. (1995) *Nursing Intimacy: an Ethnographic Approach to Nurse–Patient Interaction*. Scutari Press, London.

Seaman, L. (1982) Affective nursing touch. *Geriatric Nursing*, May/June, 162–164.

Sims, S. (1986) The effects of slow stroke back massage on the perceived well-being of female patients receiving radiotherapy for cancer. Unpublished M.Sc. Thesis, Kings College, University of London.

Smith, L. (1993) The art and science of nursing. *Nursing Times*, 89(25), 42–43.

Stevens Barnum, B.J. (1994) *Nursing Theory: Analysis, Application, Evaluation*, 4th edn. J.B. Lippincott Co., Philadelphia.

Taylor, A. (1995) Back in touch. *Nursing Times*, 91(26), 18.

Thomas, M. (1989) Fancy footwork. *Nursing Times*, 85(41), 42–44.

Tobiason, S.J. (1981) Touching is for everyone. *American Journal of Nursing*, 4, 78–80.

Tutton, E. (1991) An exploration of touch and it's use in nursing. In *Nursing as Therapy*, McMahon, R. and Pearson, A. (eds). Chapman & Hall, London.

UKCC (1992) *The Code of Professional Conduct*. The United Kingdom Central Council for Nurses, Midwives and Health Visitors, London.

UKCC (1992) *The Scope of Professional Practice*. The United Kingdom Central Council for Nurses, Midwives and Health Visitors, London.

UKCC (1992) *Standards for the Administration of Medicines*. The United Kingdom Central Council for Nurses, Midwives and Health Visitors, London.

UKCC (1996) *Guidelines for Professional Practice*. The United Kingdom Central Council for Nurses, Midwives and Health Visitors, London.

Watson, W.H. (1975) The meaning of touch: geriatric nursing. *Journal of Communication*, 25, 104–112.

Watson, J. (1988) *Nursing: Human Science and Human Care: a Theory of Nursing*. National League for Nursing, New York.

Weber, R. (1990) A philosophical perspective

on touch. In *Touch: the Foundation of Experience*, Barnard, K.E. and Brazleton, T.B. (eds). International Universities Press, Madison.

Weiss, S.J. (1986) Psychophysiologic effects of caregiver touch on incidence of cardiac dysrhythmia. *Heart and Lung*, **15**, 495–505.

Weiss, S. (1992) The tactile environment of caregiving. *Science of Caring*, **2**, 32–40.

Wise, P. (1989) Flower power. *Nursing Times*, **85**(22), 45–47.

Wright, S.G. (1995) Bringing the heart back into nursing. *Complementary Therapies in Nursing and Midwifery*, **1**(2), 15–20.

12 Positive sensations

Lee Hutchinson

KEY ISSUES

- Leisure and activity; needs and barriers
- The effects of ageing on the senses
- Assessing the sensory modalities
- Sensory environment, adaptation and enhancement of the living space, specialist and 'green' environment
- Sensory activity, generalized and specific
- Implications for carers, health professionals and managers

INTRODUCTION

The primary senses help us to understand the world that we live in. By assessing and changing the sensory experiences of caring that we offer clients we can enhance all of their daily living activities. In addition this allows the nurse to enhance their relationships with clients and provide positive direction for staff in the development of new skills. In order to achieve this objective for the older people with whom we work, this chapter will consider the value and importance of activity to us as individuals. It will explore ways in which leisure can be used to replace some of these important benefits created by work roles as well as different approaches to leisure activities. This takes the particular focus of explaining sensory stimulation and developing sensory environments, both indoors and outdoors.

The reality experienced in terms of continuing care may reflect the findings of Godlove *et al.* (1982, cited in Wynne Jones, 1984, p. 30) that for most of the time, nothing happens at all. McKenna (1993) considers the phenomenon of the psychiatric back wards, in which many of the residents are older people, dependent and demanding. Burn-out in such environments is represented by frustration in new staff and apathy in the longer-term staff. There has been disengagement on both sides from meaningful activity and inter-personal contact. Emotional distancing is a problem that many nurses experience across all settings and is often used as a coping mechanism and for personal protection (Cox, 1986).

'How many of us have opened the equipment cupboard on a Monday morning and looked in despair at the array of puzzles and tactile dominoes hoping for inspiration' (Kewin, 1991, p. 6); it is when we consider that there are five mornings and afternoons ahead of us that the despair can dampen the enthusiasm of even the most creative staff members. For nurses working in 'institutional' or long-stay environments the feelings expressed here must be only too familiar. Occupation and activity can become increasingly challenging for nurses when considering clients who have always been profoundly disabled or who are experiencing a loss of intellectual or sensory functioning. Add to this scenario requirements of interesting, stimulating, relevant, age appropriate, dignified and philosophically correct and your options appear to be reduced to the safety of television, music and craft work.

Sensory experiences and environments are about producing good feelings and good relationships. They exist to give pleasure and move us away from doing to people, to sharing with them. They enable both clients and carers to let go of the traditional tabletop and display activities and replace them with those that produce a sense of relaxation, well-being and elation. We should be overcoming the barrier inherent within our attitudes to older people and promoting the view that here are people who may have developed beyond the self and basic concerns and who are in the process of achieving the concepts of self-actualization as identified by Maslow (1987).

In order to start this process, nurses need to reappraise their approaches to care and the role of leisure within environments. It is important to strive towards a balance in activities, between therapy, education and leisure. In terms of sensory activity, leisure should be considered as the starting point. The aim of any leisure activity is pleasure and nursing needs to consider how readily this is included in the range of acceptable therapeutic activities and the professional identity of nurses.

LEISURE

Occupation and involvement are important at any stage of the lifespan. In terms of human development we seem to have an inborn desire to manipulate and investigate objects. The search for novelty and the exploration of our environment is apparent when we are just a few months old, particularly when we have moved beyond the here-and-now phase of stimulation, motivation and satisfactions of basic needs (Cohen and Salopatek, 1975).

In order to assess how important occupation can be to the individual you may find it helpful to complete the following activity.

Identify the benefits you gain from going to work.

You may well have considered some of the following areas:

■ Rewards	■ Achievement	■ Personal happiness
■ Mental stimulation	■ Confidence	■ Enjoyment
■ Opportunity	■ Individuality	■ Status
■ Purpose	■ Identity	■ Power
■ Relationships	■ Skills development	■ New experiences
■ Authority	■ Expertise	■ Choice

If we accept that older people still experience these needs, then leisure activities that are stimulating and planned for individuals can still satisfy many of the above requirements. For the older person in today's society, leisure time has expanded considerably, for some through choice, for others through ill-health, redundancy or a lifetime of disability (Stokes and Roberts, 1991). The benefits of increased leisure time could be seen as:

- Having more control over what we do
- Choosing to be alone or not
- More time to ourselves for reflection
- Reduction in stress created by work
- Relationships can have more time and be different in nature
- Development of other skills, maintenance of present skills
- New environment and experiences to be explored
- Time to support
- Time to share with others
- Time to be selfish
- Time to relax and recuperate

Throughout the lifecycle, individuals should be encouraged and enabled to participate creatively, whether actively or passively, within their environments. Nurses need to observe older people and consider how they spend their time. Hogg (1994) presents us with a model of leisure that enables us to classify and review the quality and type of leisure activities that clients engage in (Figure 12.1). In this model, activity has been broken down into five levels of involvement. The height of each box represents the perceived value of each particular activity to the individual. It reflects the possibility that those activities with little or no perceived value may increasingly encourage maladaptive behaviour from the individual. Although boredom and lack of activity can be seen as decreasing, it should be recognized that these may remain at some level and present as active choices for the person. The model includes self-determination as the basis of leisure activity. For most of us, this is an area in which we have complete freedom of personal choice, given our resources. In caring situations, the commitment to move the control of leisure activities from staff to the individual, ▶15 whatever their level of ability, could be identified as a quality of life indicator.

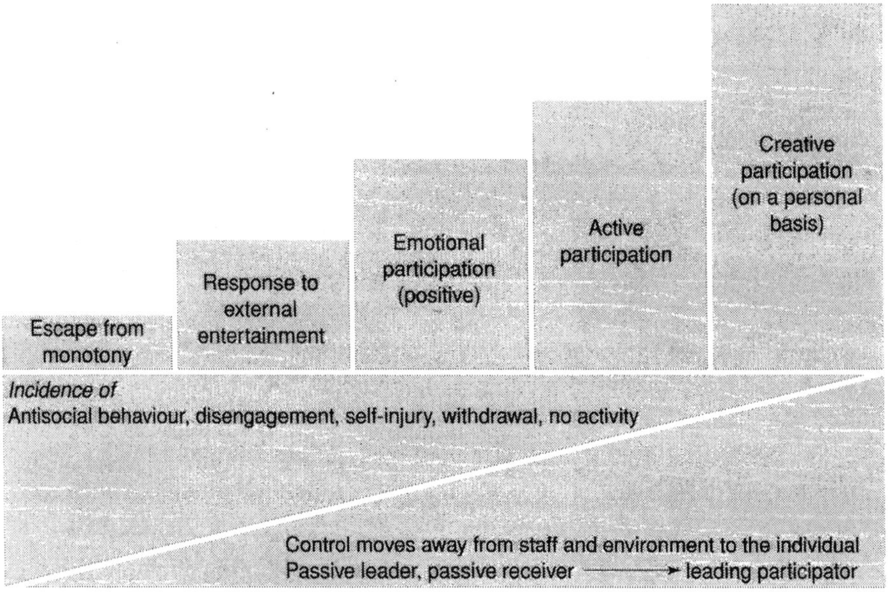

Figure 12.1 Classification of leisure activities.

Hogg's (1994) model encourages progression in activities and can be viewed as a continuum or a hierarchy. It also acknowledges that the level achieved and time spent in each area will be dependent upon:

- The ability and desires of the individual
- The nature of the activity
- The personal, material and organizational resources available to the nurse/carer

Observe the activities that individual clients are involved in within your work environment. Assess their response/level of involvement/level of control in each activity. Identify one way in which you may increase the activities or creative participation of older people.

The above activities may raise considerable discussion in terms of perceptions of the value of activities and the choices offered within the environment. In both instances, it would be relevant to involve the clients themselves. In involving clients, nurses need to accept that individuals may challenge the choice of activities. This should be seen as a positive way of involving individuals in choices about their lifestyle.

Identify one client. Record every 30 minutes what the client is doing (including nothing) on one weekday and one Saturday or Sunday.

Putting this together with the previous exercises, you can begin to develop a picture that reflects the balance and quality of activities that clients are engaged in. In smaller units, you may wish to do this for each client while in larger areas a sample would be more manageable. However, in order to plan care effectively for each individual it would be necessary in the longer term to assess each person.

Leisure is important in terms of quality of life and life satisfaction and it can fulfil needs generated or met by previous employment (Hogg, 1994). This is important for those who may have had few or no work choices as well as the replacement value for those who have retired. It allows us to be creative and use this potential to work towards self-actualization (Maslow, 1987). In order to cope with life situations we must relax and recuperate; this is equally true for people in continuing care situations. Leisure can be used to help us achieve physical and psychological well-being for clients and nurses.

Hogg (1994) suggests that both service providers and carers responsible for older people should promote active and creative leisure opportunities. Cunningham *et al.* (1991) emphasize issues which should be guiding principles when introducing and planning leisure activities:

- That they are self-selected and self-controlled and the person enjoys them
- That the focus is on the pleasure and the activity rather than any underlying therapeutic goal
- That they enable the individual to continue adding chapters of experience to their biographies.

SENSORY CHANGE

Thresholds

We start experiencing and learning about the world we are born into through the sense of smell; that first urgent breath we take. Our senses (Table 12.1) help us to recognize, understand and create our own world. They allow us to perceive time, space, dimension, depth, shape and quality. Remove or reduce the special senses and our world becomes a disturbing, limiting and dangerous place.

Most of us have been involved in exercises where we have been blindfolded. What were your reactions to losing your vision?

Did you become fearful of the environment? Did hesitation in movements become a wish to remain immobile? What happened to your time and space orientation? Was it a comfortable feeling to become totally dependent on others? The older person with a learning disability and or sensory impairment may have lived with these reactions for most of their lives. Physical and mental illness may cause these disabilities to develop in anyone.

TABLE 12.1	*The human senses and degrees of sensitivity*
Sense	Degree of sensitivity
Vision	A candle flame seen at 30 miles on a dark, clear night
Hearing	A tick of a watch at 20 feet under quiet conditions
Smell	A drop of perfume diffused into the entire volume of six rooms
Touch	The wing of a fly falling on your cheek from a distance of one centimetre
Taste	One teaspoon of sugar in two gallons of water

Source: Atkinson et al. (1990).

The negative view of ageing in relation to disease and infirmity is a stereotype that the majority of older citizens continually disprove with their lifestyles (Herbert, 1990). Disease and infirmity are not inevitable and in many cases, can be avoided by carers and clients. Table 12.2 shows the effects of primary ageing that can be expected and identifies conditions which may cause further sensory disability.

This is not a definitive list; you will need to identify the conditions relevant to the client group with which you work. However, it does show the difference between primary and secondary ageing. Primary ageing includes physical and psychological signs of ageing associated with normal wear and tear, secondary ageing being the further conditions that may occur due to ill-health. The common understanding of age is that we will all grow a little shorter, greyer and slower, that our life experiences will show in the way we look, how we feel and our overall level of health and ability. Nurses who operate from this basis are, however, at risk of ignoring additional sensory loss and disability which could be avoided and/or treated, in many cases. These are areas nurses should pay particular attention to. For example, clients and nurses need to be aware of the effects of ageing and disease in order to adapt their environment to enable them

TABLE 12.2	*Potential changes to the sensory modalities associated with ageing*	
Sense	Changes	Associated conditions
Vision	Slowing, reduction or loss of visual processing speed, adaptation to dark/light, tracking, visual search contrast sensitivity, depth perception, accommodation for near vision, visual acuity	Cataracts, diabetic retinopathy, stroke, macular degeneration, diuretics, glaucoma, arterial or venous blockage, retinitis, pigmentosa, migraine, myopia, hyperopia, astigmatism, Vitamin A deficiency, colour blindness, rheumatoid arthritis, anxiety, hysteria
Hearing	Presbycusis, location slower and less accurate, loss of high frequency, recruitment, loss of ability to tune out background noise	Wax, infections, foreign bodies, environmental, Ménière's disease, tinnitus, head trauma, otitis media, mastoiditis, prolonged exposure to loud noise, otosclerosis, facial nerve damage, anxiety, hysteria
Smell	Loss of acuteness, reduction in sensitivity to chemical senses	Zinc deficiency, head injuries, nasal cavity inflammation, anosmosis, colds, nerve damage, smoking, nasal polyps, rhinitis, sinusitis
Touch	General wear and tear, cuts, bruises, scratches, burns, dry skin, loss of heat control, skin wrinkles, folds, tactile sensitivity decreases, decrease in vibration sense, heightened cold sensation	Pruritus, dermatitis, nerve damage, scar tissue, damage to CNS, peripheral neuropathy, immobility, arthritis, HIV, rheumatoid arthritis, renal failure, trigeminal neuralgia, spinal cord lesions.
Taste	Dryness of mouth, adaptation, dentition, 50% loss of taste buds	Nerve damage, olfactory sense loss, smoking, HIV, renal failure, depression, trigeminal neuralgia, facial nerve damage, giant cell arteritis
Body sense	Reduced efficiency of vestibular and proprioceptor systems, diminished reflexes, slower voluntary movement, reduced integration of visual/vestibular/ proprioceptor systems	Vertigo, Parkinson's, sensory ataxia, cerebrovascular disease, neurological disease, spinal cord lesions, basilar migraine, drugs, anxiety, hysteria, alcohol abuse

Based on Herbert (1991), Fozzard (1990), Soloman *et al.* (1990), Kumar and Clarke (1994).

to generate new information, from other sources and in different ways. The nurse, therefore, has an extensive role to play in prevention of sensory deprivation through assessment, treatment and environmental adaptation in relation to sensory disability.

ASSESSMENT

For the older person, assessment needs to be ongoing and both formal and informal. A range of professionals may be involved, although there are many aspects that carers can test for without referral to an external agency.

Formal assessments

- Vision (opticians, ophthalmology)
- Hearing (audiological)
- Dental, oral hygiene
- General medical examination
- Neurological examination

Referral to external agencies needs to be appropriate and timely. For people with communication and/or behavioural problems, however, there may be issues with regard to acceptance, the ability to measure the response and the applicability of standard tests, for other people the problems should be minimal.

However, carers may well find that they will have to approach a number of professionals before they find a service that can adapt to the particular needs of their relative.

TABLE 12.3	Assessment	
	Sense	Changes observed
	Vision	Cannot identify position of limbs/fingers with eyes closed
		Clumsiness/accidents
		Response to passive movements of limbs
	Hearing	Proximity/position of objects/reading materials
		Clumsiness and accidents
		Reactions to changes in flooring levels
		Reactions to different colours
		Reactions to levels of lighting
		Changes in confidence levels when moving
	Smell	Loss of interest in food
		Change in diet
		Over use of perfume/aftershave
		Inability to identify/notice undesirable odours
	Touch	Response to light touch on different body parts
		Response to dull/sharp
		Response to hot/cold
		Ability to locate touch
		Ability to guess objects by touch alone
		Response to vibration
	Taste	Complaints about food
		Loss of interest in food
		Change in diet
		Excessive use of seasoning
		Reactions to/discrimination between sweet/salt tastes
	Body sense	Falls
		Cannot touch parts of body not seen
		Bumping into furniture
		Dizziness

Based on Fozzard (1990), Kumar et al. (1994), Paton and Brown (1991), Cullinan (1986).

Informal observational assessments

These can be done by nurses on an informal basis but have the potential to be formalized. The checklist in Table 12.3 requires no particular equipment but can provide nurses and carers with information on which to base the need for further investigation and referral to more formal sources. All sudden changes in behaviour, routines and habits should be investigated, as well as loss of interest in previously preferred activities.

THE RESPONSIVE ENVIRONMENT

An effective range of interventions for those caring for the older person can be developed when designing environments aimed at meeting changing needs. They range from ensuring that the normal living environment changes and adapts, through to dedicated, specialist sensory rooms. The principles for either are applicable to the person living in their own home, the resident in a nursing home or the person admitted to a formal health setting.

The living space must be adapted to take into account the sensory deficits of the person along with the distortion and overload that may occur through physical ageing or mental illness in old age. This will help the older person to:

- Reduce the effects of sensory disability
- Maintain independence and motivation
- Encourage empowerment and a sense of belonging, especially when the person has been moved to an 'institutional' setting
- Promote creativity and interest in their environment
- Reduce individual and environmental stressors in order to aid relaxation and recuperation

In this section, the following are considered:

- The adaptations that need to occur within the normal living area that will enhance the sensory abilities of the older person and limit their disabilities
- The snoezelen environment, which is a dedicated room or series of rooms and equipment
- The external environment in which we look at extending sensory activity into the gardens and areas around the buildings

The adapted environment

In order to design and use environments that will fulfil the aforementioned requirements, the nurse needs to know the person well and be able to identify their life goals (Charness, 1990).

Schiedt and Windley (1985, cited in Garland, 1990) identified ten areas in the environment which contribute to a sense of overall well-being. These areas have been adapted in order to create a checklist (Box 12.1). This can be used as the basis of an environmental audit to facilitate the creation of minimum standards.

►15 Areas requiring improvement could be highlighted and goals set to encourage and maintain change. The exercise will hopefully raise awareness within

Identify the factors that are important to you when creating your living space. Discuss these with other nurses/clients. Are there differences in the values each of you place on these factors?

Some of the issues that may have been raised are safety, privacy and aesthetic elements. For some people, changes in their environment reflect their personality or status, therefore, choice and control are valued factors. Integrate this information with a general profile of your client group, i.e. their ages, desires, abilities and disabilities and you will start to develop a picture of the range of elements that need to be taken into account.

BOX 12.1	*Checklist: environmental*

Comfort

1. Is there a choice between black-and-white and colour television?
2. Has the television been positioned to avoid glare from lights/windows?
3. Is there bright, even light throughout the environment where access/mobility/activity is required?
4. Do the illumination levels meet the following recommendations?

General	100 lux
Stairs	200 lux
Bedrooms	
Lifts	
Dining room	150–300 lux
Bathroom	150–500 lux
All changes of level	300 lux
Reading areas	300–1000 lux
Kitchen	

    (Light output requires an electrician's assessment)
5. Does the environment avoid glare by the use of window blinds/overhangs/non-reflectant materials on walls, floors, etc.?
6. Do floor and table lamps provide even illumination and coverage where access, mobility and activity is required?
7. Are floor and table lamps positioned to avoid glare?
8. Do floor and table lamps have appropriate shielding?
9. Are light switches at the right height and in a contrasting colour to the wall?
10. Do emergency lighting levels at night meet the minimum requirements (30 lux)?
11. Can the temperature be altered to suit the purpose of the room?
12. Can the temperature be altered to suit the individual?
13. Are windows overlooking stairs/hazards covered to reduce glare?
14. Are light sources indirect rather than directly above for people who spend considerable time lying down?
15. When moving from a light to a dark area, is the entrance free of level changes or obstructions to allow for slower adaptation?
16. Is unnecessary background noise avoided, e.g. by turning off TV, use of acoustic tiles?

Accessibility and safety

1. Can doors be opened with minimum pressure from the person?
2. Are signs/symbols a minimum size of 15 mm and the letters raised?
3. Are signs illuminated at a level of 500–600 lux?
4. Is the flooring non-slip in relation to shoes/walking aids?
5. Is the flooring suitable for self-propelled/electric wheelchairs?
6. Are the pathways and corridors clear of blockages?
7. Do cups/removable objects have broad bases?
8. Are stairs/hazard areas highlighted with a light colour against a contrasting background?
9. Are there bright warning strips before/on stairs/hazards?
10. Do tables/furniture have rounded/upholstered edges?
11. Are features used as landmarks for orientation, e.g. bold pictures, touch pads?
12. Are surfaces/floor coverings plain (patterns hinder depth perception)?
13. Are boundaries distinguished by colour contrasts (e.g. corners, edges of doors)?
14. Are plants and activity objects non-toxic?
15. Do fire doors and exits have specific textured cues?
16. Are floor coverings consistent and clear, i.e. no rugs, tailing wires?
17. Are stairs available (not ramps) for the ambulant older person?
18. Are ramps available for wheelchair users at a pitch of 1:20?

Layout, flexibility

1. Is the environment simple and uncluttered (e.g. furniture, plants, ornaments)?
2. Are occasional tables high and in suitable positions?
3. Are objects/furniture kept in the same position?
4. Do tables/furniture have large surfaces?
5. Do the colours used show good contrasts between light and dark (e.g. dishes and tablecloths, handrails and walls)?
6. Are the colours easily perceived, i.e. primary colours rather than pastels?
7. Can small seating groups be rearranged easily?
8. Are handrails cylindrical and the appropriate diameter (1.25"–1.25")?
9. Are stairs reduced in depth (to 4")?

Use of space and privacy

1. Do rooms have clearly defined and distinct purposes/activities?
2. Do the adaptations/aids in private spaces reflect the level of ability/disability of the individual?
3. Does each individual have enough private space?
4. Are rooms set aside for interviews/meetings/gatherings in relation to individuals?
5. Are rooms distinguished by multiple cues such as colour, texture of decoration, symbols, aroma, relevant sounds?
6. Are large rooms avoided due to noise levels/distances?
7. Are all rooms used equally by carers and clients, i.e. people spread throughout the environment through different times of the day?

BOX 12.1	*continued*

Security and control

1. Are there additional safeguards around fires, cookers, radiators?
2. Do the telephones/alarms use flashing lights, large figures and push-buttons, low frequency tones (1000–2000 Hz)?
3. Are alternative cues used to distinguish rooms/doorways/exits?
4. If self-medicating, are the bottles appropriately identified (by colour, writing symbols, shapes)?
5. Are large areas of glass easily identified (e.g. by sign/use of transfers)?
6. Are large areas of window/patio doors made of appropriate materials?
7. Do controls/remote controls have large, easily identified figures/symbols?
8. Are daily-living objects visible through use of bright colours (e.g. scissors, saucepan handles)?
9. Are daily-living objects bought in a larger size (e.g. clocks)?
10. Can individual lights/levels of illumination be controlled separately?
11. Can individual lights/levels of illumination be controlled by a remote control?
12. Are all reading materials in a minimum of 12-point font size for reading?

Special contacts

1. Are noise levels/sounds appropriate to the purpose of the room, i.e. no competing noises?
2. Are sensory aids available, working, used, checked?
3. Is seating positioned to aid appropriate visual contact?
4. Do seats have high, upholstered backs for sound absorption?
5. Are seats placed in areas where other people/activities can be watched?
6. Is the seating placed to promote social interactions, e.g. in right angles or curves?

Attractiveness and stimulation

1. Have the colours/textures/objects used in personal spaces been chosen in consultation with the individual?
2. Has the range of colours been used?
3. Has a range of textures been incorporated into the environment (upholstery, wall coverings/flooring)?
4. Have the effects of different colours been taken into consideration (e.g. cool, warm, relaxing, invigorating)?
5. Can rooms be identified through a range of cues, e.g. colour, touch, sound, smells?
6. Are there facilities/processes for removing unpleasant smells?
7. Does the environment reflect a range of appropriate smells, i.e. disinfectant in the sluice room only, coffee in the kitchen?
8. Are there a range of pleasant smells introduced in collaboration with the clients?
9. Do sound appliances have the ability to control bass/treble tones independently (e.g. bass turned up, treble down)?

Based on Paton and Brown (1991); Charness (1990); Garland (1990); Christenson (1990); Parmalee and Lawton (1990).

nurses/carers and clients in relation to their needs, changing levels of ability and the value of a responsible, well designed environment. The checklist is presented as a series of questions which require a positive answer. These questions will only form the basis of your assessment; your environment or client group may require additional elements.

Audit your living space using the checklist. Write the results as a report which comments on:

■ How you are achieving positive responses
■ The goals required to maintain these
■ The needs identified by negative responses
■ An action plan showing changes required and resource needs

The dedicated environment

The concept of the sensory environment originated in Holland. The Dutch word *snoezelen* encapsulates the two aspects of participative dynamic sensation (to sniff) and recuperation and relaxation (to doze) (Hulsegge and Verheulhart, 1987). It was developed in response to the need for quality leisure activities for people with a severe learning disability, that did not rely on intellectual ability but stimulated the primary senses, promoting pleasurable sensations. The last five years have seen an increasing and expanded use of sensory environments in relation to:

■ Care of the older person
■ Pain clinics
■ Mental health services
■ Intensive care and burns unit

Many other activities such as complementary therapies, physiotherapy, speech and language therapy can be enhanced by placing them within a sensory environment and out of impersonal clinical settings. The awareness generated by the environment can also lead to the creation of a sensory lifestyle which touches every aspect of daily living. Schooler (1990) suggests that intellectual development is sensitive to environmental stimulation and associated changes.

A lack of stimulation, leading to boredom within the environment, can result in feelings of helplessness, anxiety and poor motivation. This in turn can lead to a decrease in the person's cognitive performance and overall effectiveness. Alternatively the use of sensory stimulation to create a positive environment (Box 12.2) can create a virtuous cycle of events.

BOX 12.2	*Positive effects of sensory stimulation*			
Sensory Stimulus Novelty Intensity	$\rightarrow$	Thought Initiative Exploration	$\rightarrow$	Learning Emotional elation Motivation Flexibility Creativity

The underlying emphasis of such a sensory environment relates to the following six elements:

- Choice based on range and individuality
- Control, incorporating individuality and creativity
- Communication that is holistic and interactive
- Trust and security in relationships
- Pleasure for its own sake
- Freedom from demands and expectations

Within this, nurses must take on a facilitative and enabling role with the older person. The focus of this concept is to assist people to access and gain the maximum enjoyment from the environment, sharing the experiences and emotions of the individual (Haggar and Hutchinson, 1994). It can be difficult for nurses to give up control and the focus on outcome of care delivery and empower clients to take direction in terms of their own activity and responses. An enabling approach does, however, allow us to extend our knowledge of the individual and share the intimacy of their emotional responses through all their ordinary life experiences. Social education encapsulates these philosophies (Jones, 1992) by using sensory activity to:

- Express tensions and emotions
- Encourage choice and exploration
- Share emotions, interest and understanding

The purpose of all these interventions is the promotion of growth and development in those individuals involved. As demonstrated above, sensory environments can be used in a number of different ways by both groups or individuals. These can include a different focus in each area that concentrates on different effects and equipment, such as a pool room with a Jacuzzi that can encourage contact and equal participation from nurses and clients; dark rooms that concentrate on specific sounds and light effects that can stimulate and encourage exploration; or a white room, which could be used for relaxation or stimulation. For the purpose of this book, however, only the white room will be considered in detail.

The white room

This is a room that has been specifically designed to aid relaxation and gentle stimulation (Figure 12.2). Sudden or harsh sensory changes are avoided as this can cause discomfort. Although pastel colours or white are the basis for the environment, other colours or sensations can be used to alter or individualize the experience. What is important is that the environment inspires feelings of safety, comfort and sharing (Kewin, 1994 in Hutchinson and Kewin, 1994).

Having specified the key elements of the white room the following points identify ways in which this environment can be varied. Introduction of some or all of these elements increases the flexibility of the dedicated space and allows clients to explore more options.

- The level and colour of background lighting can be altered
- Effect wheels can be abstract (for relaxation), reminiscent (for stimulation) or created by staff and clients themselves

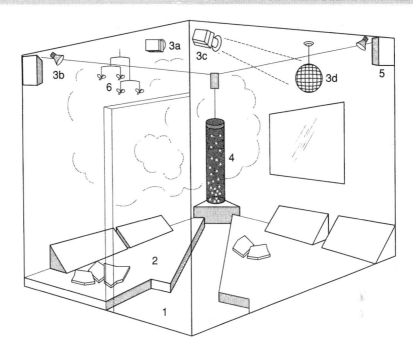

Figure 12.2 The white room: (1) access doorways and track; (2) floor cushioning, wedges, small and large chunkies and soft seating; (3a) project or with effect wheels; (3b) static spot lamp; (3c) disco spot lamp; (3d) mirror ball; (4) bubble tubes; (5) music system and speakers; (6) mobiles.

- Try a range of colours within the room to create a different atmosphere. Curtains and shapes allow you to keep the original white and experiment
- Create tents of colour using material and lights to enclose personal spaces – rooms within rooms
- Introduce bubble machines or hand-held bubble pots
- Use mirrors, prisms and mobiles to reflect lights, colours and images (mirrors may cause negative reactions to self-images)
- A fibre-optic spray can be used as a focal point as a waterfall on the wall or as a tent above a lying area
- Introduce different aromas using an aroma diffuser, joss sticks (reminiscent smells can now be bought such as lavender or new mown grass), personal perfumes, oils for massage, scented pillows and pomanders
- Consider allowing snacking in the environment. Picking themes can enhance the effect, choose a fruit and pick up the colour in throws, lighting and smells
- Music can be new age, classical, reminiscent or personal choice (be prepared for the unusual); a slow rhythm, pace and tone are important especially for those with hearing loss. Consider ways of allowing people to feel the vibrations of sound. Use windchimes and mobiles
- Introduce texture to the walls, seating, flooring. Use throws and pillows covered in different materials. Massage mattress
- Change levels and choices of seating from beanbags to rocking chairs. Consider a hammock or water bed

- Rotating effects and mirror ball (be aware this may cause nausea and dizziness), visual displays that have moving lights
- Use fans to create the sensation of wind on drapes, mobiles and around the clients

Any of these can be used in combination for reminiscence therapy, for example, seawater smell, bird mobiles, sounds of water and seagulls, seaside effects wheel, ice creams, warmth and wind, sand trays. There are no limits to the creative potential in this setting if clients and nurses/carers are allowed to exercise imagination, and practise without the inhibitions associated with the everyday living environment. However, caution must be exercised as reminiscence may also bring back unpleasant memories and emotions.

Many of the above elements can also be transferred to the normal environment, ensuring that this activity is applicable and accessible to acute care settings, nursing homes or people's own homes. Therapeutic activity can be enhanced as the older person can access the experiences at any time rather than on a purely sessional basis. The ideal would be an environment that offered a range of choices, controlled by individuals. This would allow people to experience favoured stimulation at their own pace and control the amount of stimulation offered.

The green environment

Increasingly, gardens have become an extension of the home. It can reflect the personality of the inhabitants and the house. Dressing entrances and windows not only frames the building but can distract from or enhance certain features and create a welcoming atmosphere. The sensory environment has been extended to the gardens (Weddle Landscape Design, 1995), creating rooms that reflect the seasons of the year, their moods, atmosphere and especially their memories.

It is important that the external landscape continues to encourage creativity, complexity and contemplation for the individual. Rooms that can be grown should facilitate a range of sensation activities, day and night (Table 12.4). The garden should also be designed as a series of scenes that can be viewed from each of the windows of the internal environment. The boundaries between each can be blurred by the use of conservatories, porches and decks that bridge the gap between internal and external landscapes.

The following are some ideas that you can build into any size of garden:

- Choose an evergreen background for an all-year garden and take account of the seasons
- Themes, e.g. foreign holidays, can be created by using cacti and succulents or old utensils in a kitchen garden
- Japanese gardens look at space, texture, form patterns and the use of water
- Bird baths, worm posts, housing, shade and food can attract birds; Buddleia is the butterfly bush
- Walls, screens and dense growth deaden or exclude unwanted noise and provide boundaries that create a sense of security and safety
- Water attracts people and wildlife, they both provide entertainment
- Use different flooring to associate changes in area and purpose

TABLE 12.4	*Using the garden to stimulate the senses*	
	Sense	Ways to stimulate
	Vision	Pick, press, dry, display flowers or plants; water reflects light, fountains and waterfalls; water ripples, flashes, cascades. Plants change with light, i.e. white flowers float in the dark, contrasting colours, colour themes and bands; coloured concrete and flooring; night-time lighting, floating candles on water
	Sound/hearing	Glass/wood/metal windchimes create different tones; bells hung overhead from a line; rain/water falling onto broad-leaved plants; birds; taped music; quaking aspen; grasses and bamboos; water gurgles; patters; trickles; the sound of gravel or wooden walkways
	Smell	Aromatic lawns/Corsican mint, plants that can be crushed; eucalyptus, box, lavender, jasmine, witch hazel, peony, winter sweet; good cooking; wood burning; scented candles; rosemary, thyme and mint are ideal for suntraps
	Touch	Bark of trees; pussy willow; lambs tongue; grasses; morning and evening sitting places in the sun; shade at noon; seating around trees; carvings on seats; fences; posts; different types of fencing/flooring; wood, rock, upholstered seating; sculptures; water spray
	Taste	Sweet violets, primrose, pansies in salads and soups; herbs, rhubarb, cherry tomatoes, blackberries, strawberries; tables and chairs – plan meals outside; barbecues; easy to grow – asparagus, onions, lettuce, beetroot, radish, nasturtiums
	Movement	Rocking chairs, hammocks, swings; tall grasses; running water; wind tunnels created by trees or hedging; chimes and mobiles

Based on McAllister and Smith (1994); Weddle Landscape Design (1995).

- Wide, level pathways, handrails, curves not sharp bends, turning areas, no dead ends to ensure good access
- Raised flower/vegetable beds and specialized equipment to encourage involvement
- Create shelter, privacy and intimate spaces with canopies, summer houses, pergolas, hanging lines of materials that float and change the light, fences and walls
- Use plants such as phormiums or sunflowers to create dramatic focal points
- You will be able to recreate a dining room or lounge in the external spaces that will provide as much usefulness, delight and atmosphere as the internal room

In approaching any of these options it is essential to consider safety issues, such as checking for poisonous plants, and ensuring areas with low-allergen plant choices.

EVALUATION OF SENSORY ENVIRONMENTS

Many nurses may have experienced considerable difficulty in identifying activities for older people that are relevant and stimulating. However, the white

Identify any outdoor areas you could use to create a green environment.

Using the information above, design a green environment for the older people with whom you work.

Analyze the environment in terms of the value to the individual.

Recreate it externally.

This type of activity ensures that the nurse can extend and develop therapeutic activities and experiences further, thus enabling the clients to derive the maximum benefit from the whole of their care setting.

room has specifically been found to be appropriate in terms of stimulation and relaxation for a range of mental health problems, including dementia. Evaluations by Barker and Pinkney (1994), McAllister and Smith (1994) and Pinkney (1997) have highlighted a number of important effects for clients and carers.

The effects on clients were considerable. The activity was failure free, therefore avoiding feelings of uselessness or inability to achieve a standard performance. It empowered clients in terms of independence, autonomy and control within a safe, secure and inviting environment. The need for relaxation and pleasure could become acknowledged and accepted for the purposes of care planning. Through the alternative means of communication that it offered, clients were able to share emotions, experiences and memories, allowing nurses to gain more knowledge of clients. Responses to, and awareness of, sensory stimuli generalized into the normal environment and encouraged the use of the primary senses, promoting the receipt and use of sensory information in order to meet the stresses of life. The white room combined a sense of satisfaction in people and provided a space and time in which they could re-establish their emotional equilibrium.

Nurses found the environments pleasurable and were, therefore, happy to repeat the activity. The enabling philosophy and concepts are appealing to staff members and promote a more positive role based in sharing and choice rather than directing. One of the most important elements was the satisfaction and a sense of accomplishment gained by staff from being involved in a successful activity. The quality time resulted in the development of trust and equality; therefore, the environment has a very positive healthy effect on staff in the promotion of relaxation and stress reduction. The white room appeared to enhance the counselling relationship and was instrumental in the development of rapport. Finally, it encouraged a far more creative approach to activities.

Qualitative research has also been undertaken within the areas of children (de Bunson, 1994), pain (Schofield, 1994), self-injury (Henning, 1994) and severe multiple disability (Hagger and Hutchinson, 1994). However, the studies are still very limited in terms of care of the older person both across its wider client group and within a mental health focus.

The use of snoezelen in the management of chronic pain has been the subject of a recent study by Schofield (1994). These developments have advanced, based on the move away from traditional physical interventions to a wider, more holistic psycho-social approach. The response to pain in individuals can be affected by a wide variety of factors and the management of individual care must respond to these. Sensory environments can provide a way of enabling people to cope with pain while still achieving a quality of life (Scholfield, 1994). The potential benefits that clients may experience are that it helps to promote acceptance of pain as opposed to dependence on a cure. The non-clinical environment and informal approach can pull down client/carer barriers, enabling people to interact and have fun together. The sensory environment reduces stress and promotes relaxation which may in turn help to change or reduce the pain experience. The psychical activity itself is very different and, therefore, interesting and with the stimulation can provide distraction, aiding the tolerance of pain. Individuals can control the environment and their own level of participation, whilst carers can integrate a range of other activities such as education, massage and relaxation training within the sessions.

However, in order to evaluate the effects and/or benefits of using sensory environments in the management of pain or to enhance leisure time, etc., the named nurse/key worker needs to maintain careful records of the activities used and the responses of individual clients. Elements that may need recording are:

- The responses to different sensations within each sensory modality
- Range of activities/equipment used and the older person's responses, including verbal, physical, emotional and behavioural
- Interactions noted between nurse and client, such as eye contact, touch, verbal and non-verbal
- The likes/dislikes of clients in relation to activities
- Specific pieces of equipment, specific combinations of sensations that produce positive and negative reactions
- Level of choice-making by clients
- Period of time over which positive effects last
- Whether positive feelings/relationship intensities transfer into other settings

Design an assessment and evaluation tool that you could use to inform and review the use of sensory stimulation with the clients you work with. You may find it helpful to discuss this with colleagues, carers and service users.

THE SENSORY LIFESTYLE

Having considered the mechanics of created sensory environments, it is important to look at the environments we create through our interactions.

Being aware of the senses enables nurses to start the process of overcoming sensory deprivation that clients may have experienced when placed in unstimulating environments. This is also very important when considering individuals who have impaired senses as a result of normal ageing. The aim of nursing within this situation is to ensure continuation of involvement and interaction of the client with their environment.

Imagine eating an orange. Close your eyes and visualize the process in your mind's eye. Record the experience. How did it feel?

Your experience may have included:

- The bright, smooth colour and the dimpled skin
- The feel of the roundness and the weight of the fruit
- Sliding your hands into position
- The smell of the dimpled skin
- Pushing through the skin to the moistness below
- The discomfort or pain as the pith pushes under your nails
- The sound of the flesh tearing apart
- The spray of juice against your face
- The tangy fruity smell of the juices
- The bright flesh revealed
- Pressure on your teeth, explosion of fruity, sharp taste and your mouth filling with juice

Having experienced all these sensations, the next and possibly most important step is that of anticipation of the taste and the texture of the orange.

CASE STUDY   Perhaps we should consider the situation in reality.

Mr Hughes, 70 years old, has cerebral palsy and a severe learning disability. He is unable to grasp and is partially sighted. It is dinnertime, he is being fed small pieces of orange on a spoon by a nurse. As soon as he appears to have eaten each piece, the next slice of orange is put into his mouth. The nurse is cheerful and happy, talking to the other people in the room in between mouthfuls, occasionally asking Mr Hughes to open his mouth.

Role-play Mr Hughes' experience with other members of the team.

Record your responses and feelings. Identify the senses that are being used in this situation. Identify the intensity of the experience. Which senses are not being used?

We need to be able to break the activities of daily living down into their sensory components and understand the effects of sensation, much as in the example of Mr Hughes and the orange. Developing a sensory lifestyle enables the older person to continue to remain actively involved with their environment. Analysis of this information can begin to raise the awareness in staff of the intensity of sensory information and the importance of sensation.

Considering the needs of Mr Hughes, explore how you can make bathtime a positive sensory experience. You will need to address each of the senses to create an overall experience.

You may have considered the following:

Vision

- Projector with the Deeps effect wheel
- Battery-operated spotlights with coloured bulbs or coloured filters
- Hanging plants
- Coloured cellophane over window
- Mobiles
- Candle light
- Battery wall lights/uplighters
- Changing light source/intensity/intimacy

Hearing

- Tape of tropical island/water sounds/seabirds
- Relaxation tape, wind chimes

Smell

- Battery aroma diffuser
- Joss sticks/bubble bath
- Pot pourri
- Candle fragancer and oils
- Use of client's own perfume/aftershave

Touch

- Bubble mattress/vibration
- Textures – flannel, sponge, loofah, temperature of water/room
- Massage
- Backwash
- Warm, soft towel

Taste

- Sit person in comfortable chair immediately after the bath, give a favourite drink
- Link sweet orange in the diffuser to eating/drinking orange in the bathroom

Body sense

- Movement
- Bubble mattress
- Create waves
- Massage of feet/hands/face
- Splashing/pouring

Such activities are only limited by your imagination, although you need to be aware of health and safety issues (such as candles/electrical items) this should be considered a challenge rather than a reason for not doing this type of activity. Where the client is able to, they should also be encouraged to be creative and express their preferences.

IMPLICATIONS FOR PRACTICE

For all levels of staff, there will be issues in relation to values and control. Accepting that clients will eventually provide the leadership role in this type of activity can be difficult. Enabling should not be perceived as a transitory philosophy of care, applied only to certain situations, but would need to be the focus of the management and provision of services. In addition, managers need to appreciate and accept the philosophy behind a sensory lifestyle. In so doing they need to encourage a culture that enables clients, carers and nurses to be creative.

Promoting sensation in the individual's environment will elicit emotional and cognitive responses in both clients and nurses at any time. All staff, regardless of their grade, will need to understand the concepts of sensory stimulation and have the ability to engage in and respond appropriately to each individual. In this situation therapies will no longer be the preserve of any group or grade of staff. In order to be wholly effective in this approach it will be necessary to provide education and training for all staff. This should also be supported by the provision of appropriate resources. In addition, managers and carers need to move away from task-orientated, directive interactions and plan care based on pleasure as a worthwhile alternative goal; for example, bathtime can become a relaxing sensory experience rather than a purely hygienic element of care.

Finally, sensory activity and responsive environments have many benefits for the older person. To avoid the passivity and apathy that may occur through loss of control, we need to emphasize systems of care that provide a sense of personal mastery (Parmalee and Lawton, 1990). By adapting and providing suitable environments and activities, the older person can continue to interact within environments and relationships confidently and competently.

CONCLUSION

In creating structured sensory environments it is essential for nurses to use non-directive and enabling approaches to care delivery. The concept of enabling is defined by Haggar and Hutchinson (1991) as a sensitive, caring, non-directive approach, in which an atmosphere of safety and security is created and free choice encouraged. We may interpret this as establishing a relationship based on trust and equality; that encourages mutual sharing, support, expression and participation in all possible sensory activities and opportunities. Control and direction is generated by the clients. This change may be viewed as a threat or an opportunity. The very least the sensory lifestyle may provide is a better quality of working environment and considerably enhanced relationships with clients.

FURTHER READING

Bond, J. and Coleman, P. (eds) (1992) *Ageing in Society*, 2nd edn. Sage Publications.
Overall, a useful book on ageing. Chapter 6 deals with the environment. Chapter 5 provides an overview of adjustment and theories of the process of successful ageing.

Atkinson, R.L., Atkinson, R.C., Smith, E.E., Bern, D.J. and Hillgard E.R. (1990) *Introduction to Psychology*, 10th edn. Harcourt Brace Jovanovich. *Chapters 4, 5, 10 and 11 are particularly useful in this area. The information is presented clearly and includes critical discussions.*

Birren, J.E. and Schaie, K.W. (eds) (1990) *Handbook of the Psychology of Ageing*, 3rd edn. Academic Press, San Diego. *This is one of a series of handbooks looking at the psychology of ageing. Each chapter reviews and provides a reference source for a specific area. Chapters 26 and 27 on design are particularly useful for looking at the care environment.*

Kumar, P. and Clarke, M. (1994) *Clinical Medicine*, 3rd edn. Baillière Tindall, London. *Identification of disease processes that may affect the sensory systems/perception. Clearly presented information on clinical conditions.*

Paton, D. and Brown, R. (1991) *Lifespan Health Psychology, Nursing Problems and Interventions*. Harper Collins Nursing, London. *Provides an overview of each part of lifecycle, changes and interventions. Chapters 7 and 8 specifically relate to the older person.*

Readers Digest (1995) *Good Ideas for your Garden*. Readers Digest Associated, London. *Wide ranging ideas covering all aspects of a garden, with a specific chapter relating to the sensory garden.*

Hulsegge, J. and Verheulhart, A. (1987) *Snoezelen, Another World*. Rompa, Chesterfield, 12–38. *The original book about snoezelen which covers the initial philosophy and background. It is especially useful for the section on home-made snoezelen.*

Social Education Centre. *Multi Sensory Action Pack*. Stallington Hall, Staffs. *A pack that provides a good introduction to and breakdown of sensory activities, uses of equipment and care planning records. A valuable resource for ideas.*

Hutchinson, R. and Kewin, J. (eds) (1994) *Sensations and Disability*. Rompa, Chesterfield. *Experiences of people working with snoezelen, including activities and research, from a range of backgrounds and client groups.*

USEFUL ADDRESSES

Weddle Landscape Design
27 Wilkinson Street, Sheffield S10 2GB
Tel: (0114) 2757003
A consultancy service on landscape planning, design, management and development. Environmentally aware and experienced in sensory design.

Rompa
Goyt Side Road, Chesterfield, Derbyshire S40 2PH
Tel: (01246) 211777
Design and provision of environments and equipment. The firm has considerable experience in this area.

REFERENCES

Atkinson, R.L., Atkinson, R.C., Smith, E.E., Bem, D.J. and Hildgard, E.R. (1990) *Introduction to Psychology* 10th edn. Harcourt Brace Jovanovich.

Barker, P. and Pinkney, L. (1994) *Snoezelen – an evaluation of a sensory environment used by people who are elderly and confused.* In *Sensations and Disability* Hutchinson, R. and Kewin, J. (eds). Rompa, Chesterfield.

de Bunsen, A. (1994) A study in the use and implications of the Snoezelen Resource at Limington House School. In *Sensations and Disability,* Hutchinson, R. and Kewin, J. (eds). Rompa, Chesterfield.

Charness, N. (1990) Human factors and design for older adults. In *Handbook for the Psychology of Ageing,* 3rd edn, Birren, J.E. and Schaie, K.W. (eds). Academic Press, San Diego.

Christenson, M.A. (1990) Adaptations of the physical environment to compensate for sensory changes. *Journal of Physical and Occupational Therapy in Geriatrics,* 8(3/4), 3–30.

Cohen, L. and Salopatek, P. (1975) *From Sensation to Cognition.* Academic Press, New York.

Cox, I. (1986) *Stress.* MacMillan Education, London.

Cullinan, T. (1986) *Visual Disability in the Elderly.* Croom Helm, London.

Cunningham, C., Hutchinson, R. and Kewin, J. (1991) Recreation for people with profound and severe learning difficulties. In *The Whittington Hall Snoezelen Project,* Hutchinson, R. (ed.). North Derbyshire CHCS Trust, Chesterfield.

Fozzard, J.L. (1990) Vision and hearing. In *Handbook of Psychology and Ageing,* 3rd edn, Birren, J.E. and Schaie, K.W. (eds). Academic Press, San Diego.

Garland, J. (1990) Environment and behaviour: a clinical perspective. In *Ageing in Society,* 2nd edn, Bond, J. and Coleman, P. (eds). Sage Publishers, London.

Haggar, L.E. and Hutchinson, R.B. (1991) Snoezelen: an approach to the provision of a leisure resource for people with profound and multiple handicaps. *Mental Handicap,* 51–55.

Haggar, L., Hutchinson, R. (1994) The development and evaluation of a snoezelen leisure resource for people with multiple disability. In *Sensations and Disability,* Hutchinson, R. and Kewin, J. (eds). Rompa, Chesterfield.

Henning, D. (1994) Snoezelen and self injury. In *Sensations and Disability,* Hutchinson, R. and Kewin, J. (eds). Rompa, Chesterfield.

Herbert, R.A. (1991) The Biology of Human Ageing. In *Nursing Elderly People,* Redfern, S.J. (ed.). Churchill Livingstone, London.

Hogg, J. (1994) Leisure and intellectual disability: the perspective of ageing. *Journal of Practical Approaches to Developmental Handicaps,* 18(1), 13–15.

Hulsegge, J. and Verheulhart, A. (1987) *Snoezelen: Another World.* Rompa, Chesterfield.

Hutchinson, R. and Kewin, J. (eds) (1994) *Sensation and Disability.* Rompa, Chesterfield.

Jones, H.D. (1992) *The social educator in western Europe.* In *Standards and Mental Handicap, Keys to Competence,* Matthias, P. and Thompson, T. (eds). Baillière Tindall, London.

Kewin, J. (1991) Pulling the strands together. In *The Whittington Hall Snoezelen Project,* Hutchinson, R. (ed.). ND CHCS Trust, Chesterfield.

Kumar, P. and Clarke, M. (1994) *Clinical Medicine,* 3rd edn. Baillière Tindall, London.

Maslow, A. (1987) *Motivation and Personality,* 3rd edn. Harper & Row, New York.

McAllister, P. and Smith, K. (1994) Experiences from a day hospital for adults with mental difficulties. In *Sensations and Disability,* Hutchinson, R. and Kewin, J. (eds). Rompa, Chesterfield.

McKenna, H. (1993) A long term view. *Nursing Times,* 89(41), 50–53.

Parmalee, P.A., Lawton, M.P. (1990) The design of special environments for the aged. In *The Handbook of the Psychology of Ageing,* 3rd edn, Birren, J.E. and Schaie, K.W. (eds). Academic Press, London.

Paton, D. and Brown, R. (1991) *Lifespan Health Psychology Nursing Problems and Interventions.* Harper Collins Nursing, London.

Pinkney, L. (1997) A comparison of the Snoezelen environment and a music relaxation group on the mood and behaviour of patients with senile dementia. *British Journal of Occupational Therapy,* 60(5), 209–212.

Readers Digest (1995) *Good Ideas for Your Garden.* Readers Digest, London.

Schofield, P. (1994) The role of sensation in the management of chronic pain. In *Sensations and Disability*, Hutchinson, R. and Kewin, J. (eds). Rompa, Chesterfield.

Schooler, C. (1990) Psychological factors and cognitive functioning. In *The Handbook of the Psychology of Ageing*, 3rd edn, Birren, J.E. and Schaei, K.W. (eds). Academic Press, London.

Solomon, Schmidt, and Adragna (1990) *Human Anatomy and Physiology*, 2nd edn. Saunders College Publishing.

Stokes and Roberts (1991) Maintaining Activities and Interests. In *Nursing Elderly People*, Redfern, S.J. (ed.) Churchill Livingstone, London.

Weddle Landscape Design Report (1995) Ashgate Learning Disabilities Centre, Sheffield, September.

Wynne Jones, A. (1984) The elderly person with a mental handicap. *Mental Handicap*, **12**(1), 30–31.

13 Stress and relaxation in later life

Lee Hutchinson, Christine Hunter and Jean Hankinson

INTRODUCTION

The *Concise Oxford Dictionary* defines stress as a constraining force acting upon a person. When attempting to cope, an individual exerts/strains themselves, feeling distressed or fatigued as a result. In engineering terms, stress is seen as a load or force applied to a structure until the inherent limit is exceeded, causing a collapse. We all live with stress of one form or another to different levels throughout our lives. Like engineering structures, we can operate perfectly well under certain constraints, in fact on occasions it is the arousal associated with stress that can enable us to perform at a high level and provides us with energy and motivation.

Nurses working with older people need to understand that the individual has had a lifetime of dealing with stressors and in doing so has developed a range of coping mechanisms which include cognitive, behavioural and emotional responses and methods. In caring situations, nurses should be aware of the stressors that may affect the older person and how the environment and the relationships they have with relatives and/or nurses can enhance or inhibit these coping skills.

This chapter will consider the stressors in life in relation to older people, some responses to stress, relaxation as an intervention along with other techniques that can be used to deal with stress.

STRESS

The ability of any individual to adjust and cope with major life transitions and the ways in which this impacts upon each person's environment requires significant effort and energy. A positive or negative attitude towards change will inevitably affect the way in which an individual responds and the level of stress experienced.

Definitions and explorations of stress have identified the relevance of critical life events (Holmes and Rahe, 1967), crises and transitions (Erikson, 1980), and adaptation to life crises and transitions (Moos, 1986) upon the coping mechanisms of individuals. Each of these theoretical explorations provides us with possible triggers of stress by identifying periods in the lifespan at which changes occur. In addition they are able to provide information about the impact of different types of events and the processes involved in responding to change. In healthcare of older people we need to be aware of how these concepts can inform nursing interventions, as nurses are often involved with older people at periods of stress in their lives, i.e. loss, change of environment and illness. A major role for the nurse lies in the understanding, prevention and alleviation of stress. Knowledge enables us to recognize the potential for harmful stress and intervene in order to promote healthy coping and independence.

Identify the possible causes of stress in the environment that the older person lives in.

You may have identified a range of issues:

- Financial problems
- Loss of spouse
- Losing touch with people
- Lack of ability
- Medication
- Fear of being robbed
- Lack of privacy
- Noise
- Having no choice in how the home is decorated
- Not having a job
- Losing mobility
- Eating set meals

- Eating at set times
- Poor health
- Little contact with others
- Having a mental illness
- Damp housing
- Being ignored
- Being too hot or cold
- Going to bed at a set time
- Losing abilities
- Losing senses
- Being attacked by other clients
- Being unhappy

The causal factors underpinning the range of stressors experienced will normally fall within the categories of environment, self or others. In order to meet the needs of the older person, nurses need to identify the factors that are within their sphere of influence; these are normally environmental issues. A second focus for the nurse to consider are those areas in which they can enable the older person to gain more control, e.g. decision making, or when to go out or socialize.

A single person living alone may have socialized through work and this may require new social contacts to be made outside of that environment. A whole range of activities from sports to cookery and art classes are often available at local community or education centres. Often many older people take on far

◀3 & 9 more activities in retirement than they were able to when working.

In addition, couples can look forward to spending more time together; also they may find that they can be irritated or annoyed by too much of each other's company. For those who have been in full-time employment, where most of their lives have been taken up by work, focusing on friends and family during evenings and weekends may seem hectic, but retirement highlights the number of hours in the day!

These multiple stressors may cut across physiological, economic, social and psychological areas.

Two assessments that can be used to identify the stressors being experienced by an individual are, firstly, the Holmes–Rahe Social Readjustment Rating Scale (Holmes and Rahe, 1967) which looks at a range of life events from Christmas to moving house to a divorce (Table 13.1); secondly, the Hassles and Uplifts Scale developed by Kanner *et al.* (1981), which considers the daily and cumulative impact of everyday demands (Table 13.2). The impact of life events need to be considered both in terms of the nature and quality of events.

TABLE 13.1   *Examples of stressors selected from the social readjustment rating scale*

Death of spouse	Outstanding personal achievement
Marital separation	Wife stops working
Death of close family member	Change in living conditions
Personal injury or illness	Revision of personal habits
Marital reconciliation	Change in residence
Retirement	Change in recreation
Change in health of family member	Change in church activities
Sex difficulties	Change in social activities
Gain of new family member	Change in number of family get-togethers
Change in financial state	Change in eating habits
Death of close friend	Holiday
Change in number of arguments with spouse	Christmas
Son or daughter leaving home	

Adapted from Holmes and Rahe (1967).

TABLE 13.2   *Hassles and uplifts versus major life events scale (examples from Kanner et al., 1981)*

Health

Hassles	*Uplifts*
Smoking too much	Getting enough sleep
Use of alcohol	Being rested
Planning meals	Feeling healthy
Trouble relaxing	Recovering from illness
Concerns about accidents	Staying or getting in good physical shape
Physical illness	Quitting or cutting down on alcohol
Side effects of medication	Quitting or cutting down on smoking
Concerns about medical treatment	Weight
Sexual problems that result from physical problems	Eating
Sexual problems other than those resulting from physical problems	Relaxing
Concerns about bodily functions	Think about health
Not getting enough rest	Fresh air
Not getting enough sleep	Exercising
Difficulties seeing or hearing	
Concerns about weight	

Money

Hassles	*Uplifts*
Not enough money for clothing	Buying things for the house
Concerns about owing money	Buying clothes
Concerns about money for emergencies	Having enough money for transportation
Cutting down on electricity, water, etc.	Getting unexpected money
Not enough money for basic necessities	
Not enough money for food	

Rising prices of common goods
Not enough money for transportation
Not enough money for entertainment

Relationships

Hassles

Being lonely
Not seeing enough people
Friends or relatives too far away
Problems with your lover
Problems with divorce or separation
Difficulties with friends

Uplifts

Visiting, phoning, or writing someone
Relating well with your spouse or lover
Relating well with friends
Sex
Being with older people
Being visited, phoned, or sent a letter
Socializing (parties, being with friends, etc.)
Making a friend
Sharing something
Having someone listen to you
Expressing yourself well
Getting love
Confronting someone or something
Being accepted
Giving love
Being alone
Hugging and/or kissing
Flirting

Personal

Hassles

Misplacing or losing things
Troubling thoughts about your future
Thoughts about death
Care for pet
Trouble making decisions
Home maintenance (inside)
Too much time on hands
Silly practical mistakes
Inability to express yourself
Physical appearance
Wasting time
Filling out forms
Not enough personal energy
Concerns about inner conflicts
Regrets over past decisions
Nightmares
Shopping
Yardwork or outside home maintenance
Noise

Uplifts

Practising your hobby
Not working (on vacation, laid-off, etc)
Finding something presumed lost
Completing a task
Solving an ongoing practical problem
Friendly neighbours
Having enough time to do what you want
Eating out
Having enough (personal) energy
Cooking
Having the 'right' amount of things to do
Home (inside) pleasing to you
Reading
Shopping
Smoking
Doing yardwork or outside work
Resolving conflicts over what to do
Growing as a person
Being complimented
Music
Dreaming
Having fun
Going someplace that's different
Pleasant smells
Making decisions
Thinking about the past
Praying
Feeling safe
Feeling safe in your neighbourhood
Doing volunteer work
Learning something

Both of these scales can give a picture of the amount of stress an individual is subject to, as well as what is causing that stress. Once a picture of the individual's personal situation and their experience of coping skills has been formed, the nurse is in a far better position to use the events in a positive manner as well as changing the perceptions of not being in control that the older person may be experiencing (Moos, 1986).

Effects of stress

Identify the range of possible immediate and long-term effects of stress under the following headings: physical, behavioural, psychological, emotional.

You may have considered the effects shown in Tables 13.3 and 13.4.

In the short term, stress causes the body to prepare itself for extreme physical demand, enabling you to respond on a 'fight-or-flight' basis (Table 13.3). These should be viewed as positive effects. However, eventually the constant chemical reactions in continuous stress may lead to suppression of the immune system and infections. Table 13.4 gives some signs of long-term stress. They are placed under physical, behavioural, emotional and intellectual signs and symptoms.

The range of signs and symptoms shown in Table 13.4 can aid the nurse in assessing stressors and the client's reactions to stress. As part of the assessment process it will also be necessary for the nurse to look at the individual's attitudes to or perceptions of stress as many people feel that acknowledging they are unable to cope is a sign of personal weakness. Siddell (1995) reviews social class attitudes to health where distress was viewed and experienced in different ways.

Two main views were identified; firstly, where stress is viewed as having a physical nature requiring medical treatment, i.e. it is outside the individual's control. This is identified by Siddell as characteristic of working-class people. Secondly, Siddell states the middle-class view of stress is that it is a psychological condition that is within the individual's control and therefore the individual's responsibility. These differing attitudes will have an effect on both the response to stress and subsequently to the effectiveness of nursing interventions.

TABLE 13.3	*Immediate reactions to stress*
Physical effects	Physiological effect
Dry mouth, nasal mucus decreased	Aids easier breathing
Pupils dilate	Eyes become better adapted to far vision
Digestion slows	'Butterflies' in stomach, diverting blood flow to appropriate areas
Muscle tension increases	In preparation for exertion
Sweaty/clammy hands, blushing, hotness, sweating	Cooling of body in case of exertion
Breathing rate increases	Allows for increase in oxygen production
Blood pressure and pulse raised	Allows more blood to reach muscles and brain

TABLE 13.4	Long-term signs and symptoms of stress

Physical	Behavioural	Emotional	Intellectual
Heart disease	Drug abuse	Lack of confidence	Difficulty learning
Shaking	Impairment of performance	Depression/worry/anxiety	Inattention to detail
Breathlessness	Absence	Reduction of personal involvement with others	Indecision
Hyperventilating	Avoidance	Self-depreciation/diminished initiative	Lack of interest
Difficulty in swallowing	Overemotional	Suspicious guilt blame	Preoccupation
Fatigue and exhaustion	Impulsiveness	Jealousy/apathy/tears	Forgetfulness
Restlessness	Attack	Irritability	Irrational thoughts
Insomnia	Relationship deterioration	Over confidence	Slower reactions
Lethargy	Clumsiness	Excessive sensitivity	Procrastination
Elevated blood pressure	Mispronounced words	Distress	Past orientation
Increased pulse rate	Repetition when talking	Unhappiness	Blocking
Hyperactivity	Risk taking	Despair	Mental confusion
Changes in vision	Irrationality	Despondency	Phobias
Headaches and migraine	Vigilance – looking for source	Insecurity	Decreased creativity
Backache	Overreaction	Cynicism	Slower thinking
Constipation	Mood swings	Negative attitudes	Dogmatism
Diarrhoea	Stuttering	Hopelessness	Decreased concentration
Weakening of immune system	Lack of caution	Aggression	Daydreaming
Nausea and vomiting	Phobic	Impatience	Taking the path of least resistance
Palpitations	Reassurance		
Skin complaints	Sexual problems		
Frequent and prolonged colds and Flu			
Weight loss – 10lbs			
Urinary frequency			
Narrowing of arteries			
Higher cholesterol problems			
Asthma			
Colitis			
Ulcers			
Irritable bowel problems			

Based on Benson (1975); Graham (1990); Evison (1986); Stanefoss and Prater (1990); Bailey and Clarke (1989); Soloman *et al.* (1990).

RELAXATION AND STRESS MANAGEMENT

Evison (1986) identifies a range of activities that can help to prevent or ameliorate the build-up of negative stress reactions. These are: working from strengths, changing situations, dealing with inappropriate negative feelings and thoughts; encouraging the expression of normal emotions and relaxation. In this section it is the intention to focus upon relaxation. However, the need for a wide range of interventions to be employed when looking at stress management is acknowledged.

Relaxation could be defined as a 'state of relative freedom from both anxiety and skeletal muscle tension. A quieting or calming of the mind and muscles' (McCaffery and Beebe, 1989, p. 188).

Many people may be in a state of tension without recognizing it as it may have become the norm for them in their everyday life. As we have seen, continuous anxiety or tension can contribute to physical and psychological changes that could lead to a much reduced quality of life. Nurses and the older people they work with need to be aware of signs of increasing tension and promote the use of active relaxation techniques; it is not merely a question of passively responding, for example by sleeping.

Identify the methods you use in order to relax.

Some activities you may have identified are:

- Going for a stroll
- Physical exercise
- Listening to music
- Having favourite food/drink
- Watching a good film
- Sitting in the sunshine
- Having your hair done
- Massage
- A leisurely bath
- Social activities
- Sexual activity
- The sound of water

Most of these activities require some initial effort to engage in them. Many activities will rely on the use of primary senses rather than intellectual activity. These activities can be equally relaxing for the older person particularly as they may have been part of their normal coping/recuperation repertoire of skills. If an older person is unable to engage in their normal responses to tension it is part of the nurse's role to remove or minimize the barriers they may be experiencing and promote their continued use if there is a change in environment. Alternatively consultation with clients may identify different approaches that can be used. Where illness, a loss of ability or change in circumstances seriously inhibit these activities, more formal relaxation techniques may be needed; for example, breathing awareness (Payne, 1995) or progressive muscle relaxation (Jacobsen, 1977).

Research studies examining the effectiveness of relaxation and guided imagery in older people have shown beneficial results. Yesarage (1984) used relaxation to reduce anxiety and show memory recall could be enhanced. In a sample of 39 subjects between the ages of 62 and 83 years, individuals were randomly assigned to an experimental and anti-placebo group. Those in the experimental group were shown to have decreased anxiety and perform significantly better on face and name recall compared with those in the control group.

Kiecolt-Glaser et al. (1985) demonstrated how relaxation and guided imagery improved the immune responses of older people in their study. Physical changes in the respiratory system of the older person lead to reduced efficiency in respiratory processes and increased effort within the system. Deep breathing is considered by some nurses to be an antidote for a great deal of illness or anxiety; consider how often the individual in a healthcare setting is encouraged to breathe deeply. The midwife will encourage the pregnant mother to utilize her breathing exercises. Breathing deeply is perceived as beneficial but not generally used amongst older clients in a systematic manner to improve their overall well-being or to aid relaxation in an anxious state.

Hypoxia is also common amongst older people, often due to multiple pathology. Whilst nurses may have to cope with anxiety, irritability and often a rise in 'confusion' whilst the person becomes depressed, tense and fatigued, the use of deep breathing could lead to improved oxygenation, leading to a more relaxed state within these individuals if carried out in a systematic manner (Bennett and Ebrahim, 1992).

CASE STUDY

Edith is a 76-year-old lady recovering from a stroke, having received treatment and rehabilitation in a community hospital. Prior to her illness she had reasonably good health, maintaining an active and independent life. Edith has put considerable effort into her recovery for the past three months and has reached a stage where the medical staff have started to talk to her about going home. Edith has recently become quite emotional, tearful and easily irritated.

A very quiet and pleasant lady, Edith was considered 'no trouble' by the nursing staff; now she is having trouble sleeping and becoming easily fatigued during the day. Her husband and daughters visit each day and have been talking about her discharge to try and keep her cheerful.

After talking to Edith, the nursing staff found a number of issues that were operating as considerable and conflicting stressors in Edith's situation. Edith complained that at this time she was: 'fed up! I've had enough now, I want to get home, I get bored, well you would, wouldn't you? I don't have any other worries apart from Stan [her husband] trying to manage on his own. I suppose that's playing heavy on my mind'. She was becoming anxious over her progress, putting pressure on herself to 'get better' as quickly as possible. Further discussion also revealed her concerns over her own ability to cope on discharge.

In identifying a suitable intervention for Edith we need to assess what her needs are in order to enable her to continue her progress, for example the need for:

- General calming
- Alleviation of anxiety response and muscle tension
- Information regarding support required on discharge
- A better quality of sleep
- Alleviation/distraction from boredom
- Restoration of control and confidence

In Edith's situation you may well identify a need for methods which allow for a rapid decrease in tension which will allow Edith to maintain her physical and emotional equilibrium. In addition, it may be necessary to provide a distraction which will start to alleviate the boredom within the institutional environment.

When assessing Edith, or any other individual, for nursing interventions in the area of relaxation, the following are important areas to take into account:

- Ability to concentrate and for how long
- Respiratory/musculoskeletal problems and associated contraindications
- Changes to auditory senses (pitch, volume, tone)
- Previous coping/relaxation strategies
- Comfortable physical position/posture

- Ability to use imagination
- Level of knowledge/understanding of stress and relaxation
- Frequency of intervention required

Having assessed the individual(s) concerned, it is also important to consider the environment in which the session is to take place. In doing this it becomes possible to minimize the constraints operating upon the environment and maximize the potential for an effective and positive intervention. When assessing the environment it is important to take account of the following:

- Noise levels
- Possible interruptions
- Temperature
- Ventilation
- Level of light
- Individual/group positioning
- Use of music/aromas

The assessment of the environment needs to be carried out in consultation with the individual as many of these areas will depend on personal preferences. Having identified the techniques to be used, it is important to emphasize that this process cannot be forced; this has to be based on voluntary participation. Establishing the right techniques, and the skills to use them, can take some time and effort from the nurse and the individual. Nurses must be aware that any relaxation process can become a stressor itself, especially if the person feels that they have failed to respond appropriately.

Although some techniques can be used by relatively inexperienced staff, some experience, further knowledge and training is appropriate along with consultation with colleagues before introducing these methods.

An important consideration in these discussions with respect of relaxation techniques will be the existence of contraindications within any individual. The importance of considering this area with an appropriately qualified person is reinforced by the nurse's need to operate within the bounds of the UKCC Code of Conduct (UKCC, 1992) and the Guidelines for Professional Practice (UKCC, 1996) which require nurses to place the safety and security of clients as of paramount importance.

There is, however, minimal evidence to suggest that relaxation is contraindicated for the majority of individuals. Any person suffering from a psychosis or severe depression will, however, need appropriate consideration. In addition, there are certain conditions where further assessment and medical consent should be obtained, for example:

- Inward-focusing mental health conditions may be exacerbated
- Breathing exercises may be inappropriate for people with respiratory difficulties
- Visualization may trigger allergic, phobic responses
- May increase cardiac irregularities

METHODS OF RELAXATION

There are many methods of relaxation, as outlined earlier within this chapter. This next section highlights a few methods that may be of use in practical situations.

Breathing awareness and relaxation

This is a 'quick' relaxation method that aims to change the irregular and rapid breathing associated with tension into a slow and regular pattern. An approach such as this may be helpful when considering Edith's need to decrease tension and support her in maintaining her physical and emotional equilibrium.

Payne (1995) suggests the following routine:

- Let the air out slowly
- Let the air in as slowly as possible
- Allow own rate/rhythm of breathing again for a few breaths
- Repeat sequence, until rate slows and settles
- Start to focus on expanding the lower part of the chest

This may be extended by using the following format, adapted from Benson (1975), who developed a simple technique based on meditation:

- Provide a quiet environment
- Arrange for a suitable and comfortable chair (a recliner is ideal)
- Ensure feet are on the floor, or legs are fully supported by a footstool
- Ensure clothing is not restrictive
- Invite the individual to close their eyes and focus on breathing
- Breathe in through the nose
- Breathe out through the mouth
- Allow the client to establish a regular and relaxed pattern of breathing
- **Either** introduce method of focusing attention on one word, where the individual is invited to say 'one' on breathing out, the pattern following 'breathe 'in–out–in', repeating for 10–20 minutes; **or** imagery can be introduced as appropriate for the person or group
- Ignore any intrusion of external thoughts, adopt a passive attitude

This can extend the breathing awareness for up to 20 minutes. Benson (1975) stresses that success in achieving a deep level of relaxation is not important; the individual merely needs to maintain a passive attitude and permit relaxation to occur at its own pace. The important elements within the exercise are the repetition and non-distraction.

Both of the above exercises are unobtrusive, can be practised in most environments and allow the individual to control their use and application. In order to enhance the potential success of these interventions we have provided a checklist of areas considered in this section (Box 13.1) that it is useful to consider prior to using relaxation techniques. The use of familiar routines and good preparation will reduce the changes required in any environment when introducing relaxation techniques.

When evaluating techniques and methods used it is important to consider the following:

- Has the chosen method been effective? In order to ascertain this the nurse needs to evaluate and clarify with the person any alterations or changes that would enhance the relaxation process. This would involve taking time with the older person after each session to discuss their responses
- Was the pace and presentation of the relaxation method appropriate to the individual? (Does it need to be slower, with smaller amounts of information?)

BOX 13.1	*Relaxation techniques checklist*

Breathing

Does the individual breathe normally (respiration rate, depth, rhythm)?
What factors influence the individual's breathing?
Have there been any previous breathing difficulties?
How have these been coped with?
Identify the most suitable position to ensure the individual can breathe freely.
Are there any specific problems associated with breathing?
Breathing freely is an essential criterion for the client, ensuring adequate seating and preventative methods for difficulties with breathing will need thorough assessment.

Lighting

Can lights be dimmed, curtains drawn for reduction of glare? What levels are comfortable/preferred?

Noise

Needs to be absolutely minimal. A quiet noise-free environment has to be a priority. Consider preventing access to other people once relaxation commences.

Seating

Chairs must be comfortable. Individuals need to be able to breath deeply so will need to sit upright with feet on the floor, and back well supported.
Placing chairs in a circle facing inwards may help to enhance the relaxation process. This can promote a feeling of safety, closing the circle aids privacy.

What is the most suitable environment to promote rest? Consider:

- Furniture (bed, chair, recliner, footstool)
- Temperature and ventilation of room (provision of blanket, electric fan)
- Clothing

Music

If a relaxation tape or suitable music is used, ensure all individuals can hear this, as well as the lead voice giving directions/reading the fantasy, etc. Some older people with hearing impairment may be excluded and a more individual approach such as using a personal stereo with headphones is an alternative.

Timing

Must take into account the individual's normal routine.
Eating and drinking should be assessed to ensure a preferred time for relaxation is negotiated that does not interfere with these activities.

Rest and sleep will determine difficulties in relaxing fully. Relaxation can also be utilized to aid sleep at bedtime as well as for enhancing rest during the day. Establish the normal sleeping pattern.

Elimination needs will require specific attention to ensure the individual has the opportunity to use toilet facilities or for nursing intervention to keep them clean, dry and comfortable during the relaxation process.

- Has the choice of imagery been correctly used/applied by the staff? This is essential to enable the focus of control to be kept with the person. Other areas of their life may seem out of control; facilitating techniques to empower them requires an understanding of this process
- The relevance of physiological evaluation with regard to respiration, pulse, blood pressure and the difference in muscle tension
- Weinberger (1991) strongly recommends that tape-recorded instruction is initially avoided as live instruction has proved to be more effective. This does not rule out the use of recordings later to increase personal choice and control

It is always a good idea to practise your methods on your colleagues as well as clients. Many nurses are sceptical of relaxation methods, but in our experience, having tried it out, are the first to request another session.

Some of these exercises were carried out with staff and clients in preparation for this text. Although staff were reluctant to join in at first, they obviously enjoyed the session and we were invited to return. Some of the issues staff had difficulty with were those such as learning how to 'switch off' from the pressures and concerns of their environment. This takes more than one relaxation session as we found that nurses themselves are perhaps the most difficult people to convince that caring for yourself is also about letting go of work stressors and relinquishing your 'duty'. Perhaps this is in part due to the nurse's stereotypical 'angel' image and also the praise given by older clients to nursing staff. The nurses we came into contact with for these relaxation sessions welcomed the idea but particularly the 'nurse in charge' found it hardest to relax, despite the fact she had delegated supervision of the ward to another person. This is an important consideration as such attitudes and behaviours can be interpreted negatively, indicating a lack of importance and value to such approaches.

PAIN AND STRESS

Anxiety has been well documented as a pain amplifier since the early 1950s (Hill *et al.*, 1952). It is known that environmental conditions can be an important cause of undue extra stress (Brock, 1975). Too long an exposure to unchanging sensory input produces physiological, cognitive, perceptual and affective impairments (Schultz, 1965) and it was identified that sensory restriction can lead to an increase in sensitivity for tactile and noxious stimuli which results in a lowered pain threshold. In addition Ferrell *et al.* (1990) indicates that between 45% and 80% of older people in nursing homes experience pain.

Environments that are impoverished as a result of poor design or lack of activity that engages the service user could be viewed as causing the elderly person to experience sensory restriction, this in turn leads to an increase in anxiety resulting in stress. Stress itself leads to an increase in the sensation of pain which in turn will lead to a lowered level of activity. Reduced levels of activity can place the individual in an environment that changes very little and may significantly reduce the number of social contacts available. This in turn leads to sensory restriction and boredom which can lead to stress and the cycle repeats itself and becomes self-perpetuating.

To minimize the impact of stress and manage pain it is essential to maintain activity levels, provide an environment that is interesting and changes in a way that is stimulating to the service user, and ensure that as wide a variety of social contacts as possible are fostered and maintained. The use of imagery techniques, such as the one already identified, can offer one approach to maintaining a stimulating environment whilst at the same time reducing anxiety levels.

Complete the following exercise to assess the receptiveness of your own imagination and to experience the power of mind over matter.

Describe to yourself the body movements associated with slicing a lemon and arranging it on a plate.

See yourself picking a slice of lemon up. Feel the different temperatures and textures; the hard, bumpy rind and the soft cool pulp.

Watch yourself place the lemon slice in your mouth. Feel the textures with your tongue. Suck the pulp and taste the juice as it flows through your mouth and into your throat.

When did your mouth start to water? The earlier this happened the more active your imagination and the more receptive you are to imagery. How absorbed did you become? Were you completely distracted from your current situation by the experience? How powerful was your response, did it include all of the senses as well as a cognitive process?

IMAGERY TECHNIQUES

Where the mind tends to focus, emotions and physiology are likely to follow (Pelletier, 1978, p. 252).

Anger, anxiety, fear and dread may be our responses to our worst imaginings rather than to actual reality. However, the power of the mind can also be used to work to our advantage to access other psychological processes and to provide us with a powerful intervention (Hall *et al.*, 1990). Most techniques may depend upon visualization but the best results may be achieved when all five senses are utilized within the image (Stephen, 1993a). Active imagining can be used as a coping mechanism which takes dilemmas and confusing experiences through new insights to practical solutions and reorientation to new situations for the individual. Images can be viewed as a skill procedure which can be learned and improved through practice, enhancing the individual's current coping repertoire. Imagery can be used to distract during moments of fear and boredom, promoting relaxation by being a highly absorbing activity (Graham, 1990).

Imagery for the purposes of pain relief may be defined as the use of one's imagination to manipulate some aspect of the pain experience through the purposeful development of sensory images (McCaffery and Beebe, 1994). It is based on the notion that the individual can learn specific coping skills to reappraise and acquire a sense of control over his/her experience of pain (Turk and Meichenbaum, 1994).

Guided imagery occurs when the nurse guides the individual through a scripted technique. With self-directed imagery, clients are enabled to use their own imagination to remember or create pleasant or incompatible images

(McCaffery and Beebe, 1994). The only limitation appears to be the imagination of the nurse and the client. The danger is that unsuccessful use may lead to feelings of guilt or failure on the part of the individual or the nurse. However, Graham (1992) emphasizes that, in the majority of cases, confronting the issue is considerably more beneficial than avoiding it.

Imaginative inattention can be an invaluable technique for people experiencing extreme pain, it involves focusing away from, or ignoring the pain through the use of pleasant imagery. Building upon pleasurable past experiences or fantasy, individuals can remove themselves from the painful situation simply by taking an imaginary vacation (Briebart, 1994). The nurse may guide the imagery development explicitly by leading the person through a prepared description of the scene to be imagined. Scripts have been written for this purpose and to avoid prescribing the response from the recipient (Hall *et al.*, 1990).

In the latter two approaches no overt response is required from the person as they do not have to speak or act, only listen and follow the thread of the images as they are evoked. This is especially useful for individuals who are very weak, have difficulty expressing themselves verbally or are fatigued. Self-directed strategies, for those who are able, can foster a sense of power and self-control. Briebart (1993) suggests that the aim of imaginative inattention is to distract and relax. Thus it may alleviate pain by relieving the boredom or disrupting the pain–anxiety–muscle-tension cycle which may be major components of the suffering of the person with advanced cancer. Alternatively the pain may be unchanged but the client less anxious or depressed and more able to cope.

CASE STUDY John is a 65-year-old man who has been admitted to the palliative care unit for pain control. His diagnosis is advanced mesothelioma (cancer of the lung) caused by exposure to asbestos.

He is experiencing severe pleural pain, exacerbated by nerve damage, which is extremely difficult to control. Despite increasing amounts of morphine and a complicated regime of adjuvant drugs the pain had not been controlled after one week.

John's psychological distress was increasing as conventional methods appeared to fail. Anger, anxiety and fear all started to manifest themselves as part of John's emotional state. John had been divorced for two years, and when his two daughters did not visit he felt totally abandoned by his family, but expressed guilt over the divorce and his part in breaking the family up. John expressed bitterness that his life was being cut short due to a preventable cause – asbestos. However, his anger and frustration at the situation was mainly directed at the doctors and nurses who had failed to control his pain.

One day, John said to the nurse, 'You know I wake up each morning and think – another day. Then I remember I do not have many days left. If only I could control the pain, I could go home and live each day to the full.'

In this type of scenario the pain may well be all consuming and the psychological distress a barrier to pain control. An imagery technique that looks outward and reintroduces pleasant and happy memories may be considered to be of considerable benefit. A guided imagery by the nurse would allow John time to feel comfortable with the technique and develop confidence in its efficacy.

Guided imagery

The following is an example of how you could use guided imagery to facilitate an individual to relax and reduce their stress.

Take two deep breaths . . . allow your body to relax . . . Just let the tension go . . .

I would like to invite you to imagine that you are in a park . . . Take a look around . . . There is a slight incline and at the top is a bench from which you can see the whole park . . . Walk towards the bench and sit yourself down . . . The bench may feel quite hard . . . Have a good look round . . . What is the view like? . . . Is there a playground in the park? . . . Are there swings and roundabouts? . . . Are there any people about? . . . What are they doing? . . . What are the trees like? . . . What colours are the leaves? . . . Are there any flowers? . . . Bushes? . . . What else can you see? . . . Listen carefully, can you hear any sounds? . . . Birds? . . . Little children calling out? . . . Dogs barking . . . Is there a breeze gently blowing through the branches of the trees and rustling leaves? . . .

Take a deep breath . . . Perhaps you can smell the perfume of the flowers . . . Or the recently mown grass . . . Feel the gentle breeze against your skin . . . The warmth of the sun on your face . . . How do you feel about being in this place at this time? . . . How do you feel inside? . . . Sit awhile and enjoy the sunshine . . . Feel its warmth on your face . . . Let it radiate through your whole body . . . Just enjoy the sensation of warmth.

PRACTICAL CONSIDERATIONS FOR NURSES

Assessment, planning, implementation and evaluation are obviously important first steps in introducing guided imagery into John's care package. As with Edith, it is important to consider a number of important issues (Box 13.2).

Although many of these techniques can enhance nursing care delivery it is important to consider that the imagery used will not always work as intended, or that people will be helped by the same image. This may mean that considerable time and effort needs to be invested, particularly during assessment and planning in order to find or develop an effective technique for the individual concerned.

BOX 13.2	*Guided imagery checklist*

Assessment and planning

- Conditions same as for relaxation, i.e. quiet and comfortable
- Effectiveness enhanced if preceded by relaxation techniques
- Determine the extent to which the client uses their imagination, e.g. ask them to imagine the room they slept in as a child. Then ask questions about the windows; colour of the curtains, etc.

- Lead initially, but then encourage the client to develop their own images (i.e. happy and peaceful memories). It is possible to aid the person's imagination with props, e.g. photos, aromas, music, sounds such as birdsong
- Avoid volunteering an image or scene for the client because the nurse may be unaware of associations or meaning (e.g. client may have a fear of water – beach scene may bring back feelings of fear and loss of control)
- Session may by taped, therefore can be re-used by the client
- Use permissive directions and suggestions, i.e. simply offer the image rather than force it on the client (use words/phrases such as 'Perhaps ...', 'If you wish ...')
- Try different methods/approaches to find the one that suits
- Identify time limits
- Be prepared to be flexible and individualize the script as necessary
- Assess the client's physical and psychological condition in order to choose specific techniques
- During assessment watch for spontaneous clues and images
- Assess the client's ability to concentrate, daydream, focus attention, in order to use correct techniques

It is essential when embarking upon strategies such as guided imagery that the client provides their explicit and informed consent for the use of these interventions.

Implementation

- Physical preparation is important, i.e. using the toilet, loose clothing, positioning
- Most effective to use clients' images
- Ask client to close eyes and think of an experience where they felt secure, peaceful and safe
- Ask client to give a summary of the scene
- Elaborate on the scene using their words but providing more detail
- Utilize all sensations, e.g. 'Feel the sun warm on your skin', 'Breathe in the salty/fresh air'
- Remind client to breathe slowly and evenly to increase sense of self-control
- Having started the script, do not digress, interrupt or ask questions about other subjects

Evaluation

- Following the session, it is important to allow time for silence and thought. This can be a time of deep personal insight which may be lost if talking begins too soon (Edgar, 1993)
- Successful use of imagery should never lead to the conclusion that pain is psychological in origin (Briebart, 1993). The fact that imagery works indicates that pain is present and has been temporarily relieved
- The nurse needs to explore the imagery, feelings and responses to it with the client
- Identify success of particular techniques for the individual and modifications required
- Identify how the client can gain more control over the process, e.g. taping, writing scripts

For successful use of guided imagery techniques there is a need to ensure that active co-operation and concentration by the client is achieved. If this does not exist or the person has severe emotional problems, cannot concentrate, has no time or energy to devote to using imagery or a history of psychiatric illness, then guided imagery techniques should not be used. In addition it is not advisable to use guided imagery at periods of severe pain, particularly as learning a new technique uses time and energy. Obviously should any signs of distress, restlessness or agitation be observed the session should stop. Reasons for the above will then need to be explored at an appropriate time with the individual concerned.

CONCLUSION

As in all areas of nursing, being accountable for the client's care is paramount by ensuring their safety and well-being at all times (UKCC, 1992). In order to ensure client safety, thorough assessment is recommended and discussion of relaxation methods with the client, physician and nursing staff will facilitate safety. Consent should be obtained from the client and recorded appropriately (UKCC, 1992, UKCC, 1996). LeShan (1989) observes that, if a therapy is strong enough to help, it is strong enough to hurt and as such when imagery is used to help people with advanced cancer or in chronic pain, it must be used with sensitivity and care. Imagery should provide a sense of power, control and dignity, not add stress to the person's situation.

Some people may exhibit a certain reluctance, ambivalence or doubt about imagery techniques because of fear of failure, having their hopes dashed or are sceptical about their effectiveness. Strong negative expectations and attitudes would need to be identified at the outset to avoid counterproductive outcomes. Caution does not necessarily mean non-use. Not all clients will be able to benefit from relaxation techniques for a range of reasons, e.g. mind wandering or inability to hold images may reduce effectiveness.

These techniques should not be forced on people or blame of failure attached to anyone. The nurse is not simply a conveyor of information but acts as an educator, coach, guide and assessor and must demonstrate consistent unconditional positive regard, genuineness and empathy, both verbally and non-verbally (Rogers, 1961). These are emphasized as essential conditions in the formation of a trusting, collaborative relationship in which the patient feels understood, supported and free to experiment with new ideas and activities.

FURTHER READING

Davies, M. *et al.* (1992) *The Relaxation and Stress Reduction Workbook*, 3rd edn. New Harbinger Publications, Oakland.
A comprehensive book that looks at the methodology included in a form range of stress management techniques; it ties in reactions to stress and the best methods for the individual to use to cope with stressors.

Graham, H. (1992) *The Magic Shop*. Rider, London.
Combines relevant research and theory with a series of specially focused imaginative exercises that can be practised at home or shared with others. Written in response to a series of highly successful workshops, this book introduces a wider audience to exercises which can be used to promote

relaxation, to develop physical, mental and spiritual self-awareness; and to apply these insights in the maintenance of health and the prevention and treatment of illness.

Hall, E. *et al.* (1990) *Scripted Fantasy in the Classroom.* Routledge, London.
Written as a theoretical framework and step-by-step practical guide for teachers interested in implementing imagery and fantasy in schools, the clear explanations enable easy adaptation for use by healthcare professions, provides a wide range of scripts and exercises suitable for a variety of healthcare situations.

McCaffrey, M. and Beebe, A. (1989) *Pain: Clinical Manual for Nursing Practice.* Mosby, London.
This is especially useful for dealing with patients in pain. A comprehensive handbook concerning all relevant issues and methodologies for relaxation and imagery.

Rankin-Box, D. (1995) *The Nurse's Handbook of Complementary Therapies.* Churchill Livingstone, Edinburgh.
A useful book that summarizes complementary therapies in a user-friendly format. It considers practice, policies and research. Each therapy is then described with clear contraindicators for use.

Weinberger, R. (1991) Teaching the elderly stress reduction. *Journal of Gerontological Nursing,* **17**(10), 23–27.
This article gives some background to stress and its possible causes and outcomes. It provides a good introduction to progressive muscle relaxation, including the procedure, a script and contraindicators.

Wells, R. and Tschudin, V. (eds) (1994) *Wells' Supportive Therapies in Health Care.* Baillière Tindall, London.
This book looks at a range of therapies and their uses. The case studies give clear indicators to the relevance and benefits of different approaches.

REFERENCES

Bailey, R. and Clarke, M. (1989) *Stress and Coping in Nursing.* Chapman & Hall, London.

Bennett, G. and Ebrahim, S. (1992) *The Essentials of Health Care of the Elderly.* Edward Arnold, London.

Benson, H. (1976) *The Relaxation Response.* William Collins, London.

Briebart, W. and Passik, S.D. (1993) Psychological and psychiatric interventions in pain control. In *Oxford Textbook of Palliative Medicine,* Doyle, P., Hanks, G. and MacDonald, N. (eds). Oxford University Press, Oxford.

Briebart, W. (1994) Psychological factors in pain experience. In *Textbook of Pain,* 3rd edn, Wall, P.D. and Melzack, R. Churchill Livingstone, Edinburgh.

Brock, L. (1975) The importance of environmental conditions, especially temperature, in the operating room and intensive care ward. *British Journal of Surgery,* **62**, 253.

Edgar, L. (1993) The psychological aspects of pain. In *Pain Management and Nursing Care,* Carroll, L. and Bowsher, D. (eds). Heinemann, Oxford.

Erikson, E.H. (1980) *Identify and the Life Cycle: a Reissue.* W.W. Norton, New York.

Evison, R. (1986) Self help in preventing stress build up. *The Professional Nurse,* March, 157–159.

Ferrell, B.A., Ferrell, B.R. and Osterweal, D. (1990) Pain in the nursing home. *Journal of the American Geriatric Society,* **38**, 409–414.

Graham, H. (1990) *Time, Energy and the Psychology of Healing.* JKP, London.

Graham, H. (1992) *The Magic Shop*. Rider, London.

Hall, E., Hall, C. and Leech, A. (1990) *Scripted Fantasy in the Classroom*. Routledge, London.

Hill, H., Kornetsky, C., Flanary, H. and Wilkes, A. (1952) Effects of anxiety and morphine on discrimination of intensities of painful stimuli. *Journal of Clinical Investigations* **31**, 473.

Holmes, T.H. and Rahe, R.H. (1967) The social readjustment rating scale. *Journal of Psychomatic Research,* **11**, 213–218.

Jacobsen, E. (1938) *Programme Relaxation*. University of Chicago Press, Chicago.

Jacobsen, E. (1977) You must relax (5th edn) Souvenir Press, London, cited in Rankin-Box, D. (1995) *The Nurse's Handbook of Complementary Therapies*. Churchill Livingstone, Edinburgh.

Kanner, A.D., Coyne, J.C., Schaefer, C. and Lazarus, R.S. (1981) Comparison of two modes of stress measurement: daily hassles and uplifts versus major life events. *Journal of Behavioural Medicine,* **4**(1).

Kiecolt-Glaser, J.K., Glaser, R., Wilhgier, D., Stout, J. *et al.* (1985) Psychosocial enhancement of immunocompetence in a geriatric population. *Health Psychology,* **4**(11), 24–41.

McCaffery, M. and Beebe, A. (1989) *Pain – Clinical Management for Nursing Practice*. C.V. Mosby, St. Louis.

McCaffery, M. and Beebe, A. (1994) *Pain: Clinical Manual for Nursing Practice*. Mosby, London.

Moos, R.H. (1986) *Coping with Life Crises: an Integrated Approach*. Plenum, New York.

Payne, R. (1995) *Relaxation Techniques: a Practical Handbook for the Health Care Professional*. Churchill Livingstone, Edinburgh.

Pelletier, K. (1978) *Mind as Healer, Mind as Slayer*. George Allen, London.

Rogers, C. (1961) *On becoming a person*. Houghton Mufflin, Boston.

Rogers, C. (1994) *On becoming a person. A Therapeutics View of Psychotherapy*. Constable, London.

Schultz, D.P. (1965) *Sensory Restriction; Effects on Behaviour*. Academic Press.

Siddell, M. (1995) *Health in Old Age*. Oxford University Press, Buckingham.

Soloman, E., Schmot, R. and Adragna, P. (1990) Human Anatomy and Physiology, 2nd edn. Harcourt Brace, New York.

Stalegoss, N. and Proctor, M. (1990) Stress response and illness. In *Psychiatric Nursing in the Hospital and the Community,* Wolbert Brugess, A. (ed.) 5th edn. Appleton and Lange.

Stephens, R. (1993a) Imagery: a strategic intervention to empower clients. Part I – review of research literature. *Clinical Nurse Specialist* 7(4), 170–174.

Turk, D.C. and Meichenbaum, D. (1994) A cognitive-behavioural approach to pain management. In *Textbook of Pain,* 3rd edn, Melzack, R. and Wall, P.D. Churchill Livingstone, Edinburgh.

UKCC (1992) Code of Professional Conduct. UKCC, London.

UKCC (1996) Guidelines for Professional Practice. UKCC, London.

Weinberger, R. (1991) Teaching the elderly stress reduction. *Journal of Gerontological Nursing,* **17**(10), 23–27.

Yesavage, J.A. (1984) Relaxation and memory training in 39 elderly patients. *American Journal of Psychiatry,* **141**(6), 778–781.

4 FUTURE DIRECTIONS

This section debates the response of the nursing profession to the current policy trends in order to, as far as is possible, predict the future direction of healthcare for older people. In addition, this section considers the political issues that face the nursing profession and particularly those nurses who work with older people. The dilemma of matching resources to client need is debated, as is the issue of outcome measures. In particular, with regard to outcome measures, there is a consideration of how these can affect the quality of the care delivery and therefore the experience of the client.

14 Meeting the needs of older people: resource issues

Joy Harrison

KEY ISSUES	
	■ Health versus social care
	■ Funding continuing care
	■ Inevitability of rationing: fact or fiction
	■ Needs assessment
	■ User perspectives
	■ Reality of current strategies for older people
	■ Carer consequences
	■ Opportunities for nurses as providers
	■ Evidence of effectiveness
	■ Opportunities for nurses as purchasers

INTRODUCTION

The provision of health and social care for an ageing population has become a potential arena for discourse between/amongst politicians, clinicians and managers. That this care must be provided from a finite pool of resource is an assumption accepted by much of the literature (Harrison and Hunter, 1994; Maynard, 1996; Sheldon and Maynard, 1993; Wells, 1995) and most political opinion on both sides of the British political model (Bottomley, 1989; Blunkett, 1994; Brindle, 1996). The first section of this chapter will explore different models that exist to match resources to need in a state funded health service, and will consider models from other countries where different systems of funding exist but similar problems of allocation of resources apply. The systems in two other European Union countries, Denmark and Germany, will be reviewed, with particular focus on the latter as it reflects the direction long-term healthcare in Britain appears to be going. Whatever funding model is used, finance available will not be infinite, thus the issues of 'rationing' and definitions of 'health' and 'social' care provision are considered.

To gain an insight into resources required, a clear picture of healthcare need is crucial, the concept of 'population needs assessment' will therefore be discussed with a critical review of the validity of such exercises. Nurses working with older people must have a good understanding of 'assessment of need' in order to influence this process if it does not seem to address/define nursing need; these issues will be discussed in the second section.

The third section explores detailed case studies from contemporary practice to illuminate the reality of 'needs assessment' and 'resource allocation' for older people who have problems based in multiple pathology and disability. Each case study is concluded with a brief discussion about the ethical and legal dilemmas emanating from each situation. The case studies lead into an examination of the specific relevance of rationing of healthcare for older people, the consequences of redefining individuals' need for care, and transfer of responsibility for resourcing that need to social care agencies. An analysis of how these shifts in responsibility for, and delivery of, continuing care influence the definition and practice of nursing is included here.

The chapter concludes with a section exploring the role of nurses in the whole arena of healthcare purchasing, with reference to the purchasing of nursing for older people who require continuing care.

MATCHING RESOURCES TO NEED IN A STATE-FUNDED HEALTH SERVICE

The growth of the older population on a global scale is well documented and predicted (Davis *et al.*, 1990) and the increase in frail older people, mainly those over 85, has been measured and predicted in the United Kingdom (Casey, 1997). However, not all of these people will require large amounts of healthcare, as they are generally healthier than their parents would have been at their age, but the incidence of chronic degenerative disease and malignant disease increases with age so it can be assumed that an increased older population equates with at least some increase in healthcare need.

The care of older people requires, and will increasingly take, a large share of the monies available for health and social care. The prime responsibility for providing long-term care, which includes continuing care of older people and people with chronic disability, now lies with the social services (NHS Executive, 1994). There has been a sharp fall in the number of NHS continuing-care beds and a reflected rise in the number of beds in the private nursing-home sector (Hancock, 1995); consequently, much of what was previously state-funded nursing care has now become privately funded by the individual if they can afford to pay, or by the local social services if they cannot.

The guidance on health authorities' responsibilities for long-term care (NHS Executive, 1995) implies a distinction between medical need and social need, and individual local health authorities (in conjunction with care providers and the local authority) must decide who is eligible for NHS-funded long-term care. Hancock (1995) believes that local decision making on eligibility leads to geographical variations in the provision of long-term care and challenges the principle of a national and equitable service (NAHA, 1995). A significant portion of what used to be classed as healthcare, such as the long-term care of frail, dependent older people, and respite care for older people and their carers, is now realigned as social care. Such care can therefore be purchased by the Social Services in the person's locality from whomever they choose, and increasingly from the private sector.

Currently long-term and respite nursing care for older people is therefore no longer a responsibility of the NHS, and is thus 'means tested'. A person with more than £16,000 in savings, or in property of which they are the sole occupier, is required to pay for their long-term care. In such circumstances these individuals will not receive any financial support, until capital is reduced to £10,000. At this point partial support is available, through to full support when resources are sufficiently reduced.

According to the Institute of Fiscal Studies there are other options for financing long-term care in a cash-limited health and social service:

- An increase in the threshold for 'means tested' residential care, which has now risen from £8000 to £16,000, and is set to rise again, in line with the size of a person's long-term healthcare insurance policy (Thomas, 1996)
- The Department of Health meeting the medical, but not the residential, costs of long-term care (it is assumed here that the medical costs would encompass nursing and therapy costs)
- Tax-breaks for people who take out early private insurance to meet long-term care costs

In the opinion of the consultancy 'London Economics', continuing care of older people could be funded by compulsory state insurance, requiring a contribution of 1.8% of gross earnings to meet today's needs (and 5% by 2031) (Hunter and Lyall, 1995).

There is growing evidence that the British public are not about to accept responsibility for healthcare in their old age through private long-term care insurance (PPP Lifetime Research, 1995; Hudson, 1995). Additionally, lobby groups such as Help the Aged state that the cost of insurance premiums taken out in middle or old age, which protect capital tied up in a home, are prohibitively expensive, being as much as £10,000 for a lump sum payment. Help the Aged are concerned that pensioners living on low incomes are unlikely to be able to find the money to pay for such a scheme (Kohler, 1996).

Contemporary options for funding long-term care of older people have centred on a 'public–private partnership' such as that outlined in the government consultation paper *A New Partnership for Care in Old Age* (Department of Health, 1996). The issue under proposal is that those people who insure themselves against part, or all, of the expenses of long-term care would in return be allowed to retain a larger proportion of their savings (usually mostly in the form of property equity). The two aspects of this scheme are, firstly, the provision of private insurance (by private pension providers) to cover long-term care bills for those who need it; secondly, a partnership agreement in which the government would disregard £1.00 capital for each £1.00 insurance paid and/or would entirely disregard, for the purpose of means testing, £15,000 capital, rather than the usual amount of £10,000 as was set in April 1996. This extra disregard amount would only be an option for those who had already funded at least four years of long-term care (around £80,000 of cover at current prices) either through insurance cover, personal funding, or a combination of the two.

The motivation for this partnership approach is to provide incentives for people to take out indemnity insurance to meet their (potential) long-term care costs, with the reward being extra protection against means testing once the policy has run out, that is if they outlive the policy duration. Lifelong policies are likely to be expensive due to the potential risks to the providers (the private insurers) but the 'fixed term' annuities offered reduce the insurer's level of risk and therefore the cost to the policyholders.

Clearly there remain the major philosophical arguments about the shift from the lifelong 'policy' provided by the National Health Service in its original 'cradle to the grave' format to the assumption that long-term care is no longer an automatic right.

The above options all assume that continuing care cannot be provided out of a state funded (through taxation) National Health Service, and the options seem to be centred on either a compulsory social insurance model, such as the recent German model (Chadda 1995), or an acceptance of rationing the limited state funds (which are threatened by a reduction in numbers of direct taxpayers due to demographic change and unemployment). Older people represent the largest group requiring long-term community care across the European Union (Pac-Soo, 1996); however, political and economic models to finance such care vary from Denmark at one end of the spectrum, where the state accepts total responsibility, and Germany at the opposite end of the spectrum, where compulsory insurance is the basis of funding (German healthcare is contracted through private health insurance companies). The British system appears to be moving in the direction of the German system, at least for the provision of long-term (non-acute) care, predominantly the type of care older people need, so a deeper understanding of such a system is useful to those who are working with older people, or managing resources for this group.

The German approach to the provision of care for older people is not directed through specific national legislation, but through the various initiatives of local and regional governments (Pac-Soo, 1996). Fundamentally the system relies on what are known as 'Sickness Insurance Funds' or SIF (Navarro, 1991) which are a collection of autonomous insurance companies who receive finance through equal contributions from employers and employees (with short-term supportive arrangements through shared government and individual finance for the unemployed). In the German system the purchaser of care will generally be the SIF but can also be a pension fund, a charity, or the German social services if the need is for 'home economical care' (what the British system calls 'social care'). The German social services fund 'home economical care' (that is care which is not defined as 'medical' care); the provision may be residential or at home and is means tested (similar to the current British 'social care' model). The decision on who pays for long-term care in the German community, whether insurer or social services, depends on whether the person is assessed as needing 'medical care' or 'home economical care'. The similarities to the British strategy *NHS Responsibilities for Meeting Continuing Healthcare Needs* (Department of Health, 1995a, implemented in April 1996) are clear, with similar problems of defining what is 'health'/'medical' care and what is 'social'/'home economical' care being reported (Pac-Soo, 1996).

The German system of care provision is dominated by the medical profession and what is funded through the insurance companies (and is therefore 'free' at the point of need to the consumer) is that care which is clearly a medical intervention or need. The issue of the holistic nature of nursing care is not addressed and nurses provide care under both the 'medical' and the 'home economical' banner. All non-medical care, whether in a residential home, nursing home, or the person's own home, is means tested, and people in Germany are reported as feeling that they are paying again for services which they believed would be provided by the state from the taxation they had paid throughout their lives (Pac-Soo, 1996).

Public expenditure on healthcare (i.e. from direct and indirect taxation) is over 20% higher in Germany than in Britain. Yet, along with the insurer's provision through SIF, there are still financial constraints on what can be provided to the German public. Therefore the issue of availability and distribution of healthcare resources is evident, as in Britain (Pritchard, 1992). The implementation of a quasi-market within the United Kingdom National Health Service has engendered a need to make decisions on how to distribute the 'finite' resources of a state-run healthcare system; this is commonly described as 'rationing'.

'Rationing' of healthcare has always occurred, although in the UK this has been through a system of implicit rationing, based on medical/clinical decision making behind closed doors. Some protagonists would prefer this system to continue; Hunter (1997) argues that it is efficient, commands support, and avoids damaging dispute in society. Hunter's stance may be viewed as paternalistic by the more empowered and informed in society; Sheldon and Maynard (1993) describe how both consumer ignorance and deference to medical opinion is changing. Accepting the inevitability of rationing of healthcare, the Association of Community Health Councils (1993) concurred that rationing decisions must be made explicit, and rational, to retain the support of the community for a publicly funded healthcare system. Since the NHS and Community Care Act (1990) 'rationing' decisions are made by:

- The provider (the NHS trust) of what is deemed to be healthcare (mainly acute hospital-based nursing care, and some mainly short-term, or specialized, community nursing care)
- The social services department in that locality

Responsibility for determining receipt of long-term NHS care/support is placed clearly at the door of clinicians by government policy as defined in two Department of Health documents (Department of Health, 1995a, b), which have been operational since 1 April 1996, facilitated by a prescriptive resource/training package made available by the Department of Health to all 'provider' units (NHS hospital and community trusts, social services, and private sector providers, and other interested parties).

All health authorities have been expected to add local guidelines to include:

- A local definition of 'continuing healthcare'
- Local eligibility criteria
- Key service changes
- Public consultation processes
- Local dispute and review procedures
- Local monitoring arrangements

The national guidance is clear that 'where patients have been assessed as not requiring NHS continuing inpatient care, as now, they do not have the right to occupy indefinitely an NHS bed' (Department of Health, 1995a). It is also clear that what constitutes 'requiring NHS continuing inpatient care' will vary according to local guidelines. There will clearly be a greater openness to decision making about continuing care, which is commendable given the covert, and haphazard, decision-making processes which were in evidence prior to the guidance. Older people must now receive a statement showing which elements of their continuing care will be met and funded by the NHS. The decision on eligibility will be made by the medical consultant with overall 'clinical responsibility' for their care/treatment 'in consultation with the multidisciplinary team' and with reference to local guidance/criteria.

As the long-term support for older people and chronically sick people mainly falls into the remit of nurses and therapists, they must be effectively involved in this decision-making process. It is important to ensure the potentially medical model/curative definition of healthcare does not prevail in this situation. The earlier premise is also important that healthcare rationing decisions are explicit and rational, and appropriately applied to circumstances where continuing care is required. There is an obvious trend towards a withdrawal of state-funded nursing care for older people who are long-term sick. This may create a dichotomy between acute hospital-based nursing, and 'social' care in the community which may not be nurse led. Nurses now need to show evidence of their worth to the groups of people they have historically seen as their monopoly: frail dependent older people, and those who are chronically sick. Notwithstanding the political arguments, nurses need to grasp this shift of responsibility and exhibit their skills in the new arena to whoever the purchaser may be, for the ultimate benefit of those older people requiring care. Nursing could/should be producing evidence of high-quality nurse-led cost-effective long-term care for older people with continuing care needs, the feasibility and effectiveness of which is explored by Pearson *et al.* (1988) and described in some detail by Pearson (1988). Visionary nurses will recognize that this scenario could be applied to other fields of older people's care such as rehabilitation, where the nurse may lead and coordinate a team of nurses and therapists with minimal (expensive) medical consultation and medical cover required. However, the nursing development units in Oxford have closed, despite evidence of cost effectiveness and improved quality, when compared with traditional medically led continuing care for older people (Pearson, 1988). This serves to highlight the professional political nature of such innovations, and the need for nurses to demonstrate their political acumen in addition to progressive and effective therapeutic practice. Caution must be exercised to ensure that nurse-led care is not just seen as a cheap alternative to medically led care, it must be shown to be a quality alternative too; 'evidence-based healthcare' remains on all political agendas.

The whole notion of healthcare rationing, and in particular the notion of selective availability of state-funded nursing care, creates a serious dilemma for a profession whose cultural ethos has been founded on concepts of universality of access (to nursing), comprehensive healthcare for all, and holism. Where these tenets stand in the wake of the NHS and Community Care Act and such policy initiatives as NHS *Responsibilities for Meeting Continuing Healthcare Needs* (Department of Health, 1995a) are now being debated (Wells, 1995; Timms and Ford, 1995). However, it is a dilemma which may rest on an inaccurate premise: the issue of whether rationing of nursing care is inevitable is predicated on the notion that resources are finite and demand for them unlimited (Sheldon and Maynard, 1993, Harrison and Hunter, 1994; Maynard, 1996).

There are some writers who question the inevitability of rationing, and the validity of the economic arguments. Roberts (1996) in particular describes the influence of transferring the economist's ubiquitous model of 'infinite demand, mediated through competition, for scarce resources' to state-funded healthcare without any evaluation of 'fit' (p. 19). Williams and Frankel (1993) are critical of the pessimistic assumption in healthcare policy that demand can never be satisfied: ' through the calculation of healthcare requirements of a given population and the use of resources to meet those requirements in a more effective manner, blanket decisions about healthcare rationing would be unnecessary and health needs met' (p. 14).

This leads on to another aspect of resourcing care for older people: 'that of population needs assessment'.

MAPPING THE NEED FOR HEALTHCARE: AN ANALYSIS OF POPULATION NEEDS ASSESSMENT

The ageing population, a distinguishing characteristic of the demography of developed countries, is the culmination of trends in progress over the last century. These trends include reductions in both mortality and birthrate. Concern about these changes focuses on 'dependency ratios':

- The number of older people who are not working in paid employment will outnumber those (younger) adults in paid employment (and therefore paying direct tax)
- The number of older people needing some form of care or support is increasing at the same time as the number of young adults available to provide that care is decreasing (Sidell, 1995)

In simple numerical terms, the total population of Great Britain is 57,800,900, and the number of those aged 65 years and over is 10,595,500. In terms of assessing and providing for the needs of the population it is important to remember that the proportion of older people in the community varies according to area: for example, almost half the population in some areas on the British south coast are aged over 65 years (OPCS, 1993).

The numbers of people aged over 65 years is expected to increase by 30% in the next 35 years, and those aged over 85 years are expected to increase by 66% during the same time frame (OPCS, 1993). It is important to emphasize that not every person over 65, or even over 85, requires health or social care; the health of older people has steadily improved, therefore it may be wholly inappropriate to estimate healthcare needs from numerical data based on chronological age. However, when older people require care they often require it for longer: the median duration of stay in hospital for people over 85 is twice that of people of 65 to 75, and their median stay is twice that of the 15 to 44 age group (Department of Health, 1993).

Given the above variations in health needs, it seems sensible for local providers of healthcare to make an accurate assessment of the needs of their local population, in order to plan care to meet that need. This assessment of need is fraught with methodological difficulties, but it is a crucial stage in planning a coherent strategy to meet the healthcare needs of the population. The National Health Service reforms of the 1980s and 90s put the public, the users of health services, at the centre of needs assessment. Conway (1995) describes four issues inherent in basing needs assessment on user perspectives:

- The mismatch between lay knowledge and medical knowledge
- Choosing the appropriate methodology

- Funding the needs assessment
- Feeding the results into purchasing arrangements

It is important for all healthcare professionals to remember that their understanding and perception of what people need is not necessarily the right one, and true 'population needs assessment' must genuinely respect the views of the public. For medicine, and predominantly for many nurses, the perception of needs is defined and measured in terms of the presence or absence of disease in particular, and functional ability in general; for the lay public the perception of needs is based on how health is seen to affect their everyday worlds. Population needs assessment has to reconcile these views and deliver a picture of the current and potential health and social needs of the population to enable a structured response in terms of provision.

The strategic direction of current NHS policy is towards a primary care-led service, thus assessment of local need, and subsequent resource allocation is moving into the hands of general practitioner (GP) led purchasers. Fewtrell (1991) describes the aim to be to enable GPs to influence the purchasing of all patient services against strategic commitments to a fair distribution of resources, and targeted services to those with greatest need. The stated intention of this process is to redress local health inequalities. Fewtrell describes the use of assessment tools to define 'need', such as the Jarman, and Townsend indices (Jarman *et al.*, 1991, p. 523) and local mortality, morbidity and unemployment rates (Fewtrell, 1991).

However, these tools give a retrospective view of local need and the formula now used nationally to allocate resources to regions may be preferred as a method of assessing local healthcare need. The Carr–Hill (1995) formula is arguably more reliably prospective as it uses forecast resident population figures adjusted for age, and weights them according to a 'general and acute need indices' and a 'psychiatric need indices'. In terms of making accurate and useful 'population needs assessments' for the older population chronological age adjusted forecasts may have outlived their usefulness. Their current value may be in the context of such reports as 'Getting around after 60: a profile of Britain's older population' (1996) which draws together a picture of older people in Britain from the 1991 census and the General Household Survey. The profile shows that 'in early late life' (60–79 age group) 'their mobility and task capacity are unimpaired' and they are 'well able to be involved beyond their own home and household, in work, care giving, sport and recreation'. Assessment of health and social needs of older people should therefore not focus only on long-term care needs but on short-term acute and convalescent care needs, with the potential of returning older people to their positive and healthy life at home. In order to do this it is important to consider some of the areas outlined earlier in this section.

LEGAL AND ETHICAL CONSIDERATIONS

On 7 May 1996, both major British political parties made statements which amounted to shifts in emphasis from the state as the provider of 'care' and 'welfare' to the state as an enabler of care for long-term sick and older people (Brindle, 1996). With this in mind the case studies outlined in this section reflect the experiences of older people in need of health (nursing) and/or social care in a culture of, at least partial, individual financial support (through savings or insurance) rather than of complete, state-funded, NHS-based long-term care.

CASE STUDY

Case study one

Mr Lewis is an 86-year-old married man who had suffered from Alzheimer's disease for the last ten years. His wife cared for him at home until, in 1988, he was admitted to a private nursing home due to his recent hospitalization and increasing 'intensive nursing care' needs (as defined by the hospital). Mr Lewis is unable to wash, feed, or dress himself, he is immobile, and therefore requires frequent position changes in order to maintain personal comfort and the prevention of pressure sores. Mrs Lewis has to meet the costs of care, because her husband's needs are classed as 'social' and not medical. As their assets amount to more than the £16,000 ceiling (not taking into consideration the house as this is also her home) Mrs Lewis must pay the costs in total until their savings have dropped to below £10,000 when she will be able to receive partial financial assistance.

◄6 If Mr Lewis was going into care today, from home or hospital, the new 'continuing care' criteria would be applied, and an openly rationalized decision would be made on his eligibility for funded health or social care. The said criteria would at least provide Mrs Lewis with a clear written explanation for decisions made regarding type and funding of care provided. Mrs Lewis would be aware that the decision had been made by her husband's medical consultant after taking the views of other multidisciplinary team members, and she would have a clear right to appeal against the decision. However, the 'continuing care' national guidelines (Department of Health, 1995a) make it clear that the eligibility criteria 'do not apply retrospectively' and the likelihood is that the outcome would be the same. This would depend in part on her local health authority's eligibility criteria. It would appear that an appeal could not be lodged purely on the grounds that a promise made to Mr Lewis in 1948 had been broken.

CASE STUDY

Mrs Lewis states she feels 'betrayed' by the promises of care from 'cradle to grave' made when the welfare state, and National Health Service, was established. Her husband would have been 38 years old at that time and would have been encouraged to believe that any health needs he may have in the future would be met through the welfare state system, which he was encouraged to view as paid for through taxation by himself.

It could be argued that Mr and Mrs Lewis have had their security 'stolen' from them; they have maintained their tax and National Insurance contributions during their working lives, to discover that this has little significance or value in the current economic climate.

As Green (1990) reveals, 'the greatest irony is that the vast majority of people' have paid in taxes the 'full cost of the services they receive' or should receive. Thus, tragically, by having already 'surrendered' their potential buying power to the government via taxation they have consequently surrendered their ability and freedom to choose.

This conclusion applies even more acutely to the following case study where the individuals in need of care do not have any substantial savings, or assets. This case study introduces the notion of an older person's own personal and material resources as being influential upon their health.

CASE STUDY **Case study two**

Mr and Mrs Newman have lived in their small terraced house, in a deprived area of high unemployment, since marrying in 1935. Mr Newman, due to his secure job in the steelworks, had scraped together enough to pay a deposit and secure a loan from his local 'friendly society' to purchase the house. Mr Newman was in a reserved occupation, so stayed at home during the war; however, he was seriously injured in an industrial accident in 1959, and consequently had an arm amputated, and was no longer able to work. Their only child, a son, is unemployed and lives nearby with his wife and their two young children; his wife works part time as a hospital cleaner. The whole family have spent their lives living on minimal budgets, and have had to restrict their activities to reflect their small incomes.

Mrs Newman has been getting confused and disorientated for the past two years, but Mr Newman has managed the problem by taking over all household planning and budgeting (previously the realm of his wife, as is common in this generation). Mr Newman finds that his wife is best helped by continual reassurances of who and where she is, and as few visitors as possible. She is much more disorientated, and consequently distressed, if she cannot see Mr Newman, so he now rarely leaves the house. Their son now collects their pensions, buys all their shopping, and delivers everything to them at home.

Mr Newman's own substantial personal resources have enabled him to be sensitive to, and adapt to, the changing needs of his wife. He has had to accept some fundamental changes to his own role and activities, as he used to go for a daily walk to his allotment, and play dominoes with friends, both of which he has now given up. This adaptability may be partially explained by his experiences in 1959 when he had to adapt to disability and the consequent loss/change of role and earning power. Whatever the explanation, this adaptability has enabled his wife to stay in the family home, and has prevented her from entering the 'continuing care' statistics.

The adaptability of Mr Newman may be explained with reference to researchers such as Kobasa *et al.* (1982) and Colerick (1985). Kobasa formulated a concept of 'hardiness' which functions as a stress-resisting resource, the elements being commitment, control, and challenge. Mr Newman committed himself early on to the needs of his wife and did not avoid the situation. He 'took control' of the situation rather than feeling helpless in it and transformed the very stressful events into something less harmful; he saw the 'change' in his situation as a challenge (as he may have seen his disability and reduced work opportunities in 1959, or he may have learnt through that, and other experiences, that change is best met as a challenge, not a threat).

Colerick (1985) identified a concept of 'stamina' in older people who 'demonstrate emotional resilience despite age-related losses and life change' (p. 997). Older people with 'stamina' appraise a situation which threatens their well-being, or *status quo*, and meet it with self-confidence rather than helplessness. According to Colerick (1985), older people with high 'stamina' have learned through their life years that change is 'inevitable, challenging, and manageable'. Mr Newman certainly seems to fit this picture.

CASE STUDY

Mrs Newman's mental state has got worse recently; she is now aggressive towards her daughter-in-law, whom she previously had a good relationship with, and she keeps searching for her own mother (who died in 1968). She has also become incontinent at night, and will only eat lean cuts of meat and cream desserts, all of which puts an unbearable strain on Mr Newman's careful budgeting.

Mr and Mrs Newman's son has asked the practice nurse at his parents' general practice to intervene and offer some help. She visits and finds that Mr Newman is keen to continue the care at home but needs financial assistance and continence aids (he has been padding the bed up with old newspapers to protect the mattress). However, she also discovers that Mr Newman has a very irregular pulse rate, and when pressed he admits to chest pain and dizzy spells. The GP visits and recommends admission to a medical ward as he believes that Mr Newman has treatable heart block; an assumption is made that the son and daughter-in-law, because they live very near, will step in to look after Mrs Newman in the interim period. No real assessment of the relationships involved is made, and although practical help in terms of community psychiatric nurse (CPN) referral, and weekly home help, are set up, the family are left to resolve the dilemma. The daughter-in-law cannot afford to give up her job, nor can she afford to pay for childcare for the two young children. Therefore Mr and Mrs Newman's son must take on the continuous role of caring for his mother, alongside supervising and caring for his own children. Neither house is large enough to take the family plus Mrs Newman so the son moves in with his mother, having the children there with him in the day and his wife taking them home to be with her at night. The CPN refers Mrs Newman for assessment for long-term institutional psychiatric care, but is told she is 'not demented enough' to warrant care in a specialist unit. The local nursing home, which is dual registered, will not take her because her behaviour is deemed too disruptive for their environment. Mrs Newman's son is left to manage as the family have no choice but to support Mr Newman's admission to a medical ward for potential pacemaker insertion.

This family cannot afford to pay for skilled nursing care in the home to maintain Mrs Newman whilst her husband is in hospital. Mrs Newman's 'continuing care' (Department of Health, 1995a) needs are assessed by her GP in consultation with a CPN and social worker. According to local criteria, she is deemed as requiring social care support, a laundry service, and a supply of incontinence aids is provided. This, however, is inadequate as the incontinence supply is only sufficient to meet Mrs Newman's needs for four days, consequently the family uses newspaper as they cannot afford to top up the supply themselves. In addition Mrs Newman is deemed as requiring a 'sitter' which is arranged for three nights a week. Unfortunately the social care 'sitter' varies from night to night and the lack of continuity aggravates Mrs Newman's distress, so her son usually stays in the house on these nights as well.

The 'burdens' of 'social' care have fallen on this poorly (financially) resourced family. Walker (1993) questioned the assumption that families could, should, and would, care for dependent older people: 'confidence in familism is sometimes misplaced: family care can be both the best and the worst form of support'.

By assuming that families are the soundest basis for care we may overlook conflicts within caring relationships (such as is the case between Mrs Newman and her daughter-in-law) and be 'guilty of imposing some destructive relationships on both carers and cared for' (Walker, 1993, p. 220).

CASE STUDY

Mr Newman has been hospitalized for longer than expected due to complications with the siting of his permanent pacemaker; his son and daughter-in-law, and their young children are struggling with a difficult situation which will not be resolved until Mr Newman's discharge (and then only partially).

Poverty in older people makes the challenges they face that much harder to deal with, the notion that old age acts as a 'leveller' in terms of material resources, or the lack of them, is clearly not the case. As described by Siddell (1995), financial resources can mitigate some of the problems of chronic illness and disability which can accompany old age, and lack of financial resource can exacerbate them. As nurses involved in 'continuing care' assessments we must be conscious of the effect that lack of financial resources has upon the management and resolution of chronic illness and disability. For older people in these circumstances, their freedom to provide even basic social and health needs for themselves may be severely limited.

CASE STUDY

Case study three

Mr and Mrs Burford are 86 and 79 respectively. They had one daughter who died in her twenties of 'pneumonia', and whose daughter Katherine they have brought up since the age of seven. Katherine moved away from her grandparents' home to attend university, and returned to live with them after graduating (eight years ago) and securing a job close to home so she could be near them. Six years ago, Mr Burford suffered a stroke which required hospitalization for acute care and subsequent rehabilitation; at this point Katherine decided to reduce her working hours to part-time to enable her grandfather to be cared for at home.

Two years on, Mrs Burford started to become increasingly confused and disorientated, and would wander from the house into the busy road, leaving Mr Burford unsupervised. Katherine decided to give up what had been a promising career in accountancy to care for her grandparents, who had functioned as her surrogate parents in the past.

In the past year both Mr and Mrs Burford have become increasingly frail and in need of full-time care in an institution of some sort with the relevant equipment for lifting etc. They are both currently in hospital on a medical ward for older people.

Katherine has already suffered back injury through lifting her grandfather alone at night. The minimal savings which the couple had have all been spent, and Katherine has been instructed by the hospital social worker to arrange for the sale of the semi-detached house, in which she lives, to pay for her grandparents' care in a nursing home. With nursing-home bills running at an average of £20,000 a year each, the money will not provide for their care for very many years. Additionally the state will have to fund Katherine who will now be homeless as well as long-term unemployed.

Mr and Mrs Burford have both been assessed using the national and local continuing care eligibility criteria which came into place on 1 April 1996. A decision was made that Mr Burford could be safely discharged to 'a place in a nursing home ... arranged and funded by ... the patient'. The same decision was reached for Mrs Burford, but because her needs included supervision because of wandering the local nursing home Katherine had agreed to would not take her. The likelihood of the couple being separated is now great as Mr Burford's consultant is pushing for his discharge, reminding the nursing staff who are trying to support Katherine in finding the optimum arrangement that the continuing care guidelines state very clearly that: 'patients do not have the right to occupy indefinitely an NHS bed'.

This issue will not be resolved to the satisfaction of all parties quickly, if at all. The position of the nurses is difficult due to the conflict of interests they face:

■ Their desire to support the family in coming to an optimum care arrangement, and in particular to meet the psychological and social, as well as the medical/physical needs of Mr and Mrs Burford
■ Their concern about the future health and well-being of Katherine. This relates to the wider health promotion and prevention role of the nurses (Code of Conduct, UKCC, 1983).
■ Their loyalty to the multidisciplinary team to follow the decision reached through the application of the eligibility criteria
■ Their awareness of the needs of other people both within the ward, and already in non-NHS continuing care, and the importance of applying the criteria equitably and fairly to ensure good use of allocated resources
■ The dilemma that the hospital bed is needed by someone else who may benefit more measurably from its use

The above reflection on the position of the nurse identifies some of the difficulties that this profession will face with increasing regularity, as a consequence of the implementation of the 'continuing care criteria' (Department of Health, 1995a).

 How do you feel about the above issues? What might your response be in a similar situation?

THE IMPACT OF THE PURCHASER/PROVIDER SPLIT ON THE ROLE OF THE NURSE

This chapter concludes by exploring the role of the nurse in the purchaser/provider arena, including an analysis of how the resource issues inherent in meeting the needs of older people impinge on the perceived role of the nurse, and the concept of 'nursing'.

Nurses are major providers of the care that older people currently receive, whether through community nursing in the form of district/community nurses, hospital nurses and practice nurses, or through long-term care in nursing homes. This should be seen as an opportunity for nurses to develop what they believe to be nursing, without the organizational and philosophical constraints which have constrained developments since the inception of organized, state-run, medically led, nursing services.

To be successful in utilizing this opportunity nurses will need to show that their 'nursing' care, and leadership, are beneficial to clients. Nurses must demonstrate that the nursing care delivered is in keeping with the concept of evidence-based practice. This is particularly important as nursing will be measured, by the purchaser, alongside other activities and other providers. The concept of clinical effectiveness is of importance in this context particularly in relation to efficient and effective care delivery.

The difficulty for nursing within such a quantitatively driven market is how to address the holistic nature of nursing and maintain that holism across the reductionist nature of scientific research and outcome measurement. This is where nurses need to be concentrating some research energy as the division between 'health' and 'social' care emphasized by the National Health Service and Community Care Act (1990) and the Department of Health guidelines on continuing care (1995a) is not as clear to nursing as it may be to business managers and their main informants, doctors.

Nursing is poorly defined, and in a state of flux, but there are basic tenets which are at its core:

- Holism – a consideration of the total person's needs in the context of their nursing needs: physical, psychological, social, cultural, and spiritual
- All aspects being important in the restoration and maintenance of their total health, their level of functional, cognitive and emotional ability, and their comfort and safety according to their holistic health and their position on the developmental continuum
- Humanistic intervention – based on fundamental relationships, where the nurse empowers the client through the provision of information and the evaluation of the person's understanding of their situation

Nurses must also recognize the enormous amount of care given by informal and family carers; long-term care should not be perceived as only that care which goes on within an institutional or residential setting. Nolan (1996) expresses the need for nurses to 'work more proactively' with carers, and he refers nurses to the *Carers (Recognition and Services) Act: Practice Guide* (Department of Health/Social Services Inspectorate, 1996) which provides for the right of assessment of an individual carer's needs. This assessment can be requested for an established carer or for a newly intended carer. Nurses working in any setting which involves older people who need any level of long-term care, from informal and family carers, should familiarize themselves with the *Practice Guide* and provide enabling support to carers to explore the provision of the Carers Act (1995). As Nolan (1996) suggests nurses must influence the long-term care of older people through supporting the people who provide most of that care: the family carers.

NURSES AS PURCHASERS

Some nurses are currently working in purchasing positions within the new health and social care systems. The planned reforms of the current government; handing the commissioning of health care over to 'primary care groups' (PCGs) offers significant opportunities for community nurses to be involved in planning and purchasing decisions, as do, increasingly, nursing home managers (NHS confederation, 1998). These nurses, like all purchasers of services, will wish to select the best, most effective, service for their clients. It may be assumed that nurse purchasers have a good understanding of what nurses offer, and its quality; however, they too will want, and must demand, evidence of effectiveness and quality.

'Purchasing' and 'commissioning' are concepts which differ strategically, but which are sometimes confused and used interchangeably:

- Commissioning requires planning and strategy development to meet assessed population health need
- Purchasing requires utilizing services (mainly local) to meet the needs of the specific population being purchased for

The same information should be informing the decisions of both commissioners and purchasers so that resources are not wasted on developing services which are not going to meet local need. Clearly commissioning and purchasing, although separate concepts, are inter-related activities, and the commissioning of new services, demands long-term commitment between the commissioner, the purchaser and the provider.

The next chapter explores the issue of 'outcome measurement' and the explicit link with the notion of evidence-research-based nursing practice alongside the concept of provision of care to meet client need. As nurses we need to give these measures of outcome serious regard, and use them as an opportunity to 'show off our wares' in the marketplace. This does not necessarily have to mean that we agree with a 'marketplace' approach to the delivery of health and social care, but that we are happy and secure enough in our beliefs about our own aspect of that provision to let it be scrutinized. If we truly believe that older people will suffer without access to professional nursing then we have a duty to prove this to the decision makers, some of whom are fellow nurses, for the sake of the individual people with real human needs who are getting older in this resource-limited society.

FURTHER READING

Frankel, S. and West, R. (eds) (1993) *Rationing and Rationality in the National Health Service; the Persistence of Waiting Lists.* Macmillan, London. *A useful overview of the decisions behind distribution of resources in a cash limited national health service, however, because it rests on an underlying assumption that healthcare need will always outstrip provision, this must be read alongside Williams and Frankel (1993) for a more balanced view.*

Green, D.G. (ed.) (1990) *The NHS Reforms: Whatever Happened to Consumer Choice?* IEA, London. *A critical review of the NHS users opportunities to make choices in a fundamentally cost-effective outcome-based, curative model service; this gives a broad and unemotive account.*

Hornby, S. (1993) *Collaborative Care: Interprofessional, Interagency, and Interpersonal.* Blackwell Scientific Publications, Oxford. *A useful review which introduces aspects of overlapping professsional roles, and involving users and carers as collaborators; the reader needs to consider the political implications of 'multiskilling' and the historic context behind health professional roles to get the most from this book.*

Hughes, B. (1995) *Older People and Community Care.* Open University Press, Buckingham.
One of a valuable series called 'Rethinking Ageing' which give abstract and provoking perspectives on older people's lives. Hughes defines the ideal care manager as a 'user empowerer' rather than a 'exploitative rationer'; this approach underpins her refreshing notions of resourcing older people's needs.

Jarman, B.,Townsend, P. and Carstairs, V. (1991) Deprivation indices. *British Medical Journal,* **303,** 523.
This article gives a refreshingly critical analysis of the validity of deprivation indices, and in particular their problematic application to predicting resource need.

Nolan, M., Grant, G. and Keady, J. (1996) *Understanding Family Care.* Open University Press, Buckingham.
Community care policies are only able to function due to the extensive foundations of informal care existing. Nolan et al. review the changing nature of informal care, its relationship with the resourcing of older people's care, and put forward a useful new model of caring. Professor Mike Nolan is fast becoming the national (and international) expert on all aspects of informal carers' roles, and their interaction with statutory services.

Seedhouse, D. (ed.) (1995) *Reforming Health Care: the Philosophy and Practice of International Health Reform.* John Wiley, Chichester.
A real understanding of health reform in Britain is only achievable through consideration of other health systems, their political and sociocultural basis, and their goals and outcomes. Seedhouse gives a fascinating and wide view here. Usefully criteria for success or failure of health reform are also evaluated.

Williams, M.H. and Frankel, S. (1993) The myth of infinite demand. *Critical Public Health,* **4**(1), 13–18.
The usefulness of this article lies in its critical analysis of the currently pervasive notion of infinite demand for healthcare by a growing older population; it should be read in conjunction with Frankel and West (1993, listed above).

REFERENCES

Association of Community Health Councils for England and Wales (1993) *Rationing Healthcare: Should Community Health Councils Help?* Association of Community Health Councils.

Blunkett, D. (1994) Labour opposes performance related pay. *British Journal of Nursing,* **3**(18), 923–924, Oct 13–26.

Bottomley, V. (1989) Agenda for change. *Nursing Times,* **85**(49), 16–17, Dec 6–12.

Brindle, D. (1996) The end of the welfare state. *The Guardian,* 8 May.

Carr-Hill, R. (1995) Measurement systems in principle and practice. *Journal of Advanced Nursing,* **22**(2), 221–225.

Casey, N. (1997) The problem of funding long-term care for older people. *Nursing Standard,* **11**(45), 1, July 30.

Chadda, D. (1995) Gene genie. *Health Service Journal,* **105**(5447), 10–11, April 6.

Colerick, E.J. (1985) Stamina in later life. *Social Science and Medicine,* **21**(9), 997–1006.

Conway, S. (1995) Needs assessment: All out

of perspective. *Health Service Journal*, 5 January, 22–23.

Davies, B., Bebbington, A. and Charnley, H. (1990) Resources needs and outcomes in community based care. Avebury Press. Aldershot.

Department of Health (1990) *The National Health Service and Community Care Act 1990* (Elizabeth II, Chapter 19). HMSO, London.

Department of Health (1993) *Department of Health and Government Statistical Service. Hospital Episode Statistics: England; Financial Year 1989-1990*. HMSO, London.

Department of Health (1995a) *NHS Responsibilities for Meeting Continuing Healthcare Needs*. HSG (95)8/LAC(95)5.

Department of Health (1995b) *Discharge from NHS Inpatient Care of People with Continuing Health or Social Care Needs: Arrangements for Reviewing Decisions on Eligibility for NHS Continuing Inpatient Care*. HSG(95)39/LAC(95)17.

Department of Health (1996) *A New Partnership for Care in old Age*. HMSO, London.

Department of Health/ Social Services Inspectorate (1996) *Carers (Recognition and Services Act): Practice Guide*. HMSO, London.

Fewtrell, C. (1991) The right system at the right time. *Health Service Journal*, **101**, 16–18.

Green, D.G. (1990) A missed opportunity. In *The NHS Reforms: Whatever Happened to Consumer Choice?* Green, D.G. (ed.) IEA, London.

Hancock, C. (1995) What is long term care? *Health Service Journal*, 5 January.

Harrison, S. and Hunter, D.J. (1994) *Rationing Healthcare*. Institute for public policy research, London.

Hudson, B. (1995) Nothing ventured nothing gained: long term care. *Health Service Journal*, 26 October.

Hunter, D. (1997) The challenge of health care restructuring. *Nursing Times*, **93**(39), 67–70, Sept 24-30.

Hunter, H. and Lyall, J. (1995) HAs plan to cut back on long-term care provision. *Health Service Journal*, 26 October.

Institute of Fiscal Studies (1995) Cited in Hunter and Lyall (1995).

Jarman, B.,Townsend, P. and Carstairs, V. (1991) Deprivation indices. *British Medical Journal*, **303**, 523.

Kobasa, S.C., Maddi, S.R. and Kahn, S. (1982) Hardiness and health: a prospective study. *Journal of Personality and Social Psychology*, **42**(1), 168–177.

Kohler, M. (1996) Head of Public Affairs: Help the Aged. In Thomas, R. (1996) Dorrell acts to save 'nest eggs' from state. *The Guardian*, 8 May.

Maynard, A. (1996) Lean, mean rationing machine. *Health Service Journal*, 1 February.

NHS confederation (1998) Primary Care Groups – Policy into Practice, NHS confederation, Birmingham Research Park.

Navarro, V. (1991) The West German Healthcare System: a critique. *International Journal of Health Services*. **21**(2), 565–571.

NHS Executive (1994) *NHS, Responsibilities for Meeting Long Term Health Care Needs*. Department of Health, London.

Nolan, M. (1996) Supporting family carers: the key to successful long term care? Editorial. *British Journal of Nursing*, **5**(14).

Office of Population Censuses and Surveys (OPCS) (1993) *The 1991 Census: Persons aged 60 and Over*. HMSO, London.

Pac-Soo, U. (1996) Community care: the German experience. *Elderly Care*, **8**(2), 33–36.

Pearson, A. (ed.) (1988) *Primary Nursing: Nursing in the Burford and Oxford Nursing Development Units*. Croom Helm, London.

Pearson, A., Durand, I. and Punton, S. (1988) The feasibility and effectiveness of nursing beds. *Nursing Times*, **84**(47), Occasional Paper (9), 48–50.

Pritchard, C. (1992) What can we afford for the National Health Service? *Social Policy and Administration*, **26**(1), 40–54.

Private Patients Plan (PPP) Lifetime Research (1995) *Care in the Community. Two years on*. April.

Roberts, C.C. (1996) Redefining the healthcare paradigm. *Hospital Topics*, **74**(2), 16–20.

Sheldon, A. and Maynard, A. (1993) Is rationing inevitable? In *Rationing in Action*. British Medical Journal Publishing Group, London, pp. 3–14.

Siddell, M. (1995) *Health in Old Age: Myth, Mystery and Management*. Open University Press, Buckingham.

Thomas, B. (1996) Continuing care needs for the elderly mentally ill. *British Journal of Nursing*, **5**(10), 622–624, May 23–June 12.

Timms, J. and Ford, P. (1995) Registered nurses' perceptions of gerontological nursing education needs in the UK and USA. *Journal of Advanced Nursing*, **22**(2), 300–307, Aug.

United Kingdom Central Council for Nursing Midwifery and Health Visiting (UKCC) (1983) *Code for Nurses, Midwives and Health Visitors*. HMSO, London.

Walker, A. (1993) Community care policy: from consensus to conflict. In Community Care: a Reader, Bornat, J. *et al.* (eds). Macmillan, London, pp. 204–226.

Wells, J.S.G. (1995) Health care rationing: nursing perspectives. *Journal of Advanced Nursing*, **22**, 738–744.

Williams, M.H. and Frankel, S. (1993) The myth of infinite demand. *Critical Public Health*, **4**(1), 13–18.

15 Measuring the outcomes of care

Janice Baker

INTRODUCTION

Following the National Health Service (NHS) reforms, increasing pressure has been applied to purchasers and providers to ensure that they obtain value for money within finite resources. This necessitates the requirement for the effects of care on the health status of populations and individuals to be defined and evaluated. Consequently the need for outcome measures has developed with a focus upon exploring the effectiveness of healthcare interventions in relation to value for money. Within this market culture and as a result of substantial costs associated with a large workforce, nursing has come under close scrutiny and attracted strong demands to demonstrate its effectiveness.

Against this backdrop there is a growing population of older people requiring increasing resources to address the health problems associated with the ageing process. Nurses working with this client group therefore need to develop a knowledge base and take a proactive approach to the development of outcomes. However, like so many concepts that are introduced into the NHS, no clear guidance has been given to how this might be achieved, resulting, in some areas, in confusion and a lack of action.

It is therefore the intention of this chapter to:

- Explore the need for outcomes
- Define the meaning of outcome in relation to clinical and cost effectiveness
- Identify areas that must be addressed if a culture conducive to the development of outcomes is to be created
- Identify methods that can be utilized to identify outcomes of culturally sensitive care interventions for older people
- Produce a step-by-step guide for future action

THE NEED FOR OUTCOMES

The National Health Service and Community Care Act (Department of Health, 1990) resulted in fundamental changes to the management and funding of the NHS. One consequence of this Act was the creation of an internal market. District health authorities (DHAs) and general practitioner (GP) fundholders became the purchasers of healthcare, whilst NHS Trusts and directly managed units became the providers. During the past five to six years the number of GPs joining the fundholding scheme has grown significantly. The Audit Commission (1996) reported that one in three practices in England and Wales had joined the scheme and that half of the population is registered with a GP fundholding practice. GPs have become, therefore, increasingly powerful and influential within the purchasing arena.

Purchasers receive a fixed amount of money per annum, based upon the number and category of people resident within their area or served by them. As part of the process of creating the internal market in the NHS, DHAs and GP fundholders were given responsibility for assessing the health needs of their populations and securing services to meet those needs. It is this information that forms the basis of the contracts with providers (Table 15.1). In addition a duty is placed upon purchasers, to respond to statutory policies such as *Health of the Nation* (Department of Health, 1992a) and the *Patient's Charter* (Department of Health, 1992b).

From the ever-increasing number of media reports on the NHS failure to meet individual health needs, it can be assumed that the fixed amount of money which is given to purchasers, is insufficient to enable them to respond to all identified health needs and statutory policies. As a result, areas have to be prioritized and decisions made which demonstrate efficient utilization of available resources. In order that informed purchasing decisions can be made, information is required on both the costs and benefits of interventions, packages of care and services. Although the cost element is relatively easy to determine, this is certainly not the case for measurement and evaluation of the ultimate benefits (Mellett *et al.*, 1993).

This increased focus upon the use of resources within the NHS, is not only the result of organizational and political demands but also of the increased demands upon the service. This is demonstrated by a number of factors, for example, an increase in availability of medical technology. An additional factor, of relevance

TABLE 15.1	*Commissioning process*	
	Stage	Action
	1	Identify health needs
	2	Develop commissioning objectives
	3	Explore strategic options
	4	Agree strategic plan
	5	Develop service specifications
	6	Negotiate and agree contracts
	7	Implement service contract
	8	Monitor and evaluate results

Source: P. Wobbaka (Personal communication, 1996).

to the focus of this chapter, is the change in demographic trends which is characterized by people having a longer life expectancy. The projection for the United Kingdom, which is consistent with that worldwide, is that by the year 2020, 25.45% of the population will be aged over 60 years, whilst 4.3% will be aged over 80 years (Golini and Lori, 1990).

As a result of these increasing demands being made on finite resources, especially by the older population, a need has been identified for the development of outcome measures. In this context it has become necessary for nurses to be able to clearly articulate and demonstrate to purchasers their specific contribution to healthcare delivery. Due to the historical working relationships between nursing and medical staff the input of nurses is often subsumed.

If this situation is not addressed and nurses' specific contribution is not identified then nursing will remain invisible and potentially dispensable (Bond and Thomas, 1991). It is therefore imperative that nurses involve themselves in the development of outcome measures. The need to do so was clearly identified in *Vision For the Future* (Department of Health 1993) where it was stated that 'by the end of the first year all provider units should have identified three outcome measure indicators responsive to nursing'. Although outcome measures have a clear focus within the management and purchasing context, they are also the responsibility of each individual nurse.

OUTCOMES – MEANING AND PURPOSE

It is apparent when discussing outcome measures, that the term has different meanings for people, this includes service users, nurses, managers in provider units and purchasers.

- Service users are concerned with issues such as access to services, information about their condition/illness, participation and choice in their care and treatment, pain relief, reduced disability, increased satisfaction with their abilities and improvements in their quality of life
- Nurses are primarily concerned with the direct results of their interventions with individual clients such as relief from symptoms, optimal level of functioning for the client, maintenance of mental and physical health for example through the development and support of social networks, and increased community presence and participation
- Service managers are concerned primarily with the utilization of resources to provide an effective and efficient service. Managers are therefore interested in waiting times, admission and readmission rates, community contacts, and the number of complaints and compliments that are received
- Purchasers are concerned with ensuring that the highest improvement to the collective health status of the local population is achieved with the available resources. Purchasers are therefore interested in morbidity rates, mortality rates, and incidence of issues such as pressure sores and leg ulcers

The above variations in perception of outcome measures demonstrate the fundamental tension that exists within this subject area. This is represented by the differences created between those individuals whose responsibility is to focus upon a population level, and those whose focus is the person themselves. This situation has considerable implications for deciding which outcome measures need to be selected and has the effect of creating conflict and impeding development.

CREATING A SHARED VISION

If the problems identified above are to be overcome, it is crucial that everyone has a common understanding of what is meant by outcome measures and a shared vision for their successful implementation. It is essential that a common definition is not only shared and communicated throughout an organization, but that it is also shared and negotiated with the purchasers. Additional issues that require consideration if the overall process is to be successful, are those of communication, development of the appropriate culture and involvement of users and carers.

DEFINITIONS

Last (1983) defined outcomes as 'all identified changes in health status arising as the consequence of handling a health problem'. This definition parallels the NHS Executive's definition of clinical and health outcome, which they have established as 'the attributable effect of intervention or its lack on a previous health state' (NHSE, 1996). The above definitions allude to the issue of clinical effectiveness, however little consideration is given to the issue of cost-effectiveness. Further exploration of these two concepts should facilitate greater understanding of the meaning of outcome and its value in nursing practice.

The concepts of both clinical and cost effectiveness were first introduced in the NHSCCA (Department of Health, 1990) where the attainment of predefined objectives at the lowest cost was seen as being crucial in the changing culture of the NHS. Clinical effectiveness being 'the achievement of pre-determined objectives' and cost efficiency, 'achieving pre-determined objectives at lowest possible cost' (Department of Health, 1990). Recently they have taken on a much more significant meaning with the increasing constraints on available resources and have been defined by the NHS Executive (1996) as follows:

- **Clinical effectiveness** – the extent to which specific clinical interventions when deployed in the field for a particular patient or population do what they are intended to do, i.e. maintain and improve health and secure the greatest possible health gain from the available resources. To be reasonably certain that an intervention has produced health benefits it needs to be shown to be capable of producing worthwhile benefit (efficacy and cost effectiveness) and to have produced that benefit in practice
- **Cost effectiveness** – the cost effectiveness of a particular form of health care depends upon the ratio of the costs of healthcare to its health outcomes

Of fundamental relevance to the above is the notion of health gain; in the context of working with older people it is also necessary to consider the concept of health maintenance. Failure to do so would negate the value of many health interventions and risk consigning many nursing actions into the ineffective category, which no purchaser will buy. For the purposes of this chapter it is necessary to consider outcome measures in the context not only of health maintenance and health gain but also in the context of clinical and cost effectiveness. This notion will be explored further with consideration being given to the more definable elements addressed by purchasers and managers and also to those more difficult to define and measure, that are of value to clients and nurses.

COMMUNICATION

As previously stated, the commissioning process provides the formal method of communication between providers and purchasers. This process is usually undertaken by key personnel within the purchasing organization meeting and negotiating with executive directors and contracting departments of provider units. It is possible for those individuals involved in this process to be extremely knowledgeable and skilful about population needs and about contracting processes. This expertise is not necessarily supported by current knowledge relating to good practice in the area in question. As a consequence it is important that the managers within the provider units establish effective communication mechanisms which enable nurses and other professionals to enter into valued dialogue about these issues.

How much do you know about your contract targets?
Were you informed of these formally?

What top-down/bottom-up communication exists within your organization about contract targets?

CULTURE

It is possible to identify an element of tension within the culture that currently exists in healthcare settings. This is a consequence of the converging of two very different cultures within one organization. The first of these is typically related to the situation prior to the NHSCCA (Department of Health, 1990), where professional autonomy was strong and people were only rarely held accountable for their actions and omissions, within this culture, tradition had a very strong focus. The second, which has emerged post NHSCCA, is that in which the ethos of general management has increased in momentum. Accountability both for resources and individuals' actions is much greater in this context. This is characterized by the increase in litigation and the shift towards an emphasis on risk management.

Many issues can be seen as points of conflict within this situation, not least outcome measures. To many professionals outcome measures are unfamiliar and are seen as a tool of the organization and its management, that is about stifling creativity and innovation. For this reason consideration must be given to appropriate strategies for developing a culture where professionals accept outcome measures as an integral part of their role.

USER AND CARER INVOLVEMENT

During the late 1980s the NHS was characterized by a growing emphasis on quality and customer needs. This movement was reflected in the NHSCCA (Department of Health, 1990), and has since developed momentum which can be seen for example in the production of the Patient's Charter (1992b) and its priority status within the NHS Executive targets for 1996/1997 (NHSE, 1995).

Users and carers have traditionally found themselves involved in environmental and clinical audit (Kelson, 1995). Recent directives from the NHS Executive have indicated the need to continue their involvement with particular attention to the development of appropriate outcome measures (Department of Health, 1994). This has inherent difficulties which affect overall progress in this area, these include clarity of what is actually meant by the term carer and user involvement.

In the absence of clear guidance on user and carer involvement, this phrase has been interpreted differently by providing organizations, users and carers, and their support groups. The situation has been complicated further by the variation in vocabulary currently used, for example, user and carer participation, and user and carer consultation. This has led to differences in the influence and level of involvement, by users and carers in healthcare delivery and strategy development.

It is acknowledged that in certain areas, user and carer involvement is difficult to initiate, due to the client groups involved. These would potentially include vulnerable or disadvantaged groups particularly those who have communication difficulties or whose first language is not English. Such circumstances must not be ignored and need addressing.

If organizations are to move from a culture of paying lip service and token representation, to full user and carer involvement, the healthcare strategy must include a major transfer in power base from healthcare professionals, to the user and carer. However, an unwillingness exists amongst healthcare professionals to actively involve users and carers in decision-making processes, this situation is increasingly referred to as 'professional protectionism'. To address this issue with respect to nurses, much work will be required in changing the educational systems and hierarchies within which they operate. Therefore it is essential that each nurse arduously considers and addresses their role in this area.

CURRENT SITUATION

The key areas in which purchasers are currently requesting information can be divided into two groups:

- Easily identified and measured
- Demanding significant resources from the constrained NHS

It is, however, notable that a considerable amount of overlap exists between these two groups; an example of this is in the area of pressure care management.

Although purchasers are becoming increasingly refined in the purchasing of healthcare interventions, in many instances the ability to demonstrate effective outcomes is still not sufficiently developed to be able to predict effectively the quality and cost effectiveness of care. In relation to the above example the cost of treating and preventing pressure sores in a 600-bedded district hospital was quoted by NHS Centre for Reviews and Dissemination (1995) as costing between £600,000 and £3 million per annum. As such, it is understandable that purchasers are interested in this area. The same briefing also identifies the lack of validity and rigour in relation to some of the key areas that have previously been used. These include the equipment used in this area of care and the validity of the assessment tools used to identify people at risk of pressure sores.

OUTCOME TECHNIQUES

Nurses have within their skill repertoire a number of techniques which can be used to identify outcomes of care interventions. These include standard setting and audit, development of protocols and care planning.

Standard setting and audit

The standard setting and audit cycle is well documented in many texts (see Figure 15.1) (Royal College of Nursing, 1990). The most common approaches to standard setting are the structure, process and outcome framework, postulated by Donabedian (1969) and establishing a standard and listing relevant

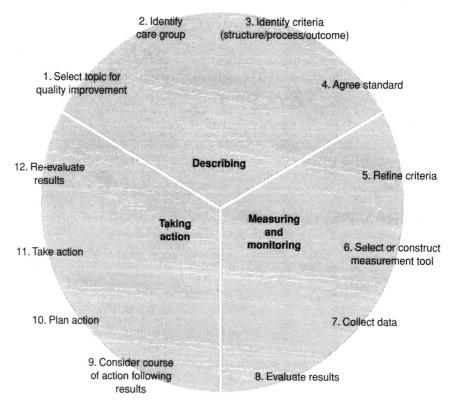

Figure 15.1 Standard setting and audit cycle.

criteria, for example as demonstrated within the King's Fund Organizational Audit Tool (King's Fund, 1993). From an outcomes perspective, it is important to utilize Donabedian's (1969) framework primarily because the outcomes section of this method is clearly separated and therefore more readily lends itself to the outcomes focus.

Protocols

The Clinical Resource and Audit Group (1993) defines a protocol as an 'adaptation of a clinical guideline to meet local conditions and constraints'. Long (1994, p. 4) further suggested that it 'represented a modification of a national guideline for local application, giving operational detail, specifying, for example, who does what, when and how, and leading eventually to the even more detailed clinical care plan'. Despite target three of *Vision for the Future* (Department of Health, 1993), clearly stating the need for nursing to identify clinical protocols, it would appear that the majority of proformas currently in existence are medically driven.

Care planning

Care planning is fundamental to the role and function of all nurses. In order to make nursing interventions more focused it is important to consider the value of constructing care plans in such a way that they meet the external demands of evidence-based practice and outcome measures in a logical and succinct manner whilst improving the quality of care delivered.

Care plans have the potential to be an extremely important tool for nurses in the negotiations with managers and purchasers. Properly constructed, care plans enable the identification of the inputs into a person's care, in the context of both material and human resources. In addition they are able to specify the process that a person can expect to experience through the interventions identified. In the current climate, this should be framed in the context of evidence-based practice, thus clearly establishing the research basis to planned interventions. They also have a purpose in the context of outcomes, as the goal identified for each individual and each intervention, should ultimately become the outcome of nursing care. The above, combined with effective baseline information should allow nurses to demonstrate the value of their input to an individual's healthcare.

Nurses need to be alert to the potential of such methods, particularly in an NHS moving towards outcomes, value for money and evidence-based practice as key determinants of what healthcare can and will be delivered. Failure to address such areas from a health and quality-of-life perspective may result in these not being key areas of nursing practice in the future.

VISION FOR OUTCOMES

As identified previously, the majority of the existing outcome measures currently being supported within the NHS are predominantly quantitative in their focus.

Although these may be of significant relevance to many older people in receipt of healthcare, this cannot be assumed to be the whole picture. There is a clear need to identify what is important to older people and hence what the nursing focus should be for outcome measures. Crucial to the success of this process and that of outcome measures, *per se*, is the need to collect effective and accurate baseline data in all areas of care intervention at individual, service, organization and population level. Failure to collate information at these levels will hinder the ability of nurses, providers and purchasers to make valid comparisons that indicate the effectiveness or otherwise of a service or intervention.

It is important to begin to address issues that are more culturally sensitive. In this chapter the cultural issues discussed will be those areas of life that are important to each individual and that are frequently taken for granted in our everyday lives. These include areas such as maintenance of social networks, participation in the local community, choice and decision making, and other areas that contribute to an overall quality of life. As such, many of these areas can be considered to have direct consequences in relation to the mental health of individuals and are potentially the business of healthcare providers. By virtue of the fact they contribute to quality of life, mental, emotional and spiritual well-being, this inevitably results in them being more difficult to quantify and hence measure.

T. Keighley (personal communication 1994) identified the need for nurses to address the following areas when considering outcome measures:

- Respect
- Concern
- Presence
- Protective care
- Anticipatory care

Respect and concern are in relation to the manner in which nurses deliver the service, in particular the attitude and behaviour in which they provide care to older people. Presence refers to the position a person holds within society and their local community. Protective care and anticipatory care can be seen as those interventions designed to meet the physical, social, biological, psychological, educational and spiritual needs of people. This is especially pertinent when they ◄3 are in receipt of longer-term intensive healthcare.

QUALITY OF LIFE

From the above it can be concluded that there is a requirement to develop techniques in relation to measuring quality of life. Although the term 'quality of life' has an apparently commonsense meaning, actually defining it has posed significant challenges for many years, to professionals from several disciplines, including nursing, medicine, sociology and psychology. No single definition yet exists but there is a consensus of agreement in relation to quality of life being a 'multi-variate' construct that is characterized by objective and subjective components. Lawton (1991) states 'quality of life is the multi dimensional evaluation by both intra personal and social normative criteria of the person environment system'.

Researchers have also made attempts to identify and verify variables that are related to, affect, or even predict quality of life. Vetter *et al.* (1988) and Francis

(1981) identified a number of variables that were perceived as important by older people. These include financial status, presence of life-long intimate friends, quality of past relationships with family, shared lifestyles of aged parents and adult children and quality of residential environment. Kayser–Jones (1981) additionally identified choice, freedom and independence as issues of importance.

One of the most recent quality-of-life models to be developed is by Felce and Perry (1995) who identify five domains:

- Physical well-being
- Material well-being (e.g. clothing, meals, income)
- Social well-being (e.g. community participation, active social networks, maintenance of friendships within these)
- Development and activity (e.g. leisure, hobbies, choice control, education)
- Emotional well-being (e.g. self-actualization, self-esteem, self-worth, status and respect)

Each of these domains can be measured objectively (for example a person's income) and subjectively (for example a person's satisfaction with their income). The model also goes one step further by recognizing that when determining a person's quality of life, it is essential to ascertain how important that domain is to them. A comparison of the variables identified by Kayser–Jones (1981), Francis (1981) and Vetter *et al.* (1988) to Felce and Perry's (1995) demonstrate significant correlation. It could be suggested therefore, that if amendments were made to the model that it could be dynamic in meeting the needs of older people.

The concept of quality of life can lead to a number of ethical dilemmas for those individuals caring for older people, especially in those services where financial resources are in short supply. For example, should an older person be given life-extending treatment when arguably they have experienced the best years of their life? Is an older person who is unable to live by themselves more appropriately accommodated in a residential home or in a family member's home? Such questions prompt widespread debate. Nurses must, however, be alert to such dilemmas and contribute to the debates from the perspective of each individual older person.

QUALITY-OF-LIFE MEASUREMENT AND TOOLS

Numerous tools exist which have been used to measure quality of life. These can be divided into the following broad categories (Bowling, 1997):

- Functional ability measures, which concentrate on mobility, activities of daily living and optimum levels of functioning (e.g. preparing meals)
- Health status measures, which generally focus on individuals' subjective perceptions of their health
- Psychological well-being measures, which are aimed at detecting common mental health problems, such as anxiety/depression, dementia and mental confusion
- Social networks and social support measures, which focus on an individual's web of social relationships and the nature of those relationships
- Life-satisfaction and morale measures
- Disease-specific quality-of-life measures

Specific examples of each type of measure are documented and discussed in greater depth in other texts, for example Bowling (1997).

However, before using any of these measures it is important to note the following caveats from both a researcher's and a practitioner's perspective.

The researcher would be concerned with the psychometric properties of the instrument, which includes degree of reliability, validity and responsiveness, whilst the practitioner would be interested in the administrative aspects of the instrument such as (Jette, 1993; Jeffrey, 1993; Long, 1995):

- Has the instrument been used in a similar setting?
- Has it been tested in a population similar to the targeted group of individuals?
- How long does it take to complete the instrument?
- Are the scores/data easy to analyze and interpret?
- Is the information that is generated useful?
- How long will it take to collate data, evaluate results and write up overall conclusions?
- What is the financial outlay with regard to manuals, computer hardware and training materials, staff training and clinical support?

AREAS FOR OUTCOME DEVELOPMENT

From the quality-of-life discussions in the previous section, considerable attention was placed upon the importance to older people of community involvement, valued activity and their physical environment. It is the intention of this section to explore each of these areas in detail, with the expectation that this will generate techniques for measuring outcomes.

Community involvement

Community involvement is of importance to the quality of life of older people. O'Brien (1980) proposed a framework that can be a way of developing this area ◄3 of care for older people. O'Brien divides community involvement into community presence and community participation. Community presence is the initial goal for services before it is possible to measure outcomes in the context of community participation. The methods for collating information regarding community presence are easy to apply and are not time consuming. Essentially they involve listing the possible areas or services within the community that a person may choose to use. These can be either established lists (Atkinson and Williams 1990; Bartlett and Cameron, 1992) or can be designed, based upon specific neighbourhood information, thus producing a tool specific to the local area.

Information required in such an exercise not only includes what facilities a person uses but the frequency with which they use them and with whom they are used. Consideration of the level of information available from this process indicates an absence of qualitative data; this is of particular relevance from the angle of choice and the quality of the experience from the individual client perspective. One method that can be used to help increase the qualitative nature of the information collected is that of social network mapping.

Social Networks

◄9 The term social networks refers to those people with whom an individual has contact, either through work, home life or leisure. Social network mapping is a method of measuring the contacts which an individual has at a specific point in time. The areas of strength and need can then be identified in order to plan care for the future. Reassessment of the person's social network, using the same process, will then allow the outcomes of interventions to be elicited.

In order to map an individual's social network it is essential that its assessment is based upon the properties and characteristics of that network (Atkinson and Williams, 1990).

The characteristics and properties of a social network have been described in more detail earlier in the book, but are listed here as a reminder. These include:

- Characteristics – family, friends, people with common interests, neighbours and acquaintances, professionals and service providers
- Properties – size or range, density, multiplexity, intensity, durability, directedness and reciprocity, symmetry

Having elicited information regarding the individual's social networks, it is important to place this in the context of the person's life experiences and personal wants, dreams and ambitions. Therefore, if a person has a lack of family contacts within that part of their network map, this may be the result of a lack of family or the consequence of family breakdown many years before. Equally, if a person makes an informed decision not to return to that relationship, then that is a choice that must be respected and documented as an outcome of the process, and no attempt to rekindle the relationship should be attempted.

Valued activity and client engagement

Client engagement in valued activities has been identified as an important consideration for older people (Vetter *et al.*, 1988; Francis, 1981).

Townsend (1962) noted that the lack of activity, lack of interaction with others and lack of opportunity for participation in activities are often the most distinctive features of institutions caring for older people with mental health needs. Despite Townsend's (1962) focus upon mental health institutions, it could be argued that the characteristics identified have equal value and importance to other institutional environments where much time and energy is often invested in meeting the physical needs of individuals. This is often at the expense of meeting emotional, social and spiritual needs of individuals. It is important to consider not only the physical needs of individuals but also the time spent meeting needs within the remaining areas.

The following section explores methods by which nurses are able to assess this area in order to establish an objective picture of an individual's level of valued activity and subsequently plan and implement nursing care.

One tool frequently used to record information of this nature is that of diaries. Within this framework, individual people in receipt of health or social care maintain, with the help of staff, a diary of their activities, stating where they went and with whom. In order to increase further the value of this process and create a rich picture of the person's lifestyle and their likes and preferences, it would be beneficial also to include their responses and reflections to the opportunities they have been offered.

To measure effectively the outcomes of activities recorded in clients' diaries it is necessary to consider methods of measuring interaction and engagement levels. This can be achieved in a number of ways, the most common of which is the use of direct observation.

Direct observation

Direct observation is, for the context of this chapter, defined as a focused and preplanned examination of a particular contact(s) within a given timescale, which takes place from a reasonable distance but without participation of the observer. In the context of engagement levels the contacts upon which the observation will focus involve not only staff–client interactions but also client–client, client–relative and client–visitor.

The nature of interaction being monitored can be either verbal or non-verbal and can be recorded as either positive, neutral or negative in its substance.

Record client engagement levels over lunchtime for positive, neutral and negative interactions.

Identify key result areas and develop a plan of action to address the negatives and develop the positives.

Previous use of this exercise by the author, in relation to observing staff–client interactions, identified that much of the interaction and engagement levels experienced by people fell into the negative category. This is particularly important information when considering the value that many people place upon mealtimes as a social event and clearly indicates ways in which service delivery can potentially be improved, in some instances without increased resources.

TABLE 15.2	*Intervention analysis framework*

Intervention	Purpose
Authoritative	
Prescriptive	Seeks to direct the behaviour of the client, usually behaviour that is outside the practitioner–client relationship
Informative	Seeks to impart knowledge, information, meaning to the client
Confronting	Seeks to raise the client's consciousness about some limiting attitude or behaviour of which they are relatively unaware
Facilitative	
Cathartic	Seeks to enable the client to discharge, to abreact painful emotion, primarily grief, fear and anger
Catalytic	Seeks to elicit self-discovery, self-directed living, learning and problem-solving in the client
Supportive	Seeks to affirm the worth and value of the client's person, qualities, attitudes or actions

Source: Heron (1990).

This method of measurement can be refined further by using the methods of intervention outlined in Heron's (1990) six-category intervention analysis framework (Table 15.2). These interventions can be used to identify the nature of the interactions older people experience that is potentially more refined and hence more useful than simply categorizing them as positive, neutral or negative. Experience of using this framework has demonstrated that many interventions within institutional settings are placed within the authoritative category, predominantly prescriptive in nature.

From the above it is apparent that the information that can be produced, is not only extremely useful but is also highly reliable and valid. The difficulty with such approaches, however, is the time consuming nature of both the planning of the observation schedule and the actual observation periods. Such an investment makes this method potentially costly and it should therefore be used with a clear remit for improving nursing practice.

Dementia care mapping

Dementia care mapping is a method devised by Kitwood and Bredin (1994) for evaluating and improving the quality of care in formal settings for those individuals with dementia. The process involves a small team of mappers (observers) tracking a group of clients and recording data at five-minute intervals for between three to five hours. The data include assigning a 'behaviour category' code which indicates the type of activity or inactivity that each client has been undergoing and a 'care value' which indicates the degree to which the client appeared to be in a state of well-being or ill-health or who was experiencing interactions conducive to either state.

The resulting map enables organizations to compare how clients fared and how care was distributed, and to compare different clinical areas and look at a clinical area at different points in time.

Physical environment

Physical environment has already been identified as an issue that many older people find important. Typically it is evaluated from an internal and an external perspective. In some instances the audit of such environments is executed in a way that not only addresses the areas previously specified but also integration of the environment to the whole area of quality of care delivery. The difficulty in this area is the ability to undertake this latter stage, thus increasing the validity of the process when using tools that have been developed locally. Conversely, the use of more universal tools means they do not always meet the needs of local populations or organizations. Examples of universal tools include Senior Monitor (Goldstone and Okai, 1986) and Program Analysis of Service Systems (PASS) (Wolfensberger and Glenn, 1977). Finally, when introducing any new concept into an organization it is essential that a strategy is formulated.

The steps necessary to introduce valid and client-focused outcomes both into the care environment and into the contracting process are illustrated in Table 15.3 (based on Long, 1995). In this plan, nurses at all levels within organizations have an important and valuable role to contribute, particularly in ensuring the provision of good quality care measured by rigourous, qualitative criteria.

TABLE 15.3	**Step-by-step plan**	
	Step	Intervention
	1	Create appropriate culture: Evaluate lines of communication between nurses, service managers and purchasers Develop user and carer involvement policy Develop in-service training programme which covers mechanisms of purchasing and contracting, user and carer involvement, methods of developing outcomes and outcome measures
	2	Choose the service, package of care, condition or intervention for review
	3	Clarify and identify the desired health outcomes from purchaser, service manager, professional, client and carer perspective
	4	Review available evidence on effectiveness to identify most appropriate method, for example, protocol or standard
	5	Select appropriate ways to measure the desired outcomes

CONCLUSION

The changes that have emanated from the NHSCCA are now embedded within the NHS and although some individuals considered that the Labour Party would reverse the situation at the time of writing, it seems unlikely. Chris Smith (1997) in his capacity of Shadow Secretary of State for Health stated that the Labour Party would 'move to a system of locality commissioning' and 'put quality and effectiveness – rather than bogus measurements of quantity – at the heart of what the NHS aims to achieve', thus intimating that the provider–purchaser split and drive towards clinical and cost effectiveness will remain.

However, this chapter has shown that outcome measures are an extremely complex issue, particularly if healthcare services are to embrace some of the more culturally sensitive areas that require consideration. The current situation has been discussed *vis-à-vis* the medical and often reductionist nature of interventions and outcomes that are currently included in contracts with purchasers. In addition the need to focus on some of the 'softer' areas that are important in maintaining a good quality of life for older people has been highlighted. Inevitably the achievement of this vision has implications for nurses and nursing practice.

The principle areas of impact are those of education/training and research, though the two are inextricably linked. Education and training is an issue for both pre- and post-registration courses and practice. Student nurse preparation needs to take on board issues relating to outcome measures and to clearly place this within a quality framework, thus allowing students to develop the appropriate knowledge base. Additionally, the inclusion of research awareness and research skills into pre-registration curricula needs to continue to develop.

Such progress will allow continued movement towards the goal of evidence-based practice. In addition to pre-registration courses, however, there is also a need to consider the educational needs of those nurses already in service who have little or no formal training in areas such as quality, outcomes, research and user and carer involvement. From a research perspective it is essential that nurses take a more proactive approach, which is clearly focused in the current agenda and demonstrates that the contribution of nursing is evidence based and good value for money.

FURTHER READING

Bowling, A. (1995) *Measuring Disease – a Review of Disease Specific Quality of Life Measurement Scales.* Open University Press, Buckingham.
Reviews disease specific measures for cancers: psychiatric, respiratory and neurological conditions and cardiovascular disease.

Bowling, A. (1997) *Measuring Health – a Review of Quality of Life Measurement Scales,* 2nd edn. Open University Press, Buckingham.
An easy-to-read text which gives a comprehensive analysis of qualitative outcomes.

Ford, P. and Walsh, M. (1994) *New Rituals for Old – Nursing Through the Looking Glass.* Butterworth–Heinemann, Oxford.
Identifies nursing rituals still in common use and their lack of benefits to clients.

Mellett, H., Marriott, N. and Harries, S. (1993) *Financial Management in the NHS – Managers' Handbook.* Chapman & Hall, London.
Explains the relevance of economic principles to the reformed NHS.

REFERENCES

Atkinson, D. and Williams, P. (1990) *Networks.* Open University Press, Milton Keynes.

Audit Commission (1996) *What the Doctor Ordered – a Study of GP Fundholders in England and Wales.* HMSO, London.

Bartlett, M. and Cameron, A. (1992) *Values into Practice for People with Learning Disabilities. A Staff Training Pack for Developing Quality Issues.* Pavilion Publishing, Brighton.

Bond, S. and Thomas, L.H. (1991) Issues in measuring outcomes of nursing. *Journal of Advanced Nursing,* 16, 1492–1502.

Bowling, A. (1997) *Measuring health – a Review of Quality of Life Measurement Scales,* 2nd edn. Open University Press, Buckingham.

Clinical Resource & Audit Group (1993) *Clinical Guidelines.* HMSO, Edinburgh. (Cited in Long (1994, p. 4).

Department of Health (1990) *National Health Service and Community Care Act.* HMSO, London.

Department of Health (1992a) *The Health of the Nation – a Strategy for Health in England.* HMSO, London. p. iv.

Department of Health (1992b) *Patient's Charter.* HMSO, London.

Department of Health (1993) *Vision for the Future. The Nursing, Midwifery and Health Visiting Contribution to Health and Health Care.* HMSO, London.

Department of Health (1994) *Improving the Effectiveness of the NHS – EL (94) 74.* NHS Executive, Leeds.

Donabedian, A. (1969) Evaluating the quality of medical care. *Millbank Memorial Fund Quarterly,* 4, 166–203.

Felce, D. and Perry, J. (1995) Quality of life. Its definition and measurement. *Research in Developmental Disabilities,* 16, 51–74.

Francis, D. (1981) Adaptive strategies of the elderly in England and Ohio. In *Dimension: Aging, Culture and Health,* Fry, C.L. (ed.). Praeger, New York.

Golini, A. and Lori, A. (1990) Aging of the population: demographic and social changes. *Aging,* 2, 319–336.

Goldstone, L. and Okai, M. (1986) *Senior Monitor.* Newcastle upon Tyne Polytechnic Products, Newcastle upon Tyne.

Heron, J. (1990) *Helping the Client. A Creative Practical Guide.* Sage, London.

Jeffrey, L.I.H. (1993) Aspects of selecting outcome measures to demonstrate the effectiveness of comprehensive rehabilitation. *British Journal of Occupational Therapy*, 56(11), 394–400.

Jette, A.M. (1993) Using health related quality of life measures in physical therapy outcomes research. *Physical Therapy*, 73(8), 528–537.

Kayser-Jones, J.S. (1981) Quality of care for the institutionalised aged: a Scottish American comparison. In *Dimension: Aging, Culture and Health*, Fry, C.L. (ed.). Praeger, New York.

Kelson, M. (1995) *Consumer Involvement Initiatives in Clinical Audit and Outcomes*. College of Health, St Margarets House, 21 Old Ford Road, London.

King's Fund (1993) *The King's Fund Organisational Audit Primary Health Care*. King's Fund Centre, London.

Kitwood, T. and Bredin, K. (1994) *Evaluating Dementia Care. The DCM Method*. 6th edn. Bradford Dementia Care Group, Bradford University, Bradford.

Last, J.M. (1983) *A Dictionary of Epidemiology*. Open University Press, Milton Keynes. (Cited in Frater, A. and Powell, M. (no date) *Managing Health Outcomes*. King's Fund, London).

Lawton, M.P. (1991) A multi-dimensional view of quality of life in frail elders. In *The Concept and Measurement of Quality of Life in the Frail Elderly*, Binen, J., Lubben, J., Rose, J. and Deutchman, D. (eds). Academic Press, New York, pp. 3–27.

Long, A.F. (1994) Guidelines, protocols and outcomes. *International Journal of Health Care Quality Assurance*, 7(5), 4–7.

Long, A.F. (1995) *Exploring Outcomes in Routine Clinical Practice: a Step by Step Guide*. UK Clearing House, Leeds.

Mellett, H., Marriott, N. and Harries, S. (1993) *Financial Management in the NHS – Managers' Handbook*. Chapman & Hall, London.

NHS Centre for Reviews and Dissemination, University of York (1995) *The Prevention and Treatment of Pressure Sores. Effective Health Care Bulletin*, Vol 2 No 1. Churchill Livingstone, Edinburgh.

National Health Service Executive (NHSE) (1995) *Priorities and Planning Guidance for the NHS: 1996/97*.

National Health Service Executive (NHSE) (1996) *Promoting Clinical Effectiveness – a Framework for Action in and through the NHS*.

O'Brien, J. and Lyle, C. (1980) *Framework for Accomplishment*. Responsive Systems Associates, Georgia.

Royal College of Nursing (1990) *Quality Patient Care: The Dynamic Standard Setting System*. Scutari, Harrow.

Smith, C. (1997) *Labour's New Deal for Nurses*. UNISON Conference.

Townsend, P. (1962) *The Last Refuge – a Survey of Residential Institutions and Homes for the Aged in England and Wales*. Routledge & Kegan Paul, London.

Wolfensberger, W. and Glenn, L. (1977) *Program Analysis of Service Systems: Handbook and Manual*, 3rd edn. National Institute on Mental Retardation, Toronto.

Vetter, N.J., Jones, D.A. and Victor, C.R. (1988) The quality of life of the over 70's in the Community. *Health Visitor*, **61**, 10–13.

16 The policy dimension: a protocol for progress

John Brown

KEY ISSUES
- Service responsibility
- Delivery settings
- Workforce planning
- Occupational standards
- Professional boundaries
- Identifying implications for practice

INTRODUCTION

Towards the end of 1996 the Joseph Rowntree Foundation published the results of a project that they had funded on establishing a regulatory framework for single registered care homes. Amongst a range of proposals the authors called for the introduction of what they called 'Gerontological Nurse Specialists' (Johnson and Hoyes, 1996). The role of such a specialist would be to allow a more flexible use of all staff in order to enable an appropriate mix of staff skills where the specialist nurse would have a particular expertise in assessment and healthcare planning for older people. Where appropriate, designated healthcare tasks would be delegated to other suitably trained staff.

Such a proposal is not unique to the care of the older person. Developments with other user groups indicate that changing philosophies of care together with evolving patterns of service design and delivery, are leading to new ways of providing support and care within a situation where specialist staff skills can be in short supply (Ovretveit *et al.*, 1997). Such developments are occurring within a rapidly changing policy situation and it is this context that provides the focus of the chapter.

The demographic dimension of social policy, especially with regard to the numbers of older people, has generated a veritable forest of statistics. In general, the increasing number of older people, especially among those aged over 75 years, is seen as having serious implications for a range of provision. The media spotlight has fallen upon various aspects of these implications. Issues around responsibilities for the provision of continuing care to meet health needs (Department of Health, 1995a), the whole arena embraced by providing long-term facilities (Department of Health, 1996a), together with heated debate over income support and pensions (Department of Health, 1996b) have all dominated the policy agenda throughout the 1990s. This has been accompanied by considerable demographic pressure upon the National Health Service (NHS).

Figures released by the Department of Health (1995b) indicate that about

42% of hospital and community health services expenditure is on people aged over 65 years, although they form 16% of the population. This expenditure reflects a dramatic increase of over 137% spent on older people treated between the period 1978/9 and 1993/4 (Department of Health, 1995b). Publication of the White Paper, *The National Health Service: a Service with Ambition* (Department of Health, 1996c), reflected such pressures when reviewing the challenges faced by the NHS in the immediate future. It is documents such as this White Paper that provide the immediate context, not just for promoting positive practice for the older person but for all user/client groups.

Ever since the introduction of the internal market with the National Health Services and Community Care Act (Department of Health, 1990) there has been an increasing volume of academic literature and commentaries that has addressed a range of issues associated with evaluating its impact. These have embraced general introductory works on the NHS (e.g. Klein, 1995) as well as those that have considered particular aspects, such as management (e.g. Morton-Cooper and Bamford, 1997), the professions (e.g. Harrison and Pollitt, 1994) rationing (e.g. Klein *et al.*, 1996), etc. In considering the policy dimension of practice, this chapter draws less upon such material than the considerable mass of official publications, such as government White Papers and circulars, that are sometimes less readily available and familiar to practitioners but are, none the less, crucial in identifying the issues that impact directly upon the situations that they confront in the immediacy of the work setting.

Foremost among these situations are those that have a direct relevance upon the development of all staffing initiatives, whether this involves advocating specific proposals such as the introduction of a Gerontological Nurse Specialist or more general debates, such has professional regulation, and the like. These issues cover a number of areas:

- Service responsibilities
- Delivery settings
- Workforce planning
- Occupational standards
- Professional boundaries

Each of these areas, considered below, has implications for practice. These implications are brought together at the end of the chapter to form the basis for identifying elements required to construct an agenda that all those involved in providing support and care for the older person need to address in the immediate and foreseeable future.

SERVICE RESPONSIBILITIES

In the spring of 1997 the former Conservative government published a White Paper on the future of social services departments, *Social Services: Achievement and Challenge*. The White Paper outlined the possibility of social services relinquishing all responsibilities for service provision, other than for children, to become primarily a purchasing agency (Department of Health, 1997a). For many years this has been the reality of local authority residential provision for the older person which shrank dramatically throughout the 1980s.

Figures quoted in the White Paper *Caring for People* (Department of Health,

1989a) show that social security support for people in independent residential care and nursing homes rose from £10m in 1979 to over £1000m in 1989 (Department of Health, 1989a). Such an expansion was accompanied by a concomitant reduction in local authority residential provision. While these figures apply to all user/client groups, and not just the older person, they indicate the dramatic shift in the location of resources away from the statutory local-authority sector that government espousal of independent, and in particular private provision, was intended to produce. This trend was consolidated and incorporated into the National Health Services and Community Care Act (Department of Health, 1990). However, when introduction of the legislation was completed in 1993, problems were apparent.

A succession of bulletins from the Audit Commission highlighted a series of concerns. Foremost among these were financial matters and the fact that the shift from a service-centred to needs-led approach, the lynch-pin of the legislation, was far from being achieved (Audit Commission, 1993, 1994a, 1996a). The Audit Commission commented succinctly,

> Critically, how are future growing expectations and needs, in the context of demographic change, to be met from limited resources? (Audit Commission, 1996a, p. 34.)

This is a key question. How it is to be answered depends as much upon central political initiatives as it does upon local concerns. In particular, with a new Labour government which is looking at the whole structure and function of the welfare state, nothing can be assumed – as the media phrase applied to the review of social security provision, 'thinking the unthinkable', indicates. What could this mean when looking at the responsibilities for the purchase and provision of services for older people? One indication is provided by a discussion document on mental health.

For over three decades, since the early 1960s, successive governments have committed themselves to the promotion of community care. This has, none the less, proved notoriously difficult to realize. Different planning cycles, funding sources and organizational cultures have contrived to limit and, at times, thwart the necessary level of co-operation required between the NHS and local government if community care was to become a substantial reality. Attempts from 1976 onwards to develop ever-more sophisticated forms of joint finance between the two sectors singularly failed to make much inroad as it was essentially making adjustments at the margins while leaving the basic structural differences between health and social care intact.

When this was allied to the Conservative government's promotion of the market economy and the private sector, together with an ideological reluctance to fund public sector services, the result was many well-publicized failures of care in the community for all user/client groups. Nowhere has this publicity been more focused than in the area of mental health. Possibly the highest profile was accorded to the case of Christopher Clunis who murdered an innocent bystander, Jonathan Zito, on a London underground platform. The Committee of Inquiry commented:

> . . . that Christopher Clunis's care and treatment was a catalogue of failure and missed opportunity. We do not single out just one person, service or agency for particular blame. In our view the problem was cumulative; it

was one failure or missed opportunity on top of one another (Ritchie *et al.*, 1994, p. 105).

Subsequent inquiry reports showed that this was far from unusual, and an Audit Commission report published later that year indicated that the failure to achieve meaningful co-operation and collaboration in health and social care was widespread (Audit Commission, 1994b). Crucially, it could be shown that the user/client, as well as carer and the community at large were offered a service that fell short of providing high-quality support and care. Against this back-cloth, the 1997 Green Paper on mental health attempted to outline a range of options that began to tackle the underlying and longstanding issues inhibiting collaboration in health and social care.

Along with proposals to identify a single responsible agency, delegate author-ity, and establish a joint body, was the suggestion that there should be created a new Mental Health and Social Care Authority independent of existing authori-ties and with its own dedicated budget (Department of Health, 1997b, pp. 23–24). Such an initiative, if it was to be adopted, would immediately get round prob-lems of collaboration between existing bodies by taking away their responsibili-ties in this area and giving them to a hopefully integrated agency charged with all aspects of health and social care for those with mental health problems.

While such an option is undoubtedly radical, and likely to be actively resisted by some, within the present political climate it is an option that cannot be dis-counted. Nor can it be ignored as irrelevant for other user/client groups, includ-ing older people. The implications of arguments for a 'seamless service', for example, do not necessarily preclude such a possibility when taken to their logical conclusion.

Many agencies are involved in promoting health and caring for people. A seamless service is one where services which individuals need are co-ordinated and integrated across the health and social care system, including primary care and social care. In a seamless service:

- organizational boundaries do not get in the way of care for patients, but it is clear who is responsible and accountable for their care at all times;
- the planning and contracting process supports practical working arrange-ments;
- roles and responsibilities are clearly defined;
- multi-professional teams come together to provide high quality services for patients, that make the best use of the specialist skills and experience of the staff involved; and
- all staff are trained to work in multi-professional teams, and there is support in working across organizational boundaries (Department of Health, 1996c, p. 28).

Such points, and the option of establishing new organizational bodies have a particular resonance when designing and developing services for the older per-son as the drive towards a primary-care-led NHS gains momentum.

DELIVERY SETTINGS

In *The National Health Service: a Service with Ambitions* (Department of Health, 1996c) five priorities are outlined for the NHS – a well-informed public;

a seamless service; knowledge-based decision-making; a highly trained and skilled workforce; and a responsive service (Department of Health, 1996c, pp. 27–31). Underpinning these priorities are a number of developments that have built up considerable momentum. Foremost among these have been the changes brought about by the introduction of general practitioner (GP) fund-holding and the emphasis upon prevention rather than cure in health provision that was signalled in the White Paper *The Health of the Nation* (Department of Health, 1992a). Both of these developments are integral to the emphasis upon a primary-care-led NHS.

Early in 1997 a Primary Care Bill was approved by Parliament. This reflects some radical departures in health provision that could not have been predicted even a few years ago. Debate is now underway to change the employment status of GPs from effectively sub-contractors to salaried employees. The implications of this are profound in that it begins to make it possible to remove the disincentives for practices 'to replace a doctor with a nurse even where this might be more efficient and provide better patient services' (Department of Health, 1996d, p. 5). While this can be seen as consolidating changes in specific areas, such as the running of particular clinics, there is the possibility of considerably expanding the role of, for example, the practice nurse.

The emergence of the practice nurse is a development that has begun to change the relationship between different areas of nursing outside of the hospital setting and has led to a situation where it is necessary to begin the look afresh at what is understood by the term 'community nurse'. There are implications for who provides what particular skills especially as the debate over continuing and long-term care for older people remains unresolved.

Attempts have been made to identify gaps in provision, along with appropriate discharge procedures, and ensuring consistency in access and treatment. The longstanding and seemingly intractable problem of split responsibility between health and social services in the public sector, and who picks up the bill for treatment, support and care, could mean that the possibility of transferring responsibility to one part of the public sector gains in credibility. Although the system of GP fundholding is not immune from criticism (Audit Commission, 1996a) it is apparent that the GP is becoming the lynch-pin in the evolving pattern of services delivered outside the hospital, whether we are considering what has traditionally been seen as falling in either health or social care.

For the older person, where it can be assumed that increasing age is likely to be associated with increasing infirmity, it is highly unlikely that any one person will not at some time have contact with their GP. In such circumstances it is possible to envisage the case being made for the transfer of all responsibility to the GP and primary care services on the grounds that eventually everyone will have to have recourse to such services. The other possibility, as with mental health, is to begin to consider the option of a totally new type of authority.

Such possibilities will inevitably be accompanied by considerable debate, which will often be heated and, at times, acrimonious. However, it is important to remember that all provision is evolving and is in a state of flux. Along with the developing role of the GP there is continuing discussion over the role and scope of the hospital sector (e.g. Audit Commission, 1996b). It is prudent not to assume that traditional practices and boundaries are immune to change. This is especially the case when the emphasis in policy documents upon multidisciplinary and interagency co-operation is considered. This has been pursued not only through considering the structure of services, but also in identifying how evolving patterns of provision require new ways of working that involve an approach to workforce planning which ensures that benefits to users/clients are not compromised and are possibly enhanced.

WORKFORCE PLANNING

The former Conservative government had a strong commitment to integrated workforce planning. This commitment was clear and unambiguous:

> The Government proposes to move to integrated workforce planning across all sectors of the NHS and professional groups (Department of Health, 1996e, p. 18).

Although relatively little headway has been made, there is no reason to suppose that a Labour administration will be any less committed. This is especially the case as one legacy of the Conservative government has been to leave in place an infrastructure for the contracting of education and training that begins to make the achievement of an integrated workforce policy possible.

Ever since the inception of the NHS in 1948, questions have been asked about the most appropriate structure for the delivery of healthcare. This has led in 1974, 1982 and 1991 to various major attempts at reorganization and restructuring. A crucial element in this has been addressing issues about staffing. Traditionally, there have been questions raised about the recruitment and retention of nursing staff, especially as they form the largest single group within the NHS. In spite of these concerns and the overall structural changes, the funding of nurse training remained largely as it had been since 1948.

Although the terminology of the committees responsible for allocating funds changed, from Regional Nurse Training Committees to Educational Advisory Groups reflecting the replacement of the General Nursing Councils by the UKCC and National Boards in 1983, the committees had a specific sum to allocate that was exclusively for nurse training. This was to change in 1994 when the Government replaced the 14 Regional Health Authorities, whose boundaries had remained largely intact since 1948, with eight Regional Offices. It is doubtful whether these changes made much impact, apart from those directly concerned, upon the majority of NHS employees. Yet this change was to introduce within each of the areas covered by the Regional Offices a new structure for delivering and allocating funding for nurse education.

Each Regional Office has a Regional Educational Development Group (REDG) that is responsible for a number of Education and Training Consortia (ETC). It is these ETC that introduce a completely new approach to the commissioning of education and training in the NHS. Their brief, unlike previous committees involved with funding nurse education and training, is now much broader and embraces all healthcare professions with the exception of medicine and dentistry (NHS Executive, 1995a, b, 1997a). For the first time, it is possible through the contracting process, and the investment plans that they are based upon, to alter the balance of education between different professional groups. For example, it may be felt that rather than contracting for ten nurses from a particular branch, it is more appropriate, given a local needs analysis, to have five nurses, three physiotherapists and two speech therapists.

While this possibility still has to be realized, the potential for such a development has been increased as various publications have clarified the role and responsibilities of the ETC. In the spring of 1997 an Executive Letter from the NHS Executive, under the heading *Devolution and Responsibilities to Education Consortia*, stated that:

> Their [ETC] focus has until now been on the main health care professions outside medicine and dentistry, but they do have an important role in relation to to workforce planning right across the healthcare workforce, including doctors and dentists ...
>
> ... Planning for the future healthcare workforce requires the assessment of staffing and development needs across the whole range of service provision, in primary and secondary care, and across professional and vocational boundaries. Over time consortia should evolve as the focal point for integrated workforce planning and development (NHS Executive, 1997a, pp. 1–2).

Such an approach is very dependent upon the quality of local information that is available upon which to base decisions and the way that ETC interpret their brief can depend upon local factors. As the development of services can vary in different parts of the country so the establishment and structure of ETCs can also vary. Clearly, for the ETCs to use their potential to 'mix and match' different education programmes within the contractual process is attendant upon appreciable political considerations both local and national. Yet within an environment in which emphasis is increasingly upon what is seen as 'value for money' and 'fitness for practice' it is probably only a matter of time before the first tentative steps are made to use and exploit this potential. Such a development complements new approaches to the terms and conditions of employment of NHS personnel.

In 1989, the key White Paper on NHS reforms was published with the title *Working for Patients* (Department of Health, 1989b). Plans were outlined for the introduction of the internal market in healthcare with particular emphasis upon the establishment of self-governing Trusts and a new GP contract. This was supported by ten specific working documents that addressed particular aspects of the plans. Taken together with the plans outlined in the community care White Paper, *Caring for People*, they were to form the basis of the National Health Service and Community Care Act, 1990. The amount of detail was considerable and the full import of many points was only to be recognized once the reforms were underway and had begun to build up momentum. This was particularly the case on the ability of Trusts to set salary levels for all staff outside the parameters set by the specific long-established National Pay Review Bodies for the different professional groups.

Working for Patients was explicit upon the ability of trusts to set their own salary levels:

> ... NHS trusts should be free to settle the pay and conditions of their staff, including doctors, nurses and others covered by national pay review bodies. Subject to their contractual obligations, NHS Hospital Trusts will be free either to continue to follow national pay agreements or to adopt partly or wholly different arrangements (Department of Health, 1989b, p. 25).

It was a number of years before the awareness of the potential impact of such provision was to be addressed by the professional bodies. It was an awareness that was heightened by the debate surrounding the Tomlinson Report on hospital provision in London (Department of Health, 1992b). The report tackled the vexed issue of hospital provision in the capital within a framework of carefully qualified statements. However, the main thrust of the report – shifting resources from secondary to primary care with the merger of some of the existing hospitals, many of which had illustrious histories in the provision of healthcare – was readily adopted by the Conservative government. Although the issues raised are still, five years on, largely unresolved and the future shape of London's hospital provision undecided, the report served to highlight problems of staff contracts when it came to mergers with the possibility of staff redundancies. This is an issue that refuses to go away.

While the Tomlinson Report (Department of Health, 1992b) specifically focused upon London it acted as a spur for similar reviews elsewhere in large metropolitan cities. The question such reviews raised was basic – is there an overprovision of hospital facilities, especially as the emphasis is now resoundingly upon primary care? Such a question was exacerbated by the functioning of the internal market with, for example, the Audit Commission questioning whether it was possible to sustain the present number of Accident and Emergency Departments throughout the country. Their conclusion was an unequivocal 'no', accompanied by the recommendation that it was possible to provide alternative, and appropriate, facilities and that at the local level, services needed to be rationalized (Audit Commission, 1996c).

Such a possibility graphically highlights the substantial changes that are about to be addressed within the NHS. In such a context contractual obligations and expectations are likely to undergo fundamental change. Although political sensitivities in the immediate short term will probably mitigate against the ready adoption of locally negotiated salaries there is the likelihood that terms of tenure will change. With managers on three-year rolling contracts this may emerge as the approach adopted for professional contracts in place of the traditional 'tenure for life' model. While this may be an anathema for the individual practitioner, from the employer's perspective it provides far greater flexibility in responding to the impact of rapidly changing services and the resulting staffing issues. Crucially, it begins to minimize the costs of meeting possible compulsory redundancies.

In such a situation, the way that performance is assessed and the criteria that are used for such an assessment begin to take on greater importance than in the past. Tentative steps have begun to be made with the introduction of clinical audit. The impact upon public perceptions and expectations brought about by the application of the Citizen's Charter (Prime Minister, 1991) to healthcare has created a more questioning environment in which performance, and crucially quality, is evaluated. The question still remains, however, of what is the most appropriate avenue by which to appraise staff performance. It is here that developments within occupational standards are most germane.

OCCUPATIONAL STANDARDS

Occupational standards, as measured by National Vocational Qualifications (NVQ), have long been approached with ambivalence by the nursing profession, especially among nurse educationalists. Proposals for the introduction of NVQs in 1986 coincided with submission to the government by the UKCC of the plans for Project 2000 (UKCC, 1986). However, the nursing profession chose to ignore this development as initial work on NVQs was to focus upon the pre-professional level. This had the effect of excluding nursing from many discussions that were held on what the content of pre-professional training was to be which, by extension, was inevitably going to have implications for what was to go into the professional level.

Initial reaction to healthcare assistants with an NVQ qualification was not welcoming, this was reinforced by the experience and concerns of those in industry, business and commerce. The administrative system associated with NVQs was seen as overly bureaucratic, mechanistic, reductionist and, at times, irrelevant (Smithers, 1993). None the less, the government was committed not only to the principle of NVQs but also to streamlining their administration and funding work to strengthen their application and relevance to the work environment (Department of Trade and Industry, 1995, p. 84). Such a commitment is to be found echoed in the NHS (NHS Executive, 1996). The drive to vocational training, as reflected in the promotion of NVQs, is one that embraces all groups in the NHS including doctors. GPs, for example, will be '... required to meet minimum standards as a condition of GP vocational national training' (Department of Health, 1996e, p. 19).

Such initiatives have been given a considerable boost with the establishment of National Training Organizations (NTOs) that are intended to assist with:

... helping employers and employees to meet their sector training and education needs ... NTOs will need to work in strategic areas of standards and National Vocational Qualification/Scottish Vocational Qualification developments (Department for Education and Employment, 1997a, p. 1).

Specifically, they are charged:

To ensure the development, review and implementation of national occupational standards, especially for NVQs and SVQs, for the specified sectors and occupations interests and sector response to national initiatives. (p. 4).

An essential element is:

To improve linkages between qualifications and progression routes from educational qualifications and programmes into employment, further training and vocational qualifications ... (p. 20).

The importance of the introduction of NTOs cannot be overstated as they build upon the increasing development and adoption of occupational standards to set standards and design qualifications that will involve professional associations, employers and higher education at the higher levels. This applies to all those groups of staff working with the older person as it does for all other user/client groups.

While NTOs cover all employment activities in the economy, with the first ones gaining recognition coming from the manufacturing sector (Department for Education and Employment, 1997b), there are specific NTOs for health and for social care. The training needs and requirements of staff working with the older person have been placed within the social care NTO, along with mental health, learning disabilities, children and young people, early years, physical disability, sensory impairment and special needs housing (CCETSW, 1997).

The establishment of the social care NTO should take place by the spring 1998 to cover five functional areas:

- Representatives of key employment organizations/sectors/services
- The four parts of the UK
- Expertise in all the work areas of the sector
- Qualification and training regulators
- Providers of education and training

These areas complement directly how the future development of activities within the ETCs is envisaged by the NHS Executive:

The future work of consortia and investment in education and development will need to support:

- The pre-qualifying education and training required to gain entry into employment as a healthcare professional;
- A commitment to continuous education and life-long learning for healthier professionals;
- Changing modes of delivery: modular, part-time programmed, open and distance learning, flexible courses delivered in a variety of forms;
- Shared learning to support team-working across professional and organizational boundaries;
- Preparing the healthcare workforce to provide a coherent service within a primary care led NHS and across health and social care boundaries; and
- Development priorities for employers and national priorities to meet service objectives (NHS Executive, 1997a, p. 6).

Taken together, the work of the ETC and the introduction of NTOs provides an important vehicle in moving towards integrated workforce planning. As was apparent with the introduction of NVQs in 1986 the role and contribution of the employer is paramount. The 1996 White Paper on the NHS recognizes this:

The NHS is the biggest employer of diploma and graduate students in the country and maintains a strong tradition of working in partnership with universities and other professional bodies. NHS employers – principally health authorities and NHS Trusts – have a key role to play in supporting this partnership and in providing direct training and development opportunities for all staff throughout their working lives (Department of Health, 1996c, p. 30).

More specifically the comment is made that further work is needed to:

Consider the deployment of NHS training and education budgets, drawing particularly on the development priorities of employers and the concerns of the professions (Department of Health, 1996c, p. 44).

The nature of this contribution is likely to be based increasingly around occupational standards using the currency of competence provided by NVQ as one way of comparing and evaluating tasks within and between different occupational groups and ensuring that practitioners are 'fit for purpose' and that preparation is 'value for money'. Such a move has already been signalled in looking at the training needs of social workers involved with children where it is proposed to develop new training that will:

... be underpinned by a national curriculum and competency framework and lead to a formal award ... The new training framework would be initially developed and launched not as a formal licence to practise but as a means through which the skills of the existing workforce are strengthened and developed. It will have a strong practical orientation (Department of Health, 1997a, p. 26).

Proposals such as this also help facilitate and reinforce the drive towards multidisciplinary and interagency work that has been promoted within government literature for over a decade. The cumulative impact is to begin to blur professional boundaries.

PROFESSIONAL BOUNDARIES

As different patterns of service provision have evolved and been introduced, so traditional boundaries of demarcation between different professional groups can become less and less tenable, especially if they can be seen to disadvantage the user/client who is intended to be the beneficiary of any particular service. Often boundaries have to be considered as result, intended or otherwise, of a particular initiative. The move, for example, to reduce junior hospital doctor hours did not mean that the work went away. It still had to be done, and provided the opportunity for nursing staff to embrace tasks that has traditionally been the province of the medical profession (Greenhalgh, 1994).

The practicalities involved in such an initiative are considerable, involving as they do personal, professional and organizational considerations that can also come to the fore when any form of multidisciplinary and interprofessional work is brokered (Ovretveit et al., 1997). In such circumstances terminology can be crucial, especially when applied to the name of a particular group – although tasks can change over time, adherence of a particular title can conjure up, in the minds of some, traditional images that current work does not necessarily support.

This is particularly the case with the professions supplementary to medicine. Here the title implies a relation to medicine which is essentially junior and possibly subservient. However, proposals to change the title of the Council for the Professions Supplementary to Medicine to the Council for Health Professions immediately conveys a different image. Indeed, the title Council for Health Professions could be seen as encompassing, for example, nursing.

While this may seem implausible, if not outlandish, to some the pace of change has been such in recent years that different groups can now overlap in a range of activities in the practice setting. The seminal report on community care by Griffith in 1988 reflected this when he called for a generic community care worker who is supported by professional specialists (Department of Health, 1988). The role of training and education in such circumstances can be crucial in preparing the practitioner to respond to, and initiate, change. The problem is ensuring that training is responsive to changing demands and expectations without sacrificing the specific and possibly unique contribution to the welfare of the user/client that is offered by a particular occupational group.

Often, there is no issue – there are no alternative groups available to carry out particular tasks. But this is not always the case, and opposition and conflict can come from within a profession as well as from outside. The Chief Nursing Officer for England has commented that for the nursing profession the particular challenge is to ensure that demarcation within the profession does not stifle and inhibit responding to challenges in a changing environment, whether the changes have implications at the pre-registration or post-registration levels (Department of Health, 1994). Confronting this issue was never going to be easy. However, changes in the environment faced by nursing are not limited to developments within the NHS as patterns of provision evolve but also now embraces a new organizational location within higher education for the main professional preparation of nursing staff.

Historically, nursing was isolated within schools of nursing separate from mainstream higher education. For those within the chronic long-stay sector training could also be geographically separate from local communities. Although there were a small number of degree courses in higher education, it was not until schools of nursing became colleges of health studies/nursing and also became affiliated or associated with universities in the late 1980s that this isolation from the mainstream began to be eroded. The announcement in 1995 that the following year all colleges were to become formally integrated into universities accelerated this process (Committee of Vice Chancellors and Principals, 1995). While integration has inevitably varied in its success throughout the country the effect has been to introduce into nurse education another agenda that has to be addressed.

Along with responding to the work of the ETC in the contracting process, assessing the likely impact of occupational standards and the work of the embryonic NTOs, keeping abreast of the training implications of service developments, there is now the added requirement of adapting to the demands of the higher education agenda. With the rapid expansion of places in higher education in recent years so that up to one-third of all 18-year-olds read for a degree, compared to some 6% in the 1960s, universities are facing fundamental questions about how to maintain quality in the face of increasing demand and diminishing resources (Department for Education and Employment, 1997c). It is increasingly likely that the United Kingdom will move towards an United States of America model with immediate implications for professional preparation for all groups across the health and social care spectrum. Such pressures compound the issues faced by the project 2000 programme of pre-registration nurse education.

Although originally conceived in the 1980s to take the profession through to the next century, the programme has, to a large extent, been overtaken by the very changes it was designed to cope with. The National Audit Office (1992) called into question the viability of the programme, which has been subsequently reinforced as the criteria for evaluation become ever sharper and emphasize 'fitness for practice' together with 'value for money'. There is a very real challenge from other groups to some areas of work traditionally carried out by the nurse that can be seen by hard-pressed managers as reasonable and viable alternatives. While the increasing momentum that is building up over evidence-based practice, clinical supervision and the reflective practitioner helps hone the nursing skills that are available, the debate over Project 2000 and its relevance to the practice setting does little to dispel managers looking for and considering such alternatives.

In such circumstances, as boundaries become blurred between groups, it is important that calls for a specialist nurse, whether it is for the older person or any other user/client group, begin to address the debates that set the context for the development of services that are intended to meet identified needs. The points raised and introduced here are but a small sample from a wide range of policy initiatives, but they begin to outline some of the elements that need to be addressed when determining the agenda to take the development of services, and the skills required by those services, forward. Some of the issues to consider when constructing such an agenda form the basis for the concluding section which follows.

IDENTIFYING IMPLICATIONS FOR PRACTICE

In conclusion, the changes outlined are considerable, and are likely to continue even with a new Labour administration although the emphasis and points of detail may vary (NHSE, 1997b). Both the pace and volume of change throughout health and social care have continued unabated for a decade, ever since the first White Paper to signal the substantial developments that were to be incorporated into the National Health Service and Community Care Act (Department of Health, 1990). Many of the developments in relation to primary care could not have been easily anticipated. For example, the increasing ascendancy of the GP over the hospital consultant, through the twin effects of promoting a primary-care-led NHS and the introduction of GP fundholding all of which flies in the face of the established medical status hierarchy that goes back over the centuries.

While this could be seen as possibly an extreme example, throughout the NHS there are many other instances of traditional barriers, and the resulting changes in relationships, being redrawn (Harrison and Pollitt,1994). The introduction of ETC and NTOs reflect such changes, not only in the detail points associated with specific change but in the underlying philosophies that inform the design and delivery of any one such initiative. In these circumstances, it is necessary for all nurses to approach situations in a manner that is both open and, to some extent, anticipates being surprised, if not always favourably! If politicians say that we should 'think the unthinkable' nurses should 'expect the unexpected'. This essentially means approaching changes in health and social care, whether for the older person or any other user/client with a specific mind set that enables nurses to:

- **Question assumptions** – it is imperative that an open mind is kept. While we are still likely to have people called 'nurse', 'social worker', 'doctor', etc. into the next century, what they actually do will be appreciably different from what their professional peers do in the mid/late 1990s. It can be irrelevant at best and dangerous at worst to project into the forseeable future contemporary patterns of discharging responsibilities and the associated expectations
- **Think laterally** – connections have to be made in ways that are not limited by taking into any one situation a set of preconceptions that blinker the perception of how things might be done better for the benefit of the user/client
- **Keep informed** – the pressures of just surviving in the workplace are such that it can be very difficult to keep abreast of developments which often appear to be distant and remote. This does not mean, however, that such developments can be ignored if the individual nurse is to attempt to provide the highest quality service possible for the user/client

- **Seek alliances** – the emphasis upon multidisciplinary work together with interagency collaboration and co-operation can mean that professionals from different backgrounds may have more in common in promoting the claims of their shared involvement with a particular user/client than they do with colleagues from their original discipline
- **Promote initiatives** – developments over the last few years indicate that groups have overwhelmingly responded to change rather than initiated change, with the result that the professions in particular have been subjected to a political momentum that does not necessarily promote the best interests of the user/client
- **Construct agendas** – not getting involved can mean that others set the agendas that ultimately influence work in the practice setting without the nurse making an input and contributing to discussion
- **Involve users/clients** – possibly the most significant developments in recent years have been the attempts to involve users/clients in decisions and services that directly affect their lives. This must be the bed-rock upon which initiatives for the future are based in ways that are not a token but a genuine and integral part of all levels of service provision and preparation for practice

Such an approach is essential if nurses are to respond constructively on behalf of users/clients to the types of developments, initiatives and proposals considered in this chapter. As the White Paper comments in a different context:

> The developments envisaged in this White Paper have implications for the skilled professionals working in the NHS. Modern health care relies increasingly on team work; the development of multi-professional teams, working not only in hospitals and primary care settings, but across the traditional boundaries of health and social care, is a key priority. The objectives of a well-informed public and responsive service also mean that the relationship between patients and professionals is changing. Professionals themselves need training and support if they are to help patients become partners in their own care (Department of Health, 1996c, p. 43).

The challenge is fundamental – to be imaginative within a changing environment and ensure that appropriate skills, whether specialist or generic, are available when required to the user/client. The danger is that without the courage to be imaginative, services are compromised on the basis of personal, professional, or organizational expediency.

FURTHER READING

The emphasis in the chapter has been upon using official government papers. All too often these are difficult to obtain, but there are two White Papers, readily available, that provide an essential introduction to the type of debate that has been introduced. There are also complemented by two academic commentaries that provide a background introduction which helps put the White Papers in context.

Department of Health (1996) *The National Health Service: a Service with Ambitions.* CM 3425. HMSO, London.
Provides a succinct and accessible introduction to the trends and priorities in healthcare policy that have emerged throughout the 1990s.

Department of Health (1996) *Primary Care: Delivering the Future*. CM 3512. HMSO, London.
Outlines, again in an accessible form, what is essentially the main policy template for promoting a primary-care-led NHS.

Harrison, S. and Pollitt, C. (1994) *Controlling Health Professions*. Open University Press, Milton Keynes.
Provides a more specific focus that will be of interest to all healthcare professionals and offers insights as to how the professions respond to various political pressures.

Klein, R. (1995) *The New Politics of the NHS*, 3rd edn. Longman, Harlow.
Provides an overview of how the NHS has evolved in response to a variety of pressures.

REFERENCES

Audit Commission (1993) *Taking Care: Progress with Care in the Community*. Health and Personal Social Services Bulletin No. 1. HMSO, London.

Audit Commission (1994a) *Taking Stock: Progress with Community Care*. Community Care Bulletin No 2. HMSO, London.

Audit Commission (1994b) *Finding a Place: a Review of Mental Health Services for Adults*. HMSO, London.

Audit Commission (1996a) *Balancing the Care Equation: Progress with Community Care*. Community Care Bulletin No 3. HMSO, London.

Audit Commission (1996b) *What the Doctor Ordered: a Study of GP Fundholders in England and Wales*. HMSO, London.

Audit Commission (1996c) *By Accident or Design: Improving A&E Services in England and Wales*. HMSO, London.

CCETSW (1997) A New National Training Organisation (NTO), 17 June 1997. Internal Briefing Document, Central Council for Education and Training in Social Work.

Committee of Vice-Chancellors and Principals (1995) *Nursing and Professions Allied to Medicine: Integration of Colleges of Health into Higher Education*, C/95/28, CVCP.

Department for Education and Employment (1997a) *A Guide to Achieving NTO Status, Promoting Sector Skills*. Department for Education and and Employment.

Department for Education and Employment (1997b) Kim Howells hails new era of training in UK as first National Training Organisations are launched. Press Release 219/97. Department for Education and Employment.

Department for Education and Employment (1997c) *Higher Education for a Learning Society (Chair: Sir Ron Dearing)*. HMSO, London.

Department of Health (1988) *Community Care: an Agenda for Action (The Griffiths Report)*. HMSO, London.

Department of Health (1989a) *Caring for People: Community Care in the Next Decade and Beyond*, CM 849. HMSO, London.

Department of Health (1989b) *Working for Patients*. CM 555. HMSO, London.

Department of Health (1990) *National Health Service and Community Care Act*. HMSO, London.

Department of Health (1992a) *The Health of the Nation*, CM 1986. HMSO, London.

Department of Health (1992b) *Report of the Inquiry into London's Health Service, Medical Education and Research (Chair: Sir Bernard Tomlinson)*. HMSO, London.

Department of Health (1994) *The Challenges for Nursing and Midwifery in the 21st Century: The Heathrow Debate – May 1993*. Department of Health.

Department of Health (1995a) *NHS Responsibilites for Meeting Continuing Health Care Needs*. HSG (95) 8; LAC (95) 5. Department of Health.

Department of Health (1995b) Department of Health supports steps to improve care of elderly people. Press Release 95/527. Department of Health.

Department of Health (1996a) *Long-Term Care: Government Response to the First Report of the Health Committee on Long-term care – Session 1995–96*. CM 3146. HMSO, London.

Department of Health (1996b) *A New*

Partnership for Care in Old Age. CM 3242. HMSO, London.

Department of Health (1996c) *The National Health Service: a Service with Ambition.* CM 3425. HMSO, London.

Department of Health (1996d) *Choice and Opportunity.* CM 3390. HMSO, London.

Department of Health (1996e) *Primary Care: Delivering the Future.* CM 3512. HMSO, London.

Department of Health (1997a) *Social Services: Achievement and Challenge.* CM 3588. HMSO, London.

Department of Health (1997b) *Developing Partnerships in Mental Health.* CM 3555. HMSO, London.

Department of Trade and Industry (1995) *Competitiveness: Forging Ahead.* CM 2867. HMSO, London.

Greenhalgh and Co. Ltd (1994) *The Inter-face between Junior Doctors and Nurses: a Research Study for the Department of Health.* Department of Health.

Harrison, S. and Pollitt, C. (1994) *Controlling Health Professions.* Open University Press, Milton Keynes.

Johnson, M. and Hoyes, L. (1996) *Establishing a Regulatory System for Single Registered Care Homes, Findings – Housing Research 200.* Joseph Rowntree Foundation, York.

Klein, R. (1995) *The New Politics of the NHS,* 3rd edn. Longman, London.

Klein, R., Day, P. and Redmayne, S. (1996) *Managing Scarcity : Priority Setting and Rationing in the National Health Service.* Open University Press, Milton Keynes.

Morton-Cooper, A. and Bamford, M. (eds) (1997) *Excellence in Health Care Management,* Blackwell Science, Oxford.

National Audit Office (1992) *Nursing Education: The Implementation of Project 2000 in England.* HMSO, London.

National Health Service Executive (1995a) *Education and Training in the New NHS.* EL (95) 27. Department of Health.

National Health Service Executive (1995b) *Non-Medical Education and Training – Planning Guidance for 1996/97 Education and Commissioning.* EL (95) 96. Department of Health.

National Health Service Executive (1996) *Education and Training Planning Guidance.* EL (96) 46. Department of Health.

National Health Service Executive (1997a) *Devolution of Responsibilities to Education Consortia.* EL (97) 30. Department of Health.

National Health Service Executive (1997b) *Changing the Internal Market.* EL (97) 33. Department of Health.

Ovretveit, J., Mathias, P. and Thompson, T. (eds) (1997) *Interprofessional Working for Health and Social Care.* Macmillan, London.

Prime Minister (1991) *The Citizen's Charter,* Cm 1599. HMSO, London.

Ritchie, J., Dick, D. and Lingham, R. (1994) *Report of the Inquiry into the Care and Treatment of Christopher Clunis.* HMSO, London.

Smithers, A. (1993) *All Our Futures: Britain's Education Revolution, A Dispatches Report on Education.* Channel 4 Television.

UKCC (1986) *Project 2000: A New Preparation for Practice.* United Kingdom Central Council for Nursing, Midwifery and Health Visiting.

Author Index

Subject Index

Printed and bound by CPI Group (UK) Ltd, Croydon, CR0 4YY

10/10/2024

01043166-0001